Praise for *Heart & Hands*

"An impressive and deeply caring book . . . reveals a shrewd and compassionate sensitivity to women's needs in pregnancy and childbirth."

—Sheila Kitzinger
Author of *The Complete Book of Pregnancy and Birth*

"Here is a book of great beauty that uniquely combines traditional midwifery teaching with the most up-to-date obstetrical theories and techniques."

—Don Creevy, M.D., FACOG
Clinical Assistant Professor of Gynecology and Obstetrics
Stanford University School Medicine

"A beautifully written and comprehensive guide . . . speaks to the need to protect the baby's rights and health."

—Mike Witte, M.D.
Board Certified Pediatrician
Medical Director for the Point Reyes Clinic

"Detailed and compassionate, *Heart & Hands* offers childbearing women, midwives, and doctors a wealth of practical information. It provides a view of pregnancy and birth not as a purely medical, mechanical event, but as a complex physical, emotional, social, and spiritual experience. Elizabeth Davis loves and respects women, and her work places childbearing where it belongs—in the strong and capable hands of mothers and midwives."

—The Boston Women's Health Collective
Authors of *The New Our Bodies, Ourselves*

"*Heart & Hands* conveys the essence of midwifery! To supplement today's abundant scientific and technological information, it literally describes the missing dimension—a commitment to the art of midwifery."

—Dorothea M. Lang, C.N.M., M.P.H.

"Provides a rich assortment of anecdotes and remedies for common problems . . . the author is to be commended for her emphasis on the fourth trimester, the important three-month period when mothers and babies are recovering from birth and becoming acquainted. It is fortunate for midwives and prospective parents that this book has been expanded and updated."

—John Kennell, M.D.
Professor of Pediatrics
Rainbow Babies' and Children's Hospital
University Hospitals of Cleveland

"Portrays well the beauty and power of birth. It honors the central role of the midwife in prenatal care, birth, and postnatal care, precisely the role recommended repeatedly by the World Health Organization for all the countries of the world. This book should be read by all birth attendants . . ."

—Marsden Wagner, M.D.
Neonatologist, Perinatal Epidemiologist
Consultant for Maternal and Child Health
World Heath Organization

"Emphasizes pregnancy as wellness . . . this book parallels the family-centered approach that I advocate in established medical and nursing practices."

—Celeste R. Phillips, R.N., Ed.D.

"The elements of *caring for* and *caring about* women are so maturely thought out and articulated that I readily recommend the book to all midwifery students of any type of educational program, for any practice setting."

—Mary V. Widhalm, C.N.M., M.S.
Director of Midwifery
Lincoln Medical and Mental Health Center
Bronx, New York

"Elizabeth Davis has done her profession a very valuable service by providing a textbook that is eminently readable and that gives the aspiring midwife the benefit of having a *friend and mentor* in the form of a book—and that is no small accomplishment! She delves into the area of judgment, which is the acid test for any midwife. She is the Wise Woman speaking, the Sage Femme who can cut through the morass of information, the current standards, and the new theories, and take us to the heart and kernel of what this work is all about."

—Tish Demmin, L.M.
Former President
The Midwives Alliance of North America

HEART & HANDS

ALSO BY ELIZABETH DAVIS

The Circle of Life: Thirteen Archetypes for Every Woman

Women's Sexual Passages: Finding Pleasure and Intimacy at Every Stage of Life

Women's Intuition

Energetic Pregnancy: A Guide to Achieving Balance, Vitality & Well Being
from Conception to Birth & Beyond

HEART & HANDS

A Midwife's Guide to Pregnancy & Birth

4TH EDITION

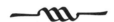

Elizabeth Davis

Photographs by Suzanne Arms / Illustrations by Linda Harrison

CELESTIAL ARTS
Berkeley | Toronto

READER PLEASE NOTE:

The medical and health procedures in this book are based on the training, personal experiences, and research of the author as well as on recommendations of responsible medical sources. But because each person and situation is unique, the author and publisher urge the reader to check with a qualified health professional before using any procedure when there may be any question as to its appropriateness. The publisher does not advocate the use of any particular birth-related technique, but believes this information should be available to the public. Because there are risks involved, the author and publisher are not responsible for any adverse effects or consequences resulting from the use of any of the suggestions, preparations, or procedures in this book. Please do not use these unless you are willing to assume these risks. Feel free to consult a physician or other qualified health professional. It is a sign of wisdom, not cowardice, to seek a second or third opinion.

CA

Celestial Arts
P.O. Box 7123
Berkeley, California 94707
www.tenspeed.com

Distributed in Australia by Simon & Schuster Australia, in Canada by Ten Speed Press Canada, in New Zealand by Southern Publishers Group, in South Africa by Real Books, and in the United Kingdom and Europe by Airlift Book Company.

Cover photography by Suzanne Arms
Cover design by Catherine Jacobes
Interior design by Betsy Stromberg
Production by Chloe Rawlins
Illustrations by Linda Harrison

Photos on pages 2, 8, 11, 18, 33, 34, 51, 58, 68, 80, 83, 87, 90, 95, 98, 105, 107, 116, 122, 124, 144, 177, 190, 191, 202, 203, 209, 211, 221, 223, 226, 231, 233, 237, 240, 243, 250, 253, and 254 by Suzanne Arms, copyright © 1981, 1987, 1992, 1997, 2004.

Photos on pages x, 59, and 137 by Stacie Nunes, copyright © 2004.

Photos on pages 53, 112, 120, and 129 by Pedro Gonzales, copyright © 2004.

Photos on pages 97 and 126 by Katy Raddatz, copyright © 1981, 1987, 1992, 1997, 2004.

Photos on pages 136 and 146 by Ed Buryn, copyright © 1981, 1987, 1992, 1997, 2004.

Photos on pages 153 and 215 by Gary Yost, copyright © 1981, 1987, 1992, 1997, 2004.

First published as *A Guide to Midwifery: Heart & Hands* by John Muir Press, 1981; mass-market edition with same title published by Bantam Books, 1983.

Library of Congress Cataloging-in-Publication Data
Davis, Elizabeth, 1950–
  Heart & hands : a midwife's guide to pregnancy & birth / Elizabeth Davis ; photographs by Suzanne Arms ; illustrations by Linda Harrison.— 4th ed.
    p. ; cm.
  Includes bibliographical references and index.
  ISBN 1-58761-221-6
  1. Midwifery. 2. Obstetrics.
  [DNLM: 1. Midwifery. WQ 160 D255h 1997] I. Title: Heart and hands. II. Title.

  RG950.D38 2004
  618.2—dc22

                                    2004012801

First printing this edition, 2004
Printed in the United States

1 2 3 4 5 6 7 8 9 10 — 08 07 06 05 04

CONTENTS

To Ryan Michael Nava, my first grandchild.

*Born to my daughter, Celeste, and her husband, Ricardo,
in a beautiful water birth at home, with grandma catching.*

We are truly blessed.

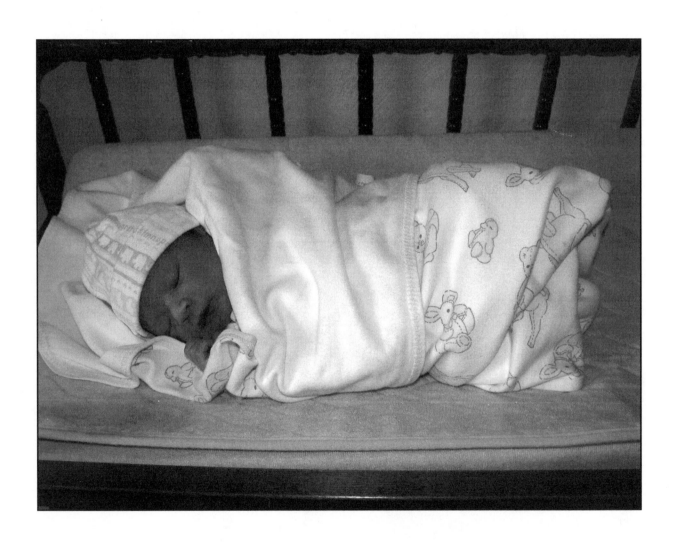

ACKNOWLEDGMENTS

I begin by thanking my teacher, Tina Garzero, for her patience and love in teaching me this wonderful art and way of being. To John Walsh, I will always remember your humor and guidance. To Anne Frye, deep thanks for many years of friendship and for sharing your outstanding manuscript for *Holistic Midwifery: A Comprehensive Textbook for Midwives in Homebirth Practice (Volume II)*.

To all my midwifery students, thank you for your inspiration, insights, critiques, and push to help me stay current.

To Shannon Anton, little sister/wise old one (and the best business partner anyone could want), thank you for your excellent sections on homeopathy and herbs in pregnancy, birth, and postpartum, as well as the unforgettable account of Liam Andrew.

Once again, I must acknowledge Linda Harrison for her stunning illustrations. And to Suzanne Arms, for the cover photo and new photos throughout, my love and gratitude.

For photos new to this edition, I also thank Pedro Gonzales and Stacie Nunes. As regards photos by Pedro Gonzales, I have included these not only because they are beautiful but to give honor to those pictured therein—my dear friend and colleague Robbie Davis-Floyd, Robert Floyd, their son Jason, and daughter, Peyton, who lost her life in a car accident on September 12, 2000. All who know Robbie can attest that even as she has enlightened us on the nature of birth, she has done the same regarding the ways of death.

For the use of photos from the first, second, and third editions, I wish to thank Suzanne Arms, Ed Buryn, Katy Raddatz, and Gary Yost.

And to all the parents and children pictured throughout the book, and to all the midwives who appear here or who assisted the families pictured, my humble gratitude.

To the staff at Celestial Arts, Joann Deck, Brie Mazurek, Catherine Jacobes, and Betsy Stromberg, my deep thanks and appreciation. And in memory of my former publisher, David Hinds—I will always be grateful for your friendship and unfailing commitment to making *Heart & Hands* as technically complete and aesthetically pleasing as possible.

At last, my thanks to my children Orion Davis, Celeste Nava, and John Shebalin, for teaching me about the Mystery of Birth and for loving me no matter what. To my sweet husband, Jim Murray, all my love—and may we share many beautiful years in the garden together.

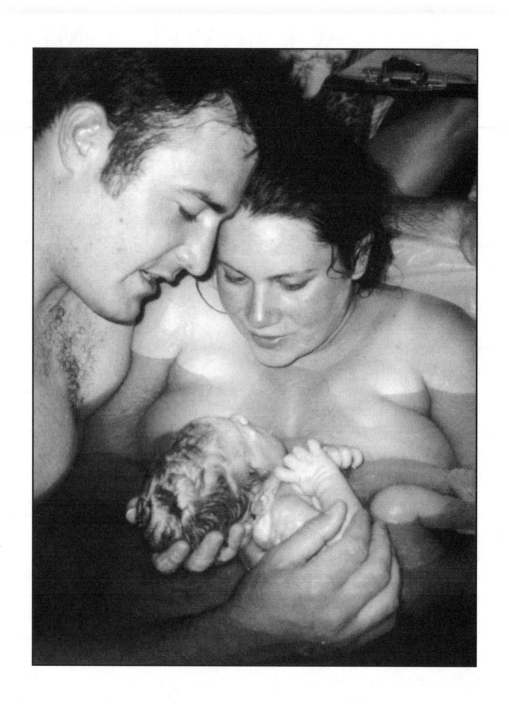

PREFACE TO THE FOURTH EDITION

How blessed I feel to have had yet another opportunity to revise *Heart & Hands*! The revision process has recast not only the text, but my understanding of, and approach to, my work. This is invaluable to me as a midwifery educator, and I hope the results benefit parent and professional readers alike.

I take the revision process seriously and can honestly state that every line in the book has been reread and reconsidered as per its timeliness and accuracy. For the first time, notes are provided at the end of each chapter. The text has virtually doubled in detail. Controversies in screening and treatment for group B streptococcus, gestational diabetes, vaginal birth after cesarean (VBAC), and postdatism are fully addressed. Details on the newborn exam have been expanded. Ways to find structure in apprenticeship have been added to chapter 7, "Becoming a Midwife." New sections in chapter 8, "The Midwife's Practice," reflect current guidelines for client confidentiality and further expand practice structure options to prevent burnout. Sections on psychosocial issues have been completely revamped, including that on postpartum depression. And as a result of increased opportunities for international teaching and learning, I have incorporated techniques from Canada, China, France, Germany, Guatemala, Italy, Mexico, New Zealand, and the United Kingdom on such topics as breech birth, shoulder dystocia, and prolonged labor.

The most sweeping philosophical changes since the previous edition have occurred in chapter 4, "Assisting at Births." As I reviewed this material, I saw that it bore remnants of the medicalized view that labor doesn't really work by itself, and therefore, someone must be on hand to suggest positions to the mother, to massage her perineum, to prevent tears, to promote bonding—in short, to manage her labor. I realized that midwifery, like any other profession, has had its developmental phases. In the early years of our current renaissance, we tended to overdo our involvement in labor so that mothers would never feel abandoned, or suffer the indignities of episiotomy, or know the pain of separation from their babies as many of us had. But with new information on what is truly natural in birth, it is clear that the less we do, the better. Calm, undisturbed birthing mothers know what to do, and when. The more we learn, the more it seems our early vision has been realized: birth works, and we can trust it!

It is interesting that while we were busy figuring this out, a new grassroots movement sprang up to point the way—the "unassisted birth" movement, which continues throughout the United States. Although financial considerations may play a part for mothers choosing this option, the stories they share of their experiences emphasize other factors, such as a desire for complete privacy, not to be told what to do, to be free to be fully intimate with their partner and other supporters, to find their own way with birth. In a health-care system such as ours, where professionalism all too often breeds complacent self-interest, underground movements repeatedly develop, comprised of both cutting-edge innovators and the lunatic fringe. The trend toward unassisted birth is such a movement, ultimately representing dissatisfaction with the available maternity-care options. In much the same way that midwives unwilling to be told what to do by medicine formed their own movement and articulated their own goals and visions, mothers unwilling to be told what to do by midwives are taking a stand, and we would be wise to take heed.

As midwifery develops its own body of research, we find foundation for our work in fascinating data on the physiology of pregnancy and birth (for both mother and baby), the benefits of water birth, mother-assisted birth, and appropriate care in the immediate postpartum. Not all of this research is new—some is so old as to be virtually buried and forgotten. I am thrilled to incorporate this material in this new edition of *Heart & Hands,* and I particularly want to thank midwife, author, and friend Anne Frye for so generously sharing her research with me.

A special word for the curious and courageous mothers who read this book. First, know that wisdom is a virtue. I have attempted to provide an entertaining and informative mixture of information, stories, and opinions, but you alone can bring this to life with your personal experience. Your intuition and innate sense of what is right for you must always come first. Midwifery means "with woman"; all honor to you for sharing this wisdom with us midwives.

I recently wrote an article for *Midwifery Today,* titled "Wild, Beautiful Birth," to express a growing sense of urgency that deep reverence for what is truly natural in birth be restored to every aspect of our work. Contrasting the beauty of a river in the rugged Alaskan wilderness with the dullness of a polluted creek in California, I urged all midwives to come out for purity and wildness—or what Native Americans call the Beauty Way—in ourselves, in birth, in the women we serve. Now that we have our professional bearings, it is time we return to our original passion and inspiration for this amazing work we are so privileged to do. Please join me in upholding the Beauty Way of Midwifery!

PREFACE TO THE FIRST EDITION

The purpose of this book is to offer a practical guide to midwifery—to instruct those women interested in becoming midwives and to convey the realities of practice. Midwifery is a lost and found art, finding its place in our time via its links to feminism and expanding consciousness. It also appeals to a growing do-it-yourself resourcefulness. Women who want to be midwives have usually experienced birth firsthand and want to share and facilitate a new awareness of the power of being female. Most are seeking to extend their relationships with other mothers and babies. Many women who think that midwifery is their calling will read this book and realize that there are many other related areas that need development, such as birth education, postpartum support, and family counseling.

This book is intended to demystify the medical elitism surrounding a very basic, natural body process. There are other books that give more detailed information on obstetrics, but none explains how to adapt this information to individual women and how to bend the rules to fit each situation. This is a book on practical midwifery, with a special focus on creative management of complications. Thus it provides some answers for parents who want more than just good quality care and are seeking to understand the various alternative solutions to problems that may arise in pregnancy and birthing. This information is also intended for midwives practicing in remote areas with little or no medical consultation.

However, this manual is only a partial guide to midwifery practice, as nothing can substitute for experience—the educated intuition that comes from attending many births. But at least the suggested practices and procedures may stimulate the aspiring midwife to question and study, and may also inspire dedicated practitioners to break ground with new, responsible methods. If this book moves parents and health professionals alike to innovative thought and humanistic understanding, the heart of its purpose will be realized.

Thanks be to the midwives—a positive, loving, bright, and pioneering bunch of women—for freely sharing skills and information without which this book would not have been written.

Chapter 1

THE MIDWIFE: A PROFILE

From the very beginning, women have helped one another give birth. One particularly attuned to this task emerged as the town or village midwife, wielding the healing skills of her time and culture. It is the midwife, not the physician, who has attended birth for most of human existence, certainly in indigenous societies. And in the modern-day cultures of Denmark, Holland, and Sweden, midwife-assisted birth remains the norm. In fact, the six countries with the lowest perinatal mortality rates in the world all make generous use of midwives, who attend 70 percent of all births in these countries. In the United States, where midwives assist only 5 percent of births due to political constraints, perinatal mortality is alarmingly high: worldwide we rank twenty-sixth.[1]

Despite the efficacy of the midwifery model, midwives have been persecuted throughout history, particularly in the West. During the Inquisition and the subsequent period known as the "burning times," the main targets were the midwives. Healing by way of nature and aligned with the wisdom of the body, it's no wonder the *Malleus Maleficarum,* handbook of the Inquisition, declared: "No one does more harm to the Catholic church than do the midwives."

In the United States, attacks against midwifery accelerated in the early 1900s, when medicine became a profession for profit and the newly emerged male physician became eager for the revenues of childbirth.

Women were barred from university, thus those wanting to attend childbirth could not acquire the requisite credentials. Midwifery was nearly eradicated at this point, so vehement was the campaign of male physicians to discredit midwife practitioners, who were portrayed as slovenly, immoral, drunken, promiscuous, and perverse, "whores with dirty fingers." In medieval times, midwives were branded consorts of the devil; now they became "loose women" intent on their own ways of healing, in contrast to "good girls" who pursued nursing and accepted roles subservient to the physician.

Predictably, physician-attended birth proved to be both expensive and unsafe. For example, note the high incidence of childbed fever linked to hospital birth in the early 1900s, which not only cost women their lives but also cost their families a tidy sum. Still, women who could not afford to be in hospital continued to rely on the midwife's skill in preventive medicine, benefiting from her emphasis on cleanliness, good nutrition, and the use of herbs. Thus midwives of the past fostered their clients' strength by providing education and counseling on a variety of health-related issues, much as they do today. The midwife's scope of practice has traditionally been care "from womb to tomb," with a holistic, community health approach to treating a spectrum of women's diseases and afflictions.

For midwives to continue to assert their time-honored scope of practice meant war with the increasingly powerful medical profession—a war that continues to this day. Left to themselves, midwives would have never survived; they were poor, politically powerless, and disorganized. Midwifery is alive today for one reason only: women's insistence on midwifery care. Midwifery is simply a fact of life, perpetuated by the needs and desires of birthing women and their supporters.

Although traditional midwives trained by apprenticeship have practiced almost continuously in the United States, the development of nurse-midwifery is fairly recent. The Frontier Nursing Service began training midwives in 1939, using a model developed in England. There are now more than forty programs preparing nurse-midwives, although barriers to practice are considerable. Physician reactions to the nurse-midwife are mixed—on the one hand, she can be a valuable adjunct to a busy practice; on the other, if she seeks to practice independently with her own case load, she is little more than a threat, an economic competitor. That the physician expects the nurse to be subordinate is rooted in

our culture's suppression of women healers and its technocratic model of medicine. But the midwife's responsibilities require that she have the autonomy to make her own decisions and use interventions, maneuvers, and procedures in case of emergency that inadvertently cross into the physician's self-proclaimed scope of practice.

The question of how to forge legitimacy within the medical system has caused sharp divisions among nurse-midwives. There are nearly even ranks in the **American College of Nurse-Midwives (ACNM)** of those who align more strongly with nursing than midwifery, and vice versa. The debate continues as to whether training as a nurse is truly relevant. It is noteworthy that in the Netherlands (where midwifery has long been established), midwifery applicants lose points for having a nursing background, for it is well understood that a nurse must follow orders, whereas a midwife must be able to think and act independently. The United States is the only country in the world that utilizes the title

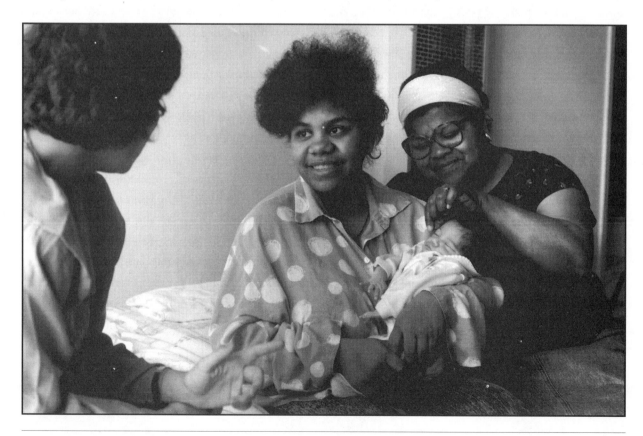

"nurse-midwife"—everywhere else, a midwife is simply a midwife.

Nurse-midwifery does enjoy fully secure legal status nationwide, whereas traditional midwifery remains illegal in many states. Although traditional midwives have struggled to reanimate old midwifery laws, or create new ones if necessary, they continue to meet with bitter opposition from the wealthiest and most powerful lobby in the country, the American Medical Association (AMA). In California alone, seven attempts at legalization were made over a ten-year period, during which more than fifty midwives were investigated, with a number arrested and prosecuted. Practicing traditional midwives once numbered three hundred and fifty in the Golden State, but a decade later, their ranks had dwindled to sixty or so.

How did this happen? In 1974, a pregnant agent from the District Attorney's office visited midwife Kate Bowland. Wired for sound, she garnered evidence to the effect that Bowland was found guilty of practicing medicine without a license. Thus in California (as in other states), the mere practice of midwifery was defined as a misdemeanor. Misdemeanor practices resulting in death or injury (regardless of whether the death or injury was unpreventable or accidental) are further subject to felony charges of manslaughter or murder. It has cost midwives a tremendous sum—tens of thousands of dollars—to defend themselves and their colleagues against unfounded counts of murder. This money has been hard to come by, and it would have been better used to fund midwifery schools or educate the public regarding midwifery care. We do not exaggerate in calling this modern-day war against midwives a "witch hunt."

Yet the continued threat of criminal prosecution has strongly motivated the effort to legalize midwifery. It is a testament to the fortitude and vision of traditional midwives that they have been able to survive the costs—not only financial, but personal as well—of these seemingly endless and agonizing legal battles. We owe the evolution of midwifery's legitimacy to the persistence of our contemporary founding mothers, who encouraged the next generation to take up the banner of self-regulation.

And so, by 1980, traditional midwives began creating standards of practice and mechanisms for certification state by state, even in jurisdictions where legislative efforts appeared futile. In 1982, the **Midwives Alliance of North America (MANA)** was founded to enable midwives "of every stripe" to articulate their goals and visions and to find support in their struggle for legitimization. Now licensing or legal certification for traditional midwives is available in twenty-two states, and the practice is legal but unregulated in another sixteen states. This has led to a somewhat confusing barrage of professional titles: licensed midwife (LM), certified midwife (CM), and direct-entry midwife (DEM). (The latter pertains more to educational preparation than professional status, denoting a midwife who has been trained to the profession directly, without a nursing background.)

Several historic events bear mentioning at this juncture. In 1985, MANA members first considered the possibility of national certification. But the notion was shelved for fear that setting national standards might negatively impact states just beginning to self-regulate. Then, in 1991, the Carnegie Foundation funded a task force of both nurse- and direct-entry midwives to address the future of midwifery education. This group produced a document entitled *Midwifery Certification in the United States,* which outlined identical competencies and scope of practice for all midwives, regardless of training route. Before long, there was renewed discussion of national certification for direct-entry midwives.

Some years earlier, in response to members desire to have a means to demonstrate their competence, MANA had established the **North American Registry of Midwives (NARM),** charged with developing and administering a national registry exam. In light of recent events, NARM now considered administering a national certification process. To facilitate this, I called together a group of state leaders, many of whom had formulated and passed midwifery legislation in their respective jurisdictions, to form the **Certification Task Force (CTF),** with dual purposes of developing a prototype certification process and providing technical assistance to NARM. After numerous meetings at both state and national levels, a process was approved by the MANA membership, and in 1995, the first **certified professional midwife (CPM)** was recognized by NARM.

NARM certification is **competency-based**. The student chooses her educational pathway, but to be certified she must demonstrate entry-level midwifery knowledge and skill. This process is comprised of the following components found in state licensing and certification mechanisms: (1) verification of requisite clinical experience, (2) verification of requisite skills and caregiving abilities, (3) verification of character/letters of recommendation, and (4) verification of knowledge via a comprehensive written examination. Once certified, the midwife must agree to fulfill continuing educational requirements, keep CPR and neonatal resuscitation training updated, work within the confines of the MANA core competencies, and uphold MANA standards and ethics of practice. In contrast, the ACNM offers certification only to those who have completed an accredited program before passing the national exam.

How does the CPM interface with state licensure or certification? In time, it seems likely that national certification will be adopted state by state as the universal process for assessing direct-entry competence. Midwives in states with unduly restrictive practice guidelines might use national certification as a rationale for regulatory changes. Many states already utilize the NARM test as their licensing or certification board exam. As more and more states adopt the national process in its entirety, reciprocity will be increasingly available for midwives wishing to relocate, and the entire profession will benefit from increased self-regulation.

Self-regulation remains the point where battle lines are drawn between midwives and the medical profession. Many nurse-midwives believe that higher education—that is, masters-level midwifery—is the key to greater professional autonomy. Conversely, most direct-entry midwives believe that no credential will be enough as long as physicians are the ruling class, and that midwives must define midwifery on its own terms rather than continuing to jump through endless legitimacy hoops. In spite of these differences, I predict that midwives will one day unite behind the issue of independent practice. This day may come sooner than later, as the fight for autonomous midwifery now rages internationally; in fact, there is not a country in the world where midwives are not somehow restricted in caregiving. For example, German midwives assist deliveries but cannot give prenatal care; Italian midwives can give prenatal care but must call the physician when birth is imminent. In order to address the worldwide struggle of midwives to meet their communities' needs and take their rightful place in the health-care system, the **International Confederation of Midwives (ICM)** drafted the *International Definition of a Midwife,* which was adopted in 1972 by both the World Health Organization and the International Federation of Gynecologists and Obstetricians:

> A midwife is a person who, having been regularly admitted to a midwifery educational program duly recognized in the country in which it is located, has successfully completed the prescribed course of studies in midwifery and has acquired the requisite qualifications to be registered and/or legally licensed to practice midwifery.
>
> She must be able to give the necessary supervision, care and advice to women during pregnancy, labor and the postpartum period, to conduct deliveries on her own responsibility, and to care for the newborn and the infant. This care includes preventive measures, the detection of abnormal conditions in mother and child, the procurement of medical

assistance and the execution of emergency measures in the absence of medical help.

She has an important task in health counseling and education, not only for the women, but also within the family and the community. The work should involve antenatal education and preparation for parenthood and extends to certain areas of gynecology, family planning and childcare. She may practice in hospitals, clinics, health units, domiciliary conditions or in any other service.

This definition is remarkable not only for what it says, but for what it leaves unspoken. Nowhere do we find any stricture regarding the risk status of our clients, nor any attempt to limit our practice to childbearing women, "well" women, or "interconceptional care": terms commonly used in statutes to restrict scope of practice. Particularly powerful are the assertions that the midwife "conduct[s] deliveries on her own responsibility" and executes "emergency measures in the absence of medical help." Unfortunately, the description of educational preparation leaves traditional midwives out of the loop (which reflects an ongoing controversy within the ICM). More inclusive, pivotal documents have been generated by the MANA membership, including *MANA Statement of Values and Ethics, MANA Core-Competencies for Midwifery Practice,* and *MANA Standards and Qualifications for the Art and Practice of Midwifery* (see appendix A).

Yet another organization that has contributed to the professionalization of midwifery is the **Midwifery Education Accreditation Council (MEAC),** now fully recognized by the U.S. Department of Education. MEAC was founded by a group of midwifery educators who wanted to promote better learning experiences for students by linking their educational programs to the accountability mechanisms and funding opportunities of accreditation. MEAC's primary goal is to preserve a variety of educational routes to midwifery practice, particularly that of apprenticeship.

Addresses for MEAC, MANA, ACNM, and NARM may be found in appendix B. At the grassroots level, **Citizens for Midwifery (CFM)** is the consumer arm of these organizations.

Numerous educational organizations have also cropped up in recent years. Of these, **Midwifery Today**—with magazine, e-zine, conferences worldwide, and an international section—plays a critical role in fostering the next generation of midwives while drawing on the wisdom of those already in practice. As an active participant on the Midwifery Today conference circuit, I can attest to the outstanding work of this organization and the deep inspiration to be found in learning about midwifery by sharing knowledge and skills in a supportive, international environment. (Again, see appendix B for more information.)

Considering the troubled past and the challenging present of midwifery, its survival is something of a miracle. What makes midwifery so desirable to birthing women? Simply put, midwifery promotes well-being. It is an art of service, in that the midwife recognizes, responds to, and cooperates with natural forces. In this sense, midwifery is ecologically attuned, involving the wise utilization of resources and respect for the balance of nature.

Midwifery care is *personalized* care. Within the parameters of safety the midwife upholds, she recognizes wellness as an amorphous state with periodic deviations from normal; her task is to decipher the unique and fluid patterns of each mother's well-being. The more thorough and continuous her care, the more likely she will be to detect a complication at its inception. And the better she and the mother communicate, the more readily will they develop and implement a solution. She and the mother are a team, but the locus of responsibility is always with the latter. As the *MANA Statement of Values and Ethics* states, the mother is "the only direct care provider for her unborn child." The birth itself is merely the culmination of a deeply intimate relationship between the midwife, the mother, and her supporters. Every birth has some potential for complications, and the midwife is trained to deal with these, but her ability to do so is greatly enhanced by foreknowledge of the mother's physical and emotional nature and by the mother's trust in her midwife's competence.

The essence of midwifery is staying in the moment: humble and fully attentive. But this seemingly simple approach is the antithesis of the modus operandi in our culture, particularly in medicine. Early in training, physicians learn to control themselves through the rigors of residency, and then to control their patients and outcomes through standardized procedures. They learn little of the art of caregiving, being taught instead to forgo personal involvement, to mistrust their intuition, to rely only on hard evidence, to expect pathology, and to fear death. It's no wonder they seek control, and as they do, there is no room for nature to take its course.

Such standardized, fear-based care has never appealed to women. What women really want is competent, sensitive attention to their entire condition—care from the inside out. We define our health as more than physical; we seek care that will enable us to be fully ourselves, at our greatest potential. This is precisely what midwives offer. Midwifery has been dubbed an art of invisibility because it is noninterventive, except to do what is needed to promote or restore harmony.

Who is today's midwife? Whether a nurse or empirically trained, working openly or underground, doing hospital or home births, she is a woman ready and willing to go against the grain—that is, if she intends to practice true midwifery. Illegal practice is especially difficult, for she must risk her own welfare to maintain that of her clients. This takes a strong, independent, freethinking woman. And herein lies the secret to the midwife's notoriety: she is a rebel, and a female one at that!

It is ironic that feminism has not more strongly aligned itself with the midwifery issue, especially since reproductive self-determination is central to the feminist vision. Truly, what could be more feminist than the practice of midwifery? The most potent lesson of childbirth is the revelation of essential feminine force. Giving birth calls on a woman to shed her social skin and discover her ability to cooperate with and surrender to elemental forces. Birth can profoundly transform a woman, strengthen her faith, and deepen her identity. Hence the midwife, guardian and facilitator of this process, is intrinsically feminist by the very nature of her work. She knows that women who labor on their own terms and triumph in spontaneous birthing will mother in a fiercely independent fashion, with strength and inner certainty spilling into every other aspect of their lives.

Clearly, the transition of childbirth is more than having a baby; it is a pivotal event in a woman's personal development. In their full capacity, midwives care for women in a whole life context, facilitating physiologic milestones of menarche, birth, menopause, and death. These times of transition are more than biological; they are our Blood Mysteries. In them, we gain wisdom through our bodies that utterly transcends any rational process. Many indigenous cultures have deliberately created rites of passage for men involving pain and suffering (such as the Native American Sundance) to replicate the growth and transformation rendered naturally to women through the Blood Mysteries.

Thus the cultural/evolutionary aspect of midwifery is to motivate women to extend the power and joy of giving birth, to reach beyond the isolation of the nuclear family, to network and share their resources, and to raise their children cooperatively. Midwifery can be readily linked to social innovations in childcare, renewed emphasis on extended family, and holism in other health-care modalities acknowledging factors of nutrition, lifestyle, rest, and support as crucial to well-being. Client and practitioner alike, those who choose midwifery seek connection, they long to rise above divisiveness and competition, they yearn to establish support systems and create community.

Above all else, midwives advocate choice. They vigorously defend a mother's right to choose the place of birth, as they fight for their own right to practice in various settings. Hospital privileges are frequently denied to midwives, or to physicians who support them. We have lost some of our finest obstetricians since the advent of the malpractice crisis: those who could not, in good conscience, perform a requisite battery of tests or procedures at odds with their patients' well-being. It is more than unfortunate that our malpractice system fails to differentiate between acts of fate and those of misconduct; our trial lawyers, posing yet another threat to midwifery and choice, stand to profit whenever there is an unhappy outcome in childbirth, regardless of fault. For midwives, this has meant a dearth of good backup and more urgency than ever to advance a woman-centered model of maternity care.

No wonder most women who choose care with a midwife also choose to give birth at home; they instinctively seek the comfort, privacy, and opportunity for family participation inherent in their own environment, with minimal intervention. Research has shown that the more relaxed and at ease a laboring woman feels, the more efficiently her body will function. If she becomes stressed or frightened, she releases hormones (catecholamines) that inhibit cervical dilation. All birthing mammals behave thus; if they are moved, threatened, denied privacy, or otherwise disturbed, an arrest of progress occurs. This is why pitocin—a synthetic form of oxytocin, the hormone that causes uterine contractions—is so frequently used in hospital births. Unfortunately, pitocin also makes contractions abnormally strong and painful, so many women hoping for natural childbirth end up requesting pain relief. To make matters worse, pain medications may interfere with labor so that more pitocin is needed. But if the uterus is pushed too hard, it will

not relax enough between contractions for healthy circulation, fetal distress ensues, and a cesarean becomes necessary. This cascade of interventions has resulted in a cesarean rate of 26 percent or more in most hospitals, whereas midwife practices average only 3 percent. *When women are in charge of their environment, when they have the privacy to labor undisturbed, when they feel completely at ease and supported, outcomes are always superior.*

Thus the midwife's most basic task is to do everything she can to promote a mothers' relaxation and peace of mind. Beyond her repertoire of medical techniques, her skills encompass less concrete abilities to intuit, evoke, and channel energy. Her hands are her most precious tools, as she senses, heals, and blesses with her touch. Ever attentive but infinitely patient with the process of birth, she waits, and waits, and waits some more. Quietly aware, she serves as a mirror, striving to reserve judgment but speak the truth as the need arises. Above all else, she keeps the following dictum in mind: "It's not my birth." Upholding this tenet of woman-centered care means surrendering her expectations to whatever the mother and her supporters need or desire.

In this regard, experienced midwives often speak of a laboring woman's extraordinary ability to know what is best for herself and her baby. We must never forget to ask the mother's opinion in crisis situations, nor her perceptions of how best to facilitate progress. Put simply, miracles happen in childbirth. The midwife must keep her senses ever alert, and then stand back, let birth happen, and gratefully bear witness.

If we hope to create a maternity-care system that implements midwifery and is truly woman-centered, mothers and their supporters need better access to information, so they can choose both the place of birth and a practitioner with the personal qualities and competence to suit them. Midwives have an urgent obligation to educate the public and to stand firm in their support of woman-centered birth. Why? Because whenever a

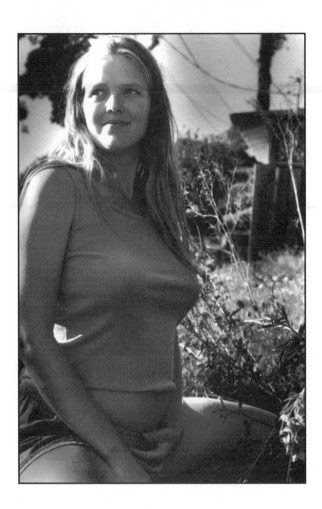

woman reclaims her right to experience birth exactly as she desires, she opens the door to unprecedented joy and fulfillment, while firmly reestablishing the primacy of motherhood in our culture.

Let us wait no longer to heed society's call for midwifery care!

Note

1. United Nations Statistics Division, www.unstats.un.org.

For Parents: Choosing a Midwife

1. How was she trained? In a home or hospital setting? Is she licensed/certified? If not, why not? Are former clients and community members available who can vouch for her? Is she active in, and well regarded by, her local midwifery community?

2. What is her experience? How many births has she attended since completing her training? Has she worked in a variety of settings and practices? Has she completed neonatal resuscitation? Does she regularly attend midwifery conferences, seminars, and workshops to further her education?

3. What do her services include? Complete prenatal care? How long are the appointments? Does she do home visits (how many)? Sibling preparation? Postpartum follow up (how much)? Lab work? Prepared childbirth classes?

4. What are her fees? Does she accept insurance, and what portion of her fee will be paid by your plan? What does her fee include? What if you move or change your mind during the pregnancy? Is her fee competitive? How does she want it to be paid?

5. Does she work alone, with a partner, or with assistants? If there are several assistants involved in the practice, can you choose one to be at your birth? What, exactly, is the assistant's role?

6. Does she have a ceiling on the number of births she attends per month? Is this in keeping with the amount of assistance she has? What would happen if two or more births were running simultaneously? Has she ever missed a birth? If so, what were the circumstances?

7. Who would back her up in case of personal emergency? A midwife outside the practice? Will you have a chance to meet her before the birth?

8. What is her communications system like? Is she available twenty-four hours a day at all times? Is she planning to go on vacation during your pregnancy? If so, who will be on call, and how reachable is she? Can you get the same information on this backup midwife as you are now requesting in this interview? (This is especially critical if her vacation will take place during your third trimester.)

9. What experience has she had with complications? Which ones? Has she ever had to resuscitate a baby? How would she handle a hemorrhage? A stillbirth? Under what circumstances would she transfer care during pregnancy, or transport during labor?

10. What equipment does she bring to births? Oxygen, IV fluids, ambu-bag for baby? Medications for hemorrhage? Homeopathy and herbs? Vitamin K for baby? What does she offer for pain relief?

11. What is her medical backup like? Does she have a particular backup physician and hospital? Is this covered by your insurance? If not, what would be approximate costs to you? Do you have the option of transferring to a hospital that does take your insurance? If so, how is this arranged? If she has a particular backup physician and hospital, what are her privileges in that setting? If you do not have insurance, is there any type of retroactive coverage (state aid) available? What about pediatric backup?

12. What is her philosophy of care? Why is she a midwife? What are her basic beliefs about birth? Does she encourage family participation? Father or partner participation? How? What are her expectations of you regarding self-care in pregnancy?

13. Do you like her? Feel comfortable in her presence? Can you be honest with her? Will she be honest with you? Can you trust her, and yet feel free to make your own decisions? Do you want her at your birth? ■

Chapter 2

PRENATAL CARE

Midwives typically provide comprehensive, continuous prenatal care. By doing so, they get to know clients well enough to have some sense of what to anticipate at the birth. Careful prenatal assessment is the cornerstone of effective midwifery practice; the better we do our work prenatally, the less we are surprised by long, drawn-out labors. Every mother's condition is unique and can only be appreciated by regular contact. Thus we build rapport and a solid working relationship in what we call **continuity of care.**

Assessment is important throughout pregnancy but becomes particularly crucial during the last six weeks. At this point, the midwife can identify certain factors regarding the baby's position, growth rate, and size, and relate these to the mother's condition. On this basis, she can more realistically prepare the mother (and herself) for labor, offering suggestions to prevent complications and make the birth easier. On a technical level, knowing the baby's and mother's norms enables the midwife to determine acceptable range during labor. For everyone concerned, prenatal care definitely proves its worth in terms of time, energy, and anxiety spared at births.

Prenatal care really means wellness care and as such involves nutritional counseling, exercise recommendations, nonallopathic healing options of herbology or homeopathy, and mind-body integration techniques like yoga and meditation. It also includes essential tests and procedures that screen for complications. Routine urinalysis, blood pressure evaluation, uterine/fetal palpation, fetal heart ausculation, and assessment of fundal height/fetal growth are detailed later in this chapter, as are lab work and interpretation of results. If any significant abnormality arises, medical consultation should be sought for guidance and prognosis.

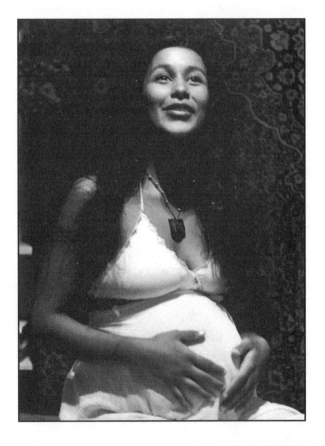

Your first contact with a woman seeking your services will probably be by phone. If you know each other already, you must put aside preconceived notions and be open to new impressions in this preliminary discussion of her pregnancy. Ask her how she became interested in having her baby at home, and what she is looking for in a midwife. This will help you see how well founded her interest is and whether it is worth pursuing further.

If the initial information checks out well, go ahead with questions about her general state of health, her relationship with her partner (if applicable), previous pregnancies, or any history of medical problems. Hopefully, she will have questions regarding your philosophy, experience, backup, and so on. If you decide to meet, an initial visit should be scheduled within the next week or so, preferably at a time when her partner can also attend. Plan to spend at least two hours on this visit, as there will be plenty to discuss and physical examinations to perform if she decides to have you care for her.

Whatever you do, never try to talk a woman into giving birth at home or selecting your practice. She must make the decision on her own to come to you. To uphold principles of woman-centered caregiving, it is crucial that the mother's responsibility for her experience be established from the very beginning.

THE INITIAL INTERVIEW

This very personal, in-depth meeting is your opportunity to understand the mother's ideals surrounding birth and parenting. If she has had other children, she will probably share her previous birth experience(s). If this is her first baby, she will be full of questions.

Your most important task in the initial interview is to determine whether you and the mother are suited to work together. The best way to do this is to relax and be as open as possible. Follow the mother's energetic leads and physical pacing, matching her timing and conversational style so she feels sufficiently at ease to disclose her true beliefs and concerns. Unless she is in charge of the exchange, this will not happen, and your most sage advice will fall on deaf ears. But if you gain her trust, any suggestions you make are apt to be taken seriously. Stay in a receptive mode as much as possible, receiving the mother body and soul, and notice how this contact affects you. If you feel uneasy, apprehensive, or distracted after the meeting, you may not be a match. Having twenty-five years in the field has given me ample opportunity to hear midwives recount their unhappy outcomes, and in each and every case, they ruefully recalled feeling uncomfortable with the mother at the initial visit. Pay attention to your first impressions.

Elicit reasons for choosing home birth from both the mother and her partner (if present). Notice priorities. Ask about the response of friends and family. Factors that go into choosing the place of birth are many, but in order to support mothers in doing what is best for them, we must first understand the role of social and biological instincts.

Social instincts include the need to belong, to be a member of a group and to be recognized by that group. These instincts lead us to make socially recognized choices. Biological instincts are more deeply rooted than social instincts and include those for survival and self-realization. These instincts connect us to our innermost feelings and biological competencies.[1] Problems can develop if biological instincts and social instincts are in conflict, for example, if a woman wants a home birth but none of her friends or family approve. Women with strong biological instincts can break away from their group for a short time, but not without a certain amount of stress.[2]

On the other hand, women with weak biological instincts need more social structure and approval. If planning home birth, they may end up in the hospital and later feel very distressed because they couldn't satisfy their biological instincts. Social and biological models are rarely aligned in hospital birth, thus women birthing within these systems experience this conflict inherently.[3]

To satisfy both instincts, a woman needs a group with similar values to her inner model. This is why support of other home-birthing parents is so critical. It also explains why birth centers offer an effective middle ground for some women; they lessen the conflict because they are more accepted by society.[4] Draw on this perspective to understand the mother's response to questions on how her friends and relatives feel about her plans, and if they are not supportive, how she will deal with this.

Along the same line, who will be at the birth? The mother's response will give you insight into her emotional nature: Is she private or highly social? Ask to meet the birth team as soon as possible, to see whether her projections are realistic and to identify any gaps in her support system. Some women initially plan on having quite a party at the birth and then whittle down participants as pregnancy advances; you can certainly help her choreograph the event as it draws near. But do encourage her to speak to everyone interested in being at the birth about committing to specific tasks of postpartum assistance. It is never too early to start lining up some take-in dinners, or help with laundry, housework, and so on for the first few weeks after the baby comes.

Try to get a clear sense of how the mother defines your role in pregnancy, labor, and postpartum. Does she want lots of guidance, or will her partner be her main support? If she wants help primarily from her partner, do her expectations seem realistic? Does her partner want to catch the baby? If they want to do most of the birth themselves, do they accept the necessity of routine checks from time to time? As the mother expresses her hopes and desires, it becomes easier for you to anticipate her needs and tailor your level of participation to suit.

Throughout this discussion, there may be appropriate moments for passing along information, suggesting resources for further study, or providing referrals to groups or individuals. Help the mother and her partner realize that there is a lot to learn, and that it is up to them to explore their options. Recommend books, magazines or newsletters, websites, videos, or prenatal exercise or support groups. Generate a reading list to provide at this first meeting, including referrals to local chapters of organizations like La Leche League (see appendix B).

You must also disclose your training, philosophy, style of practice, and expectations of clients. The easiest way to do this is with a take-home document, a "Professional Disclosure and Consent to Care," to be returned and signed in your presence. Include conditions that require consultation or referral, your relationship to the medical community, risks of home birth, and complications that might result in damage or death to mother or baby. Of course you should stress that thorough prenatal care and careful monitoring in labor will go a long way toward preventing these, but make clear that some complications are unforeseeable. In California, licensed midwives are required by law to disclose whether they have malpractice insurance; in any case, you must disclose your legal status. The consent-to-care language should state that clients, in full knowledge of your limitations, voluntarily agree to work with you, and with their signature, release you and your associates from all liability. It is also wise to include a statement that in the event of a dispute, parents agree to seek nonbinding arbitration before filing suit.

As you review and discuss this form at the next visit, watch for nervous or negative reactions. Note resistance to hospital transport or apprehension regarding life-threatening complications. If the mother (or her partner) seems unusually fearful, ask for her or his worst nightmare regarding the birth. This gives you an opportunity to evaluate the depth of commitment to home birth, and a chance to provide some explanation of how complications occur. Also emphasize the preventive role of prenatal care, hopefully impressing the mother with the importance of keeping appointments and informing you of any unusual developments.

Early in caregiving, the two most serious emergencies—hemorrhage and fetal distress—require detailed discussion. Explain possible causes of hemorrhage and your procedures for handling it. Discuss your methods for dealing with a depressed baby, including training, tools, and techniques for resuscitation. Most of the time you will go out of your way to inform the mother and her supporters of any unusual developments during labor, taking pains to thoroughly explain treatment options. But there may not be time for this in emergency situations, so get the basics across as soon as possible.

MEDICAL HISTORY

Medical history can be taken by interview or provided by the mother via a take-home form (see appendix C). It should survey for all conditions and diseases that might impact this pregnancy. Preexisting diabetes or hypertension, thyroid disease (hyperthyroidism), chronic lung disease, severe asthma, epilepsy, clotting disorders, congenital heart disease (grades 2–4), and kidney disease contraindicate home birth. Conditions arising in pregnancy that rule out home birth include Rh– with antibodies, severe anemia unresponsive to treatment, and acute viral infections (depending on when they occur) such as rubella, cytomegalovirus, toxoplasmosis, chicken pox, or herpes. Preexisting conditions of unresolved sexually transmitted disease, malnutrition, drug addiction, moderate to frequent alcohol use, and smoking are also contraindications. Have a comprehensive obstetrical text available to evaluate any irregularities in the medical history, and seek the consultation of peers or medical backup whenever in doubt.

Obstetrical history is of foremost importance. Note any history of transport, or obstetrical emergencies of placental abruption, fetal distress, postpartum hemorrhage, shoulder dystocia, or neonatal asphyxiation. Investigate thoroughly and consider implications for the current pregnancy. History of previous childbirth losses requires attention to physical factors and the mother's emotional recovery. Perceived losses due to disappointing birth outcomes should also be discussed. Is there anything that the mother experienced with previous birthing that she wants to avoid this time? Or is there something she had hoped for previously that she would like to experience this time? Don't forget the issue of child spacing; if she has had a child within the past two years, explore the impact of close-set childbearing on her physical and psychological health.

Any history of abortion should be discussed as soon as the mother is ready. What type of procedure was used? Was there a problem with excessive bleeding or infection afterward? Suction is less traumatic to the uterine lining than dilation and curettage, which involves scraping the endometrium and may cause scarring that can interfere with placental implantation (as may postabortion sepsis). How was the decision to have an abortion reached? What, if any, were the emotional side effects? Many women feel great loss after an abortion ("like tearing your heart out," one woman said) and need to talk it over, either with you or with a specialist. The same is true of women with a history of repeated miscarriage. If the mother had a saline-, Cyotec-, or prostaglandin-induced abortion, she experienced a version of labor and may link negative emotions with contraction sensations. Do your best to forestall difficulties in labor by discussing this thoroughly in advance.

What about **previous cesarean birth**? Now here is an area of controversy. Until recently, the data on vaginal birth after a cesarean (VBAC) with low transverse incision showed no significant dangers to mother or baby. But in the past decade, the use of the labor stimulant Cytotec (an ulcer medicine unapproved for this purpose) has increased the rate of uterine rupture to as much as 6 percent.[5] Consequently, the medical standard has changed from support for VBAC to recommended repeat cesarean. This is maddening, as midwives in the home setting don't use Cytotec.

Nevertheless, midwives in some states are now forbidden to assist VBAC at home; in others, midwives may do so, depending on medical backup and hospital policy. In New Hampshire, the following VBAC guidelines were recently instated in legal practice code:

A midwife shall accept as a client a woman who has had a previous birth by cesarean section only if:

a) The potential client has had only one previous cesarean section;

b) The midwife can confirm through a review of the records of the previous delivery by cesarean section that the section was performed through a low transverse uterine segment incision;

c) The potential client has had no other uterine surgeries;

d) At least 18 months' time separates the date of the potential client's previous cesarean section and the due date of the current pregnancy;

e) An obstetric ultrasound documents that the placenta is not in a low-lying anterior position;

f) The potential client plans to give birth in a location no more than 20 minutes' drive from a hospital with obstetrical and anesthesia services on call 24 hours a day.

There is also evidence to suggest that single-layer suturing of the cesarean incision (in contrast to the more thorough double-layer repair) quadruples the risk of rupture.[6] But single-layer repair has been practiced for years, and medical records seldom specify the method of incision closure, so the point is somewhat moot. Bottom line: the healthier the mother, and the greater the interval between cesarean and subsequent pregnancy, the less she is considered to be at risk.

Psychological issues for a mother desiring a VBAC are formidable. She may have been told she needed surgery because her bones were too small, her hormone levels too low, or she simply failed to progress. Such comments leave devastating scars, and before vaginal birth is attempted, some healing must take place. Veterans of cesarean birth may need hypnotherapy, eye movement desensitization and repro-

cessing (EMDR), or other mind-body therapy to regain a sense of confidence in themselves and their body. Support is also available through organizations like the **International Cesarean Awareness Network (ICAN)** (see appendix B).

Plans for an out-of-hospital VBAC definitely require that the mother and her partner sign a detailed consent form. But because of all she must do to prepare herself, assisting a woman with a VBAC is truly a privilege.

Gynecological history is also of great significance in pregnancy. Check for history of fibroids, the prime symptom of which is painless bleeding with intercourse. These benign uterine masses vary in size but tend to grow considerably during pregnancy. Depending on whether they are external or internal, pregnancy may be affected by reduced intrauterine space or disrupted placental implantation, and the immediate postpartum may be complicated by hemorrhage. A sonogram is advisable to determine the exact size and location of fibroids.

Gynecological surgeries can complicate pregnancy, depending on the procedure. If the mother has had a cone biopsy (to remove abnormal cervical cells), considerable scarring may retard dilation. Cervical cauterization and cryosurgery are less traumatic, but the cervix should still be checked for scarring. Scar tissue may be softened by evening primrose oil massaged gently onto the cervix in the last few weeks of pregnancy. LEEP, a laser procedure similar in effect to cone biopsy, has been correlated to incompetent cervix and premature labor. Some midwives feel that any woman with a history of this procedure should be checked for cervical changes throughout pregnancy and should be educated regarding signs of premature labor.

Contraceptive history is also important. If the mother had an IUD prior to conception, she may be anemic because of excess menstruation and should be checked for this as soon as possible. The IUD can also cause scarring of the uterine lining, which predisposes to ectopic pregnancy, irregular implantation of the placenta, and third-stage hemorrhage. Pelvic inflammatory disease (PID) has the same effect. Scar tissue may also form at the cervical os (see earlier suggestion regarding evening primrose oil). If the mother used oral contraception immediately prior to pregnancy, she may be deficient in folic acid and should be advised to begin supplementation at once.

Family history is important to determine a propensity for hypertension, diabetes, cancer, or other diseases that could impact pregnancy or require additional screening from a specialist.

Spend plenty of time at this visit reviewing symptoms experienced with this pregnancy. Any incidence of **bleeding or spotting** is significant and should be closely tracked by both mother and midwife. If combined with nonrhythmic pain, immediately consult with backup to rule out tubal pregnancy (the window for rupture is ten to thirteen weeks). If bleeding becomes chronic, missed abortion and molar pregnancy must be ruled out, or, if late in pregnancy, placental problems (see chapter 3). Generalized edema experienced before conception or prior to twenty-four weeks should be medically evaluated; if occurring later in pregnancy, rule out preeclampsia (see chapter 3). In either case, immediately have the mother eliminate heavily processed foods, and suggest plenty of high-quality protein, fresh vegetables, salt to taste, and ample fluids. Hormones and circulatory changes may cause occasional headaches, but a persistent headache, particularly in combination with signs of preeclampsia, indicates a medical crisis and the need for immediate referral. Visual problems, upper abdominal pain, or epigastric pain—especially on the right side—are urgent warning signs of preeclampsia (see chapter 3).

Any history of flu-like symptoms such as swollen glands, extreme fatigue, or generalized body aches should be noted, although the most devastating viral infections of pregnancy are frequently asymptomatic. **Cytomegalovirus** is a fairly common infection—60 per-

cent of the general population has antibodies—and is most damaging in the first trimester. **Toxoplasmosis** is known to cause severe neurological damage to the fetus, but only if contracted after ten weeks. Mothers can minimize their chances of contracting toxoplasmosis by avoiding uncooked meat and any contact with cat feces (let someone else change the litter box). Even viral infections like **varicella (chicken pox)** can be extremely dangerous in pregnancy, so encourage all mothers to avoid possible exposure.

Any report of painful vaginal sores combined with flu-like malaise in early pregnancy may indicate an initial outbreak of **herpes.** Check the mother's history, do a visual inspection, and take cultures. An initial outbreak in the first trimester can have serious consequences for the baby and requires immediate consultation with backup. Barring this, protocol for managing preexisting herpes is ever changing and has yet to catch up with the research. The standard of care is to perform a cesarean if there are active lesions at the onset of labor, as neonatal infection can lead to central nervous system damage and death. But studies show the rate of neonatal infection to be much less with a recurrence at the onset of labor (3 percent) than with an initial outbreak (41 percent).[7] It appears that mothers who suffer nonprimary herpes while pregnant pass antibodies to their unborn fetuses. Nevertheless, medical management for women with a history of herpes remains conservative.

If there is a recurrence in pregnancy, the cervix should be cultured, as herpes at this site can be asymptomatic. If cervical shedding is noted, plan to do a slide test (or at least a visual inspection) at the onset of labor to rule out current infection. If lesions are present externally (not in the immediate path of the baby), some midwives do permit vaginal birth. Lesions must be covered with surgical adhesive film or spray-on bandage.

Any history of vomiting with the pregnancy should be carefully explored to rule out **hyperemesis gravidarium.** A mother with this condition has more than occasional nausea-related vomiting; instead, it is chronic and self-perpetuating. This so disrupts her electrolyte balance that she cannot retain either food or liquid and must be restabilized with intravenous replacement therapy before she can eat or drink again. It bears mentioning that hyperemesis gravidarium is one of the only conditions for which conventional medicine acknowledges emotional underpinnings, and some midwives do note a correlation between hyperemesis and psychological conflicts or difficulties regarding the pregnancy. Another theory is that elevated estrogen levels may cause liver irritation sufficient to engender the condition in some women. With emotional factors outstanding, suggest counseling. Otherwise, have the mother immediately take ginger root three times daily, either fresh grated in tea or ground in capsules, as you continue to monitor her condition. If vomiting persists beyond the first trimester, consult with a colleague or physician backup.

Fatigue is certainly common in early pregnancy (due primarily to elevated hormone levels), but fatigue combined with dizziness or nausea beyond the first trimester may indicate anemia (more on this condition in chapter 3).

Any report of **urinary tract problems** must be addressed immediately. During pregnancy, characteristic signs of urinary tract infection (stinging, urgency, pain after urination) may be nearly absent, due to progesterone's softening effect on the urethra. This can lead to kidney infection, or **pyelonephritis,** which in turn can lead to premature labor. Any woman with a history of bladder infection must be alerted to these facts and should be told to call for screening with even the subtlest symptoms. Pay close attention, too, to any report of **vaginal discharge** or signs of infection. Depending on her symptoms, arrange for her to be screened for sexually transmitted diseases (STDs) that could negatively impact pregnancy (see the section on "Lab Work," later in this chapter).

It is also crucial to note the **use of any prescription or over-the-counter medications** (OTCs) with this pregnancy. Thirty percent of mental retardation is of unknown etiology. The fetus has an underdeveloped blood-brain barrier, which ordinarily protects the brain from harmful substances. Thus pregnant women should avoid OTCs with the same vigilance they do alcohol or recreational drugs.

The same is true of many household chemicals, substances used in the workplace, and environmentally based chemicals found in drinking water and food. Any substance that can harm the fetus or cause fetal anomalies is called a **teratogen.** The midwife can research teratogenic side effects of medications in a current copy of *Physician's Desk Reference*, or may consult Anne Frye's *Holistic Midwifery (Volume I)* to investigate risks of certain environmental or work-related chemical exposures. The Organization of Teratology Information Services (OTIS) has extensive information on teratogens: contact them at (866) 626-6847 or at www.OTISpregnancy.org. Information is also available from the March of Dimes, at www.marchofdimes.com.

Take note of the mother's response to the question regarding ethnic, cultural, or religious preferences. If you have not yet had diversity training, consider taking a class or workshop on the subject. It is particularly difficult to realize cultural bias if you are white and thus part of the dominant culture. As Professor Peggy McIntosh has stated in her article "White Privilege: Unpacking the Invisible Knapsack": "As a white person, I realized I had been taught about racism as something which puts others at a disadvantage, but had not been taught to see one of its corollary aspects, white privilege, which puts me at an advantage. . . . Many, perhaps most of our white students in the U.S. think racism doesn't affect them because they are not people of color: they do not see 'whiteness' as a racial identity."[8] For specific information on cultural and religious beliefs and preferences regarding pregnancy and birth, see the outstanding section on this subject in Frye's *Holistic Midwifery (Volume I)*.

A bonus in the take-home format of the medical history is that the final set of questions prompts both the mother and her partner to make definitive statements regarding their hopes, fears, and expectations. How they respond to the possibility of damage or death to mother or baby speaks to their perception of responsibility in the event of an unexpected outcome, their level of emotional preparedness, and ultimately, their commitment to home birth. Responses regarding hospital transport are also important, as anything less than full willingness to consider the midwife's directives precludes establishing a healthy working relationship. Likewise, responses regarding the midwife's role may reveal incompatibility with her style of practice.

Occasionally you will encounter a woman unwilling to fill out take-home forms. She may profess enthusiasm for home birth, yet in nearly every case I can recall, this stance has borne out an unwillingness to take responsibility. If any part of the history is incomplete, send it home to be finished up before accepting her into your practice.

PHYSICAL EXAMINATION

Every woman should have a complete physical examination early in her pregnancy, unless she has had one within the past year. This is to rule out any conditions that might negatively impact her pregnancy or the baby's health. As competency in performing physical assessment requires considerable hands-on training, I will not attempt to present this here. A physician or other practitioner can always perform the physical, whereas breast exams, pelvic exams, and the routine assessments described in this section are essentials of midwifery care. Learn more about physical examination from a comprehensive midwifery text, such as Frye's *Holistic Midwifery (Volume I)* or Helen Varney's *Varney's Midwifery*.

The initial exam provides an opportunity to ascertain the mother's general state of health. Beyond that, a core purpose of this assessment is to earn her trust.

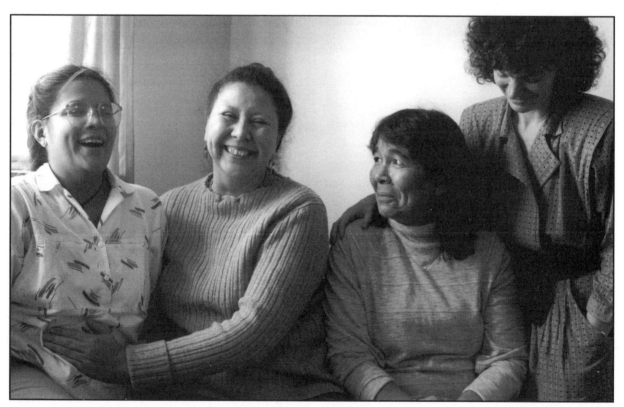

Native American pregnant woman with aunties and midwife, right.

Do this by establishing physical intimacy at a pace that is comfortable for her. And record your findings as you go (see the "Prenatal Care Record" in appendix D).

Begin by establishing her **estimated date of delivery (EDD)** or, if you prefer, **estimated date of birth (EDB)**. Take the first day of her **last menstrual period (LMP),** count back three months and add one week—this formula calculates ten lunar months, or 40 weeks, and is known as **Naegele's Rule.** Also record her **previous menstrual period (PMP),** note the interval between that and the LMP, and compare with her average cycle length. A short interval (less than three weeks) suggests that the LMP was implantation bleeding, not a true period. Recalculate the EDD accordingly.

A word of caution—don't take the EDD too seriously. The Mittendorf study showed the average length of human gestation to be forty-one weeks plus one day.[9] No wonder only 5 percent of women give birth on their due date! Frustrated by the confines of Naegele's Rule, midwifery professor Carol Wood Nichols developed a method of calculating the EDD that takes into account variations in cycle length as well

---

High Risk Factors in Pregnancy

Medical and Health Factors

1. **Diabetes.** Preexisiting diabetes is a definite contraindication to home birth.

   Dangers: Fetal demise after thirty-six weeks, five times the normal incidence of fetal abnormalities, increased polyhydramnios, 30–50 percent higher incidence of preeclampsia, increased incidence of prematurity and newborn respiratory difficulties.

2. **Thyroid disease.** Particularly hyperthyroidism. Slight enlargement of the thyroid gland is normal in pregnancy, but persistent tachycardia or elevated levels of circulating thyroid hormone are symptoms of disease.

   Dangers: Thyroid medication has potential for causing severe fetal complications. Hyperthyroidism can cause miscarriage, premature labor, and fetal anomalies. Untreated hypothyroidism can lead to cretinism in the newborn.

3. **Active tuberculosis.** Refer to physician backup. If under treatment, prognosis for mother and baby is good, although the baby must be immediately separated from the mother if she is infectious.

   Dangers: Slightly higher risk of miscarriage or premature labor.

4. **Chronic lung disease.** As diagnosed by medical history.

   Dangers: Mother at risk for pulmonary complications, baby for fetal acidosis and hypoxia.

5. **Severe asthma.** As prediagnosed.

   Dangers: Respiratory infections and stress may intensify attacks. Cardiopulmonary function could be reduced, affecting fetal growth and well-being. Certain medications used to treat asthma are contraindicated for pregnancy.

6. **Epilepsy.** There is controversy over whether or not this condition is exacerbated by pregnancy.

   Dangers: Anticonvulsant drugs may cause folic acid deficiency, which when treated with folic acid may cause seizures. The infant may develop deficiency of coagulation factors.

7. **Clotting abnormalities.** Afibrinogenemia, hypofibrinogenemia, excessive fibrinalytic activity, or a combination of these.

   Dangers: Can lead to maternal blood loss, shock, or death.

8. **Rh– with antibodies.** Refer to physician backup.

continued →

Dangers: Hemolytic anemia, fetal or neonatal death (although intrauterine transfusion can avert this).

9. **Severe anemia.** Hereditary anemias such as Thalassemia B or sickle cell, as well as nutritional anemias (iron, B-12, and folic acid deficiencies) unresolved at term.

Dangers: Maternal infection, prolonged labor, hemorrhage, intrauterine growth restriction, fetal hypoxia during labor.

10. **Acute viral infection.** Rubella, mumps, cytomegalovirus, herpes, coxsackie virus, pneumonia, hepatitis B or C, smallpox, severe influenza, and polio.

Dangers: Possible birth defects, fetal or maternal death.

11. **Congenital heart disease (grades 2–4).** Refer to physician backup.

Dangers: Increased blood volume and weight put strain on impaired heart. Condition requires clinical, electrocardiography, and radiological surveillance.

12. **Renal disease.** Impaired kidney function necessitates close medical surveillance in pregnancy. Signs of renal disease include protein in the urine, hypertension, edema, and elevated blood urea all before the twentieth week.

Dangers: Acute renal failure.

13. **Extreme obesity.** Preexisting, with history of medical problems.

Dangers: Nearly two-thirds of extremely obese women have obstetrical complications, including diabetes, hypertension, pyelonephritis, uterine dysfunction, and hemorrhage.

Lifestyle and Personal Factors

1. **Tobacco use.** More than ten cigarettes daily, although no amount can be considered without risk.

Dangers: Associated with intrauterine growth restriction, miscarriage, congenital heart disease, and fetal hypoxia in labor.

2. **Malnutrition.** Extreme dietary deficiencies (may be correlated to substance abuse, debilitating illness, eating disorders).

Dangers: Intrauterine growth restriction, preeclampsia, maternal or fetal infection, prematurity, stillbirth, dysfunctional labor, and hemorrhage.

3. **Drug addiction.** Chronic substance abuse.

Dangers: Intrauterine growth restriction, fetal hypoxia, respiratory distress syndrome (RDS), maternal malnutrition, infection, preeclampsia, dysfunctional labor, hemorrhage. Newborns whose mothers are addicted to cocaine, crack or crank, heroin, or barbiturates will go through withdrawal within the first three days of delivery.

4. **Moderate to heavy alcohol use.** Periodic binging, or more than two drinks per day of alcohol may cause damage or defects.

Dangers: Fetal alcohol syndrome—fetus has 50 percent chance of mental retardation, 30 percent chance of anomaly, impaired eyesight, behavioral problems, and stillbirth.

5. **Heavy caffeine use.** In excess of ten cups per day of moderately strong coffee, black tea, cola, or other caffeine-containing beverages.

Dangers: Fetal malformations, heart defects, reproductive problems. ∎

as previous childbearing. Here is her formula, known as **Nichols' Rule:**[10]

First-time moms with 28-day cycles: LMP + 12 months − 2 months, 14 days = EDD

Second-time moms or more with 28-day cycles: LMP + 12 months − 2 months, 18 days = EDD

Cycles longer than 28 days: EDD + (days in cycle − 28 days) = EDD

Cycles shorter than 28 days: EDD − (28 days − days in cycle) = EDD

Before proceeding to physical assessments, ask the mother's permission and clearly obtain her consent. This may seem a formality to you after a while, but it is crucial in upholding her role as director of her care, and yours as assistant.

Begin by **checking her weight,** noting her prepregnant norm and total gain thus far. Assuming that her starting weight was normal for her height and frame, an average gain is about a pound per week. Many women are sensitive about their changing figure and should be reassured that an ample weight gain is both desirable and essential for the baby's health and their own endurance, particularly during labor and the immediate postpartum. It is noteworthy that most European midwives do not routinely check their prenatal clients' weight, relying instead on hemoglobin levels, general vitality, and the baby's rate of growth as better determinants of well-being. Considering the degree to which women in the United States tend to be obsessed about their weight, easing up on this routine evaluation might benefit both mother and baby.

Then **check her urine** with a testing strip, looking for protein and glucose. Many midwives encourage clients to test their own urine and have cups and testing strips available in the rest room. If using a broad-spectrum strip, check for blood, ketones, and nitrates. Ketones signal inadequate food intake or dehydration (more details in chapter 3). Findings of blood or protein require another, clean-catch sample to rule out contamination from vaginal discharge. Anything over a trace of protein may indicate preeclampsia; blood or nitrates are suggestive of urinary tract infection. Always explain any unusual findings to the mother immediately.

Next **check her blood pressure,** which may be somewhat elevated due to tension or excitement. There are two assessments made when taking blood pressure: the systolic reading (high number), which indicates the pressure in the arteries when the heart is actively pumping, and the diastolic reading (low number), which indicates the pressure when the heart is at rest. Normal blood pressure during pregnancy ranges from 90/50 to 140/90, although readings higher than 130/80 or a steady rise from baseline are cause for concern.

In essence, diastolic pressure assesses baseline intravascular tension, whereas systolic pressure indicates cardiovascular tolerance for exertion. Medical texts claim that only the systolic reading is influenced by emotional state, but I have found elevation in both to be fairly common at the initial visit, particularly if the mother is nervous. If so, I reassure her for the moment and take her blood pressure again before she leaves. If still high, I schedule a recheck in a few days. Women with consistent readings of 130/80 or more in early pregnancy may have undiagnosed essential hypertension (see chapter 3). But if readings later climb to this level, begin stress-reduction or other therapies in earnest. Additional symptoms of generalized edema or proteinuria may indicate preeclampsia, for which the mother should be immediately referred to a physician backup.

Along with the blood pressure, **check her pulse and temperature** to establish baselines. Since heightened reflexes can be a signal of preeclampsia, it's also wise to **establish baseline reflexes** as soon as possible. Use a reflex hammer and note degree of reflex irritability.

You should also **perform a breast exam.** Your goal is to determine the overall structure of breast tissue and identify all lumps within it. The norm is bilateral symmetry, which nevertheless allows for dramatic variation in structure from woman to woman. On occasion, I have been alarmed to find something quite unusual in one breast, only to be reassured by discovering the exact same tissue formation in the other. Of the several standard techniques for performing breast exam, I prefer the following:

1. *Begin by observing the woman's breasts while she is sitting upright.* Look for symmetry, note nipples pointing in an unnatural way, any puckering or pull around the areola, or irregularities in skin texture. Also have her place her hands on her hips and push against her hipbones, and observe as above.

2. *Have her lie down, and continue your exam by pressing your fingertips across the entire surface of the upper chest, collarbone down to the breasts.* Some women have accessory breast tissue in this area, so check thoroughly. Normally, all you feel is a layer of muscle tissue with ribs beneath.

3. *Continue the same pressing motion as you explore the breast tissue, quadrant by quadrant.* It is okay to lift the breast and move it slightly to one side or the other to accomplish this. Try using a combination of light, medium, and firm pressure in each area, sliding (rather than lifting) your fingers to the next spot to be sure you don't skip an area. If at any time you find a lump or mass, immediately check the same spot in the other breast (if structures match, everything is fine).

4. *Focus on the upper, outer quadrant of the breast, as this is the area that contains the most tissue and is therefore the most likely site for abnormal growth.* Feel more deeply into this area by using thumb and forefingers to reach in and grasp underlying tissue, rolling it to assess structure. In small- to moderate-sized breasts, the tissue forms a bar extending from armpit to nipple; larger breasts will have an extension of this bar down from the nipple to the bottom edge of the breast. Use this lifting and rolling motion on any area of the breast that has thick (or unusual) tissue. Again, if you find anything unusual, compare it with the other breast.

5. *Be sure to feel directly beneath the nipple, and then squeeze it gently to check for any secretion.* Colostrum, recognizable as a thick yellow discharge, may be evident after the first months of pregnancy. Occasionally women have greenish or bloody discharge that proves perfectly normal but should still be evaluated by an expert.

6. *Finally, feel along the outer edge of the breast and into the armpit, feeling deeply for any lumps* (likely to be enlarged lymph nodes).

7. *Repeat the entire procedure on the other breast to establish symmetry.*

Explain what you are doing step by step, and then have the mother repeat the exam in your presence. Many women give up on self-exam because they feel the technique is too complicated, or because they are alarmed to find their breasts lumpy instead of smooth. Reassure the mother that every woman's breasts are lumpy, so her best bet is to identify the lumps in one, and then compare with the other to be sure the lumps match. If her breasts are particularly dense or large, have her try leaning forward to palpate. This new technique is thought to allow better access to deep breast tissue much the way mammogram screening does.

Some midwives postpone **pelvic assessment** until the second visit. As you and the mother have had little contact thus far, this may be the best approach. If she has been a victim of sexual abuse, she will probably have a strong reaction to internal examination. (Although questions on the medical history form address this issue, you will not yet have this information if using the take-home format.) Every midwife should be fully aware of signs of sexual abuse and how to respond appropriately. More information on this subject can be found in chapter 3.

In any case, always ask the mother's permission before beginning pelvic assessment. If she has not already put her shirt back on after breast exam, see if she would like to do so or would like a blanket or sheet to cover up. If her partner is present, don't assume the mother wants him or her there for this portion of the visit. Take your lead from the mother; she will invite her partner or ask if he or she can be present if this is what she desires.

Internal exam is an intimate experience, and most women have had enough rough, insensitive exams to feel more than a little nervous. Explain what you are going to do and proceed gently. Ask her to position herself with knees bent, legs apart, and feet flat on the bed or exam couch. (Stirrups are unnecessary, but it helps if she can get the small of her back flat so that her pelvis tips slightly upward.) Wash your hands, put on a glove, apply lubricating jelly to your index and middle fingers, and ask permission to begin. As you do so, let yourself be guided by her muscular reaction—never ever force your way. Make eye contact if she is open to it and continually reassure her by sharing your findings.

Once you and she are comfortable, **check her cervix.** Note its condition (consistency, length, patency), position (central, posterior, or anterior), and any growths at or from the os, which may be respectively cysts or polyps. If the cervix feels irregular, insert a speculum and do a visual inspection. Depending on what you see, you may wish to do a Pap smear—although you should postpone this temporarily, as lubricating jelly can contaminate results (see "Lab Work" in this chapter).

If she is sixteen weeks or fewer, you may confirm the EDD by doing a **bimanual exam** to size the uterus. Press up firmly on the cervix while using your other hand to palpate the fundus (top of the uterus). If this is difficult, place a finger on either side of the cervix and press up that way. As you bring your hands together, you will get an idea of how large the uterus has grown. At ten weeks, the fundus barely clears the pubic bone; at twelve weeks it is generally a few centimeters above the pubis; at sixteen weeks it is midway between the pubic bone and the umbilicus.

If uterine size does not seem to conform to the EDD, reevaluate the menstrual history. Women with irregular cycles may have incorrect dates, as may breast-feeding mothers who conceive before ever having a period. Others are uncertain of their dates because they have continued to bleed after conception, perhaps for several months at the time menstruation would ordinarily occur. If the uterus does not seem to be enlarged, do a pregnancy test before proceeding further. Also consider scheduling a prenatal visit at the time the woman would be twenty weeks, according to the current EDD (for details, see page 28).

Now you are ready to **perform pelvimetry.** As you make your assessments, be sure to explain to the mother what you are doing (perhaps your partner can show points on a model pelvis). And remember that the pelvis will expand as pregnancy progresses.

Certain measurements of your hand must be taken prior to practice. Measure first from the inside of your thumb joint to the tip of your middle finger. Then make a fist and measure across your fingers. Note both these measurements in centimeters.

Pelvimetry has five basic steps. The first is **assessing the depth of the sacral curve.** Begin by finding the coccyx: place your fingers (pad side down) a few inches inside the vagina, lift your wrist, and press down as far as you can reach. Do this slowly but steadily, with fingers perpendicular to the vaginal floor. When you feel the hardness of bone, keep pressure on this point as you rotate your thumb up (so it faces the mother's chin). Keeping your fingertips firmly on the bone, trace the sacral curve upward toward the sacral promontory (see illustration "Measuring the Diagonal Conjugate," page 26). The sacral curve should feel deep and rounded, like a half-circle, although usually you can only trace it for several inches. If it feels flat, note the possibility of an android pelvis. If you can feel the entire curve (and your fingers are not exceptionally long) note the possibility of a platypelloid or smaller gynecoid pelvis. Occasionally, a strong bulbocavernosus muscle (located about an inch or so inside the vagina) presents an obstacle to this maneuver. In this case, go in a bit further initially, then press down and draw your fingertips back toward you to find the coccyx.

Next, **assess the size of the pelvic inlet.** If the sacral curve is deep (no bone can be felt after a few inches), the inlet is clearly adequate. Otherwise, follow through until you reach the sacral promontory (your fingers should be at a horizontal plane). You are now in position to measure the **diagonal conjugate.** For example, if your span from thumb joint to fingertip is 13.5 cm, and a centimeter of your span remains outside the mother, you estimate the diagonal conjugate to be 12.5 cm. From this, subtract the 1.5 cm thickness of the pubic bone to obtain the actual inlet dimension the baby must negotiate, termed the **obstetrical conjugate.** A measurement of 10.5 cm or greater is considered adequate.

Next, **assess the contour of, and distance between, the ischial spines.** Withdraw your fingers until they are only a few inches inside, then bend them directly sideways, pressing all the way to the pelvic sidewall, that is, until you feel bone. Move slightly downward (if right handed, from nine to eight o'clock), then hook your fingertips toward you. The ischial spine feels like a mass of ligamentous tissue. A definite indication that you have found it is the mother's response; she will flinch as you touch nerve attachment points in close proximity. Disregard the inclination to pull your fingers away, and press a bit more deeply (without poking) to see whether the prominence is blunt and barely noticeable, or sharply pointed and protruding. Note the contour of one spine, then turn finger pads down and repeat the procedure for the other (at the four o'clock position).

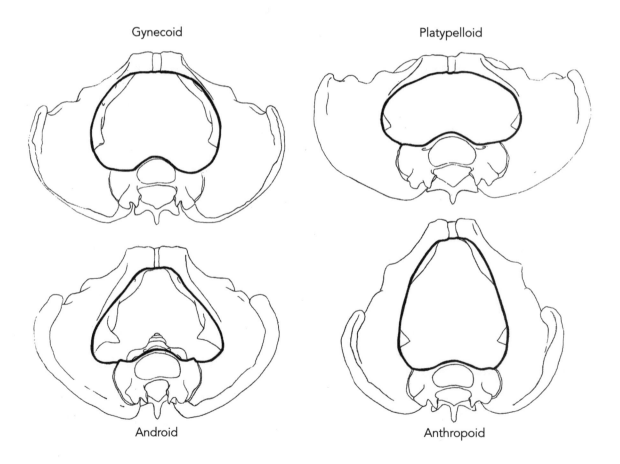

Gynecoid

Platypelloid

Android

Anthropoid

Basic Pelvic Types

Sometimes one spine is prominent, and the other is not. Complete your assessment by opening your fingers to measure the distance between the spines, or **interspinous diameter,** which should be at least 10.5 cm.

Next, slowly turn your fingers pad side up and withdraw to about an inch. Lift your palm up to an angle of about 45 degrees, press your fingers up under the pubic bone, and **assess the angle, or width of the pubic arch.** You should be able to fit two fingers beneath the arch and spread them slightly apart. Finally, take your fingers out and **assess the outlet dimension or intertuberous diameter** by making a fist and gently pressing it between the lowest point on the ischial tuberosities (somewhat below the introitus). If your fist is of average measurement—around 8.5 cm—it should fit comfortably, with some play side to side.

This completes the pelvic exam. Chart your findings, as these may have relevance in labor. Women occasionally ask if the shape or size of their hips has any bearing on labor. Explain that there is a difference between the **true pelvis,** which includes all dimensions from the inlet downward, and the **false pelvis,** which includes the illiac crests or hip bones, above. Though disconcerting, this terminology serves to illustrate that hip size is unreliable in predicting pelvic capacity.

In terms of pelvic type, refer to the diagrams on page 24. Basically, it all comes down to depth (of sacral curve and inlet dimension) in relationship to width (between spines, of pubic arch, and between ischial tuberosities). The **gynecoid** provides a round space, equally deep and wide, and is by far the most common. The **anthropoid** is notably deeper than it is wide, a tall oval with great depth in the sacral curve, but more narrow in width than the average gynecoid. The **platypelloid** is wider than it is deep, a wide oval, with less depth in the sacral curve but more width than the average gynecoid. The **android** has all the quirks: prominent, close-set spines, tapering sidewalls, narrow pubic arch (less than 80 degrees), and close-set tuberosities. The android is sometimes called the funnel pelvis because

it gets more and more narrow toward the outlet. Fortunately, pure android types are quite rare, although a woman may have a single android characteristic, like one prominent ischial spine.

Some midwives prefer to wait on pelvimetry until the last trimester, when hormone-induced softening of the four pelvic joints—**the symphysis pubis joint, the sacrococcygeal joint, and the two sacroiliac joints**—may dramatically increase any borderline aspect of the pelvis, particularly the transverse or outlet dimensions. I personally think doing pelvimetry early helps assuage women's nearly universal fear of being "too small" to give birth vaginally. And because an adequate pelvis is ultimately determined by the size of the baby, you can truthfully reassure any woman at this point that there is plenty of room. Just don't worry if the tissues feel tight in early pregnancy, as changes during the third trimester are really quite remarkable.

Beginning midwives often find the **Three Ps** context of passage, passenger, and powers helpful for appreciating the relative significance of pelvimetry. The **passage** is defined as the bony pelvis and musculature, the **passenger** is the baby and how it is presenting, and the **powers** refer to uterine activity during labor (which reflect the mother's emotional and physical well-being). Note that the passage is not just the pelvis, but includes vaginal muscles as well. In light of new research compiled by Frye in *Holistic Midwifery (Volume II)*, it is clear that progress in labor is determined as much by flexibility in these tissues as by bone structure. Thus the importance of healing from vaginal or sexual trauma cannot be overestimated. Particularly if you find that the mother tightens as you do the exam, or that the sacral curve is impossible to access because of tension in the pelvic floor, ask the mother about history of abuse and refer for counseling if indicated. As soon as seems appropriate, offer to teach her pelvic floor exercises and vaginal awareness practices (see page 56).

The significance of the Three Ps is based on their interrelationship. Thus a woman with a small passage and

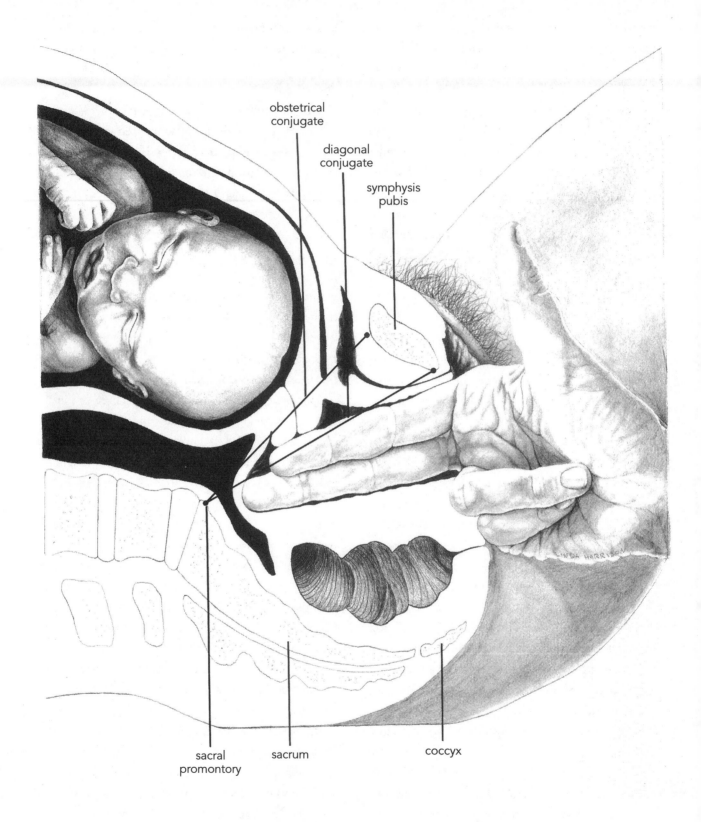

Measuring the Diagonal Conjugate

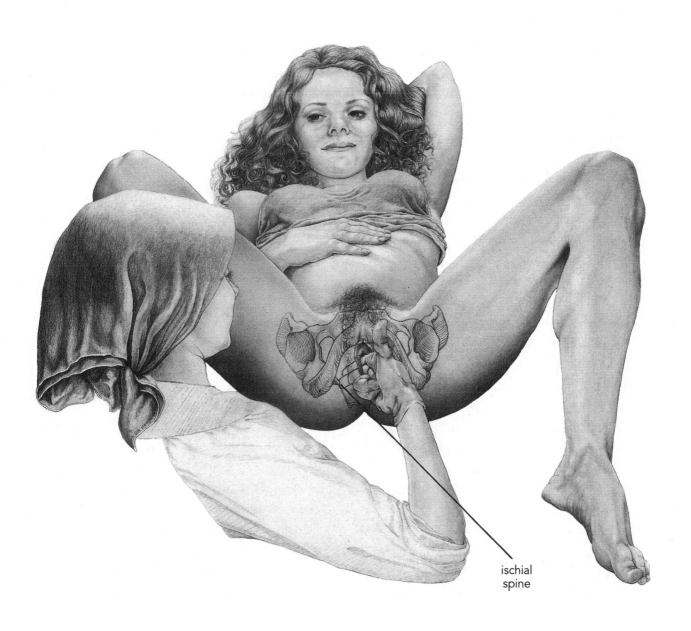

ischial
spine

Finding the Ischial Spines

medium-sized baby may nonetheless birth with ease if her tissues are relaxed and her powers are strong. Then again, a woman with ample passage and average-sized baby might have difficulty if her powers are weak because of poor health, history of abuse, or lack of support. In just a few decades, obstetrics has replaced pelvimetry with forceps delivery, vacuum extraction, and cesarean section—that is, "If the baby doesn't deliver in time, we'll just pull or cut it out." And due to the relativity of pelvimetry's significance, some midwives have chosen to discard it altogether. Yet certain traditions in midwifery practice, such as the skill of manually repositioning a mal-presenting baby, or safely assisting a breech at home, depend largely on the mastery of pelvimetry. Midwifery is based on limiting the use of technology and artfully facilitating vaginal birth, so let us uphold our competencies in this regard. Pelvimetry is rapidly becoming a lost art—midwives must seek to preserve it.

If the mother is at least eighteen weeks pregnant, also **assess fundal height.** Using a soft tape measure, place one end at the upper edge of the pubic bone, then stretch the tape to the top of the uterus (the fundus). Record your measurement in centimeters. Make sure to dip in deeply at the very highest point, which may be slightly off-center, depending on the baby's lie. Give or take a couple of centimeters, the fundal height matches the baby's **gestational age (GA),** which is simply the number of weeks pregnancy has progressed since the LMP.

One of the midwife's "tricks of the trade" is to **schedule a prenatal visit at twenty weeks to confirm the EDD,** particularly if the LMP is in question. If the dates are correct, the uterus will be round and exactly at the level of the umbilicus, no matter if the mother is carrying twins, a baby destined to weigh six pounds, or one that will be twelve pounds at term. If dates are off a month either way, it will be easy to tell. At sixteen weeks, the uterus is halfway between the umbilicus and pubic bone, a tall oval. At twenty-four weeks, it is sev-

eral centimeters above the umbilicus, a wide oval reaching all the way out to the illiac crests. Palpate the uterus, then adjust the EDD if necessary (and avoid an unnecessary ultrasound).

Performing uterine/fetal palpation is a most pleasurable and relaxing aspect of the visit for everyone involved. Your evaluations of the uterus and baby (from twenty-four weeks on) include determinations of fetal lie, presentation, position, and attitude as well as assessments of fetal growth, fetal responsiveness, and amniotic fluid volume. The maneuvers used to palpate the baby are commonly known as **Leopold's maneuvers.**

Fetal lie—the relationship of the baby to the long axis of the mother's body—will be longitudinal, oblique, or transverse. Begin by observing uterine contour: Is it taller than it is wide, or vice versa? Then feel the fundus to see if any obvious part can be identified—the head feels very hard and very round, and the butt is softer and more irregular in contour. If nothing is immediately apparent in the fundus, feel along the sides of the uterus. If the poles of the baby's body (head or butt) are at the sides, the baby is in a transverse or oblique lie. Although common at twenty-four weeks, the baby finds this lie increasingly confining as it grows and will generally seek the roomier, longitudinal aspect of the uterus by twenty-eight weeks.

If you've found either the head or the butt in the fundus, palpate the sides of the uterus for the location of the back and small parts (which you will use in a moment to determine position), and then feel above the pubic bone to find the **presentation.** If the lie is longitudinal with the butt at the pubic bone, the presentation is breech; if the head is at the pubic bone, the presentation is cephalic. If the lie is transverse, the shoulder presents. Whatever the presentation, the part of it used to determine the position of the baby is called the **denominator.** For example, with a longitudinal lie, cephalic presentation, the denominator is the

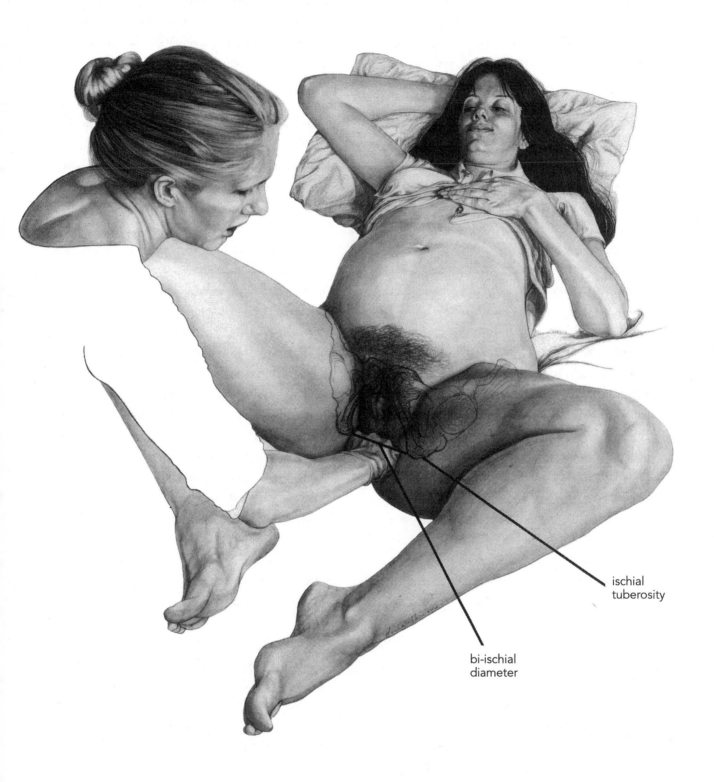

ischial
tuberosity

bi-ischial
diameter

Checking the Outlet Dimension

occipital bone at the back of the baby's head (see illustration "Fetal Skull," on page 115). In breech presentation, the denominator is the sacrum, and with shoulder presentation, the acromion process.

We base **fetal position** on the relationship of the denominator to the front, back, or side of the mother's pelvis. For example, if the baby is head down with its occiput and back on the mother's right side, this position is right occiput transverse (ROT). Babies in transverse position are quite easy to feel; the back is distinct on one side with small parts on the other, and often a foot can easily be seen or felt. If the baby is head down with occiput and back on the mother's left but near her sacrum, we call this left occiput posterior (LOP). Posterior babies are more challenging to palpate; there are lots of small parts and little more than an edge of back, but you may find a shoulder just above the pubic bone that will tell you more conclusively which side the baby is on. If the baby is breech with sacrum on the mother's left and back near her pubic bone, we call this position left sacrum anterior (LSA). Anterior babies are "all back," with small parts tucked against the mother's back and out of range of feeling. See illustration "Fetal Presentation and Position," on the opposite page, for more examples.

Less commonly used is the term **presenting part,** which refers to the part of the presentation lying directly above the cervix. This is determined not by palpation, but by internal exam.

Attitude is a more subtle assessment of the degree of fetal head flexion. A well-flexed cephalic presentation will manifest a continuous curve of back and head from fundus to pubic bone. This is obviously more difficult to determine if the baby is posterior. Deflexion of the head can be corrected most effectively around thirty-five weeks gestation (see diagram on page 55).

Palpation is obviously an art learned by experience. Among women of the Yucatán peninsula, the word for *prenatal visit* is the same as that for *massage.* I've noticed that midwives spend much more time on palpation than physicians do; it is yet another of our endangered arts for which technology (ultrasound) has become a substitute. If combined with continuity of care, careful palpation renders precise evaluations of fetal growth, responsiveness, and amniotic fluid volume easy to track week-to-week. These assessments are especially critical if factors predispose to fetal growth restriction, if the uterus is large for dates, or if pregnancy is prolonged (see chapter 3). Teach the mother how to palpate herself, and if her partner is present, encourage him or her to feel the baby too.

Next, **take fetal heart tones (FHT)**. The fetal heart should be audible by twenty weeks with a fetascope; if you cannot hear it, use your Doppler (ultrasound stethoscope). Normal range is 120–60 beats per minute (BPM), but younger babies are considered normal up to 170 BPM (the heart rate tends to be higher in early pregnancy, slowing ten to fifteen points as the baby grows). In addition to the BPM rate, **check for variability** by listening for several fifteen-second increments, determining the FHT rate for each and charting the overall range (for example 132–48 BPM). Variability occurs in response to palpation, uterine contractions, or the baby's own movements and is considered a sign of neurological health. It should be documented by twenty-eight weeks. Don't forget to invite the mother's supporters or other children to listen to the baby—it is a nice way to end the first visit.

To consolidate this overview of **lost midwifery arts,** it is noteworthy that since the first edition of *Heart & Hands* was published in 1981, the skills of pelvic assessment, fetal and uterine palpation, fetal heart auscultation, and fundal height assessment have been almost entirely replaced by ultrasound. Yet research has demonstrated repeatedly that neither maternal nor fetal outcomes are improved by routine use of this technology.[11] In fact, serial ultrasound has recently been shown to pose significant risks of fetal growth restriction.[12] In cases with clear risk, ultrasound can be helpful, even

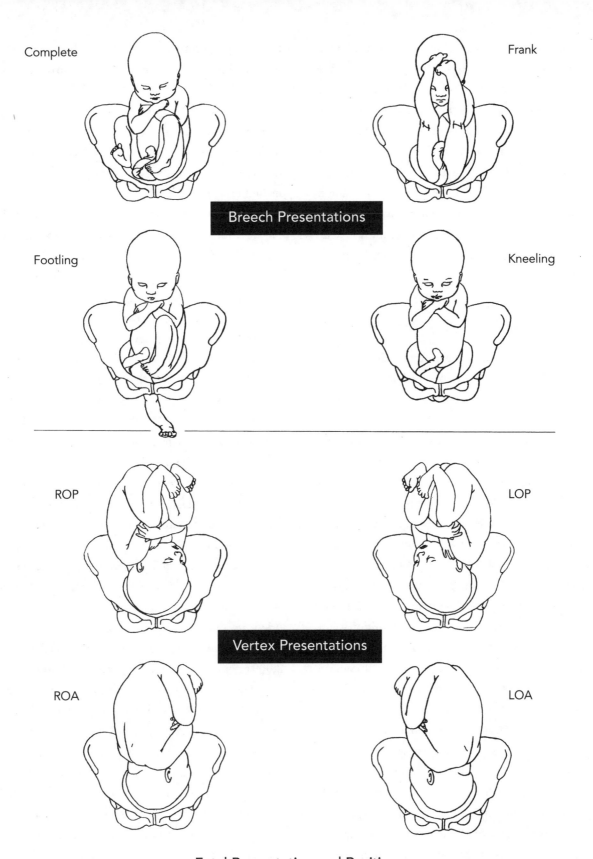

Complete

Frank

Breech Presentations

Footling

Kneeling

ROP

LOP

Vertex Presentations

ROA

LOA

Fetal Presentation and Position

lifesaving. But in general, it is grossly overused for reasons that have nothing to do with good care—to have hard-copy records in the event of a lawsuit, to generate office revenues, or simply because the skill to do otherwise has been lost. Now, new studies are demonstrating what midwives have known all along—that palpation, fundal height assessment, and fetal heart auscultation as described in this chapter are just as efficacious in determining fetal well-being as the use of ultrasound.[13, 14] Once again, midwives must take the lead in preserving and teaching these traditional skills and competencies.

NUTRITION AND EXERCISE

Base your **nutritional recommendations** on the mother's three-day record of her food and fluid intake, including all supplements. Don't forget to ask for this when you schedule the initial visit, so she can bring it with her. Nutrition is the trunk of the tree of health as regards pregnancy and postpartum—there is hardly a perinatal complication that cannot be forestalled or mediated to some degree by good nutrition.

There are innumerable theories concerning optimal nutrition, but it is not my purpose here to survey them. My own method of determining whether the expectant mother's diet is adequate does not involve adding up micrograms of this mineral or that, but I do have a good working knowledge of the nutritional content of most foods and herbs and so can appraise a diet at a glance. It is helpful to have on hand a comprehensive reference such as the U.S. Department of Agriculture's *Composition of Foods* (also available online at www.nal.usda.gov/fnic/etext/000020.html). This will aid you in settling disputes about how much zinc is in mushrooms, calcium in tofu, and so on.

If the mother has symptoms that indicate deficiencies, begin by helping her improve the quality of her diet. Assimilation of supplements is unpredictable, and as normal doses for the mother are extremely high

for the fetus, many must be taken with caution. Supplemental iron is routinely labeled with toxicity warnings, so doses should remain below 100 mg daily. The only safe quantities of vitamins A and D are nonpregnant minimum daily requirements. Although nontoxic, high quantities of vitamin C taken near the time of delivery can cause newborn withdrawal symptoms, including scurvy. Similarly, if the mother ingests large amounts of calcium near term to raise her pain threshold in labor, neonatal hypocalcemia can result. Supplements should be supplemental! Food comes first—but do encourage the mother to buy organic whenever possible, as the nutritional value of most organic fruits and vegetables is much higher than that of those commercially grown.

Above and beyond a good-quality, well-balanced diet, the following daily supplements may help compensate for devitalized soil, stress, air pollution, and so on: (1) vitamin E—400 units; (2) vitamin C—500 mg; (3) folic acid—800 mcg; and (4) iron—75 mg of a chelated, organic brand. Key minimums for the prenatal diet are 80 g protein and at least two quarts of fluid daily. A calcium intake of at least 1,200 mg daily is important, but the best sources are not necessarily dairy products; sesame butter (tahini) is excellent, as is orange juice "plus calcium" (acidity facilitates absorption). Iron can be readily obtained from organ meats, but pumpkin seeds, dried fruits, and almonds are also good sources. Adequate intake of calories is crucial for accelerated metabolic functions; pregnant women need at least 3,000 calories daily, and nursing mothers, 4,000 per day.

The vegan mother must be careful to ingest adequate B-12, without which a serious form of anemia may develop and cause neurological damage to both her and the baby. The best way for vegans to get B-12 is by supplement, with the vitamin in active form, that is, cyanocobalamin or hydroxocobalamin. Although fermented soy products, shiitake mushrooms, seaweed, and spirulina have been touted to contain lots of B-12, they actually contain analogs of the vitamin that can block absorption of the real thing. Fortified soy products or fresh juices can be excellent sources (look for cyanocobalamin or hydroxocobalamin on the label). Sublingual tablets are another option.

Mothers who eat organic foods, raw or lightly steamed vegetables, freshly squeezed juices, and high-quality protein generally feel and look better than those who eat commercially grown produce or "fast food." Quality counts—but beyond that, how food is selected and when it is eaten also make a difference. Every mother has a natural, inner voice of hunger telling her what to eat, how much, and when. This may lead her to devour six oranges at one sitting, or to crave a particular protein source to the exclusion of all others. Mothers with several children often recall that certain foods felt central to their well-being with each of their pregnancies (and not the same ones each time). Keep

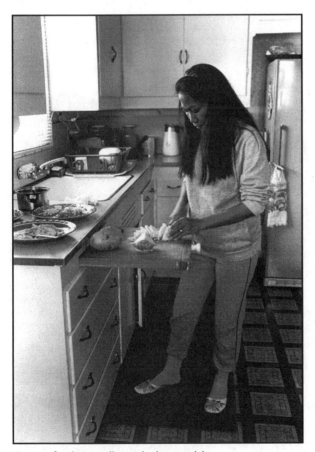

Eating fresh is well worth the trouble.

in mind, though, that this natural voice of hunger only operates in women free of addictions to sugar, caffeine, alcohol, or marijuana.

When confronted with a diet lacking essential nutrients, remember the cardinal rule of nutritional counseling: always begin with praise for whatever is outstanding. In terms of making improvements, base your suggestions on the mother's likes and dislikes. For example, if breakfasts are missing on her report, survey which breakfast foods she enjoys, then point out those with the greatest nutritional value.

Although nausea may be a factor in the first trimester, consider a diet greatly lacking in variety an indication of inadequate resources. Any woman who has been pregnant will tell you she would never limit herself to just a handful of foods, unless she was ill or had no choice. If obtaining food is a problem, refer the mother to public assistance. Sometimes a letter from the midwife verifying pregnancy and stating that the mother is at risk due to inadequate weight gain is necessary to help her qualify. Every midwife should be knowledgeable regarding social services available in her community. Once funding is obtained, have the mother dictate a list of everything she likes to eat, and then help her formulate meals based on her best choices.

If dealing with ethnic or regional dietary preferences, here is an important tip: Do not attempt to replace core foods or ingredients with other, albeit healthier, selections. For example, it would be foolish to suggest that an Asian woman substitute brown rice for white rice—if you are concerned about her need for whole grains and B vitamins, find an altogether different source. The same goes for sweets or treats; asking a woman fond of chocolate to substitute carob is probably a waste of time. In short, work around the less-than-perfect, emotionally based aspects of the mother's diet. If your recommendations are unrealistic, she will become evasive, and should some complication or concern necessitate another diet report later in pregnancy, she may not be fully truthful.

Before you attempt nutritional counseling, analyze your own three-day diet. You might also contemplate (or journal on) this question I ask my midwifery students: *What is your relationship to nourishment?* These tasks can help you find compassion for clients struggling with food issues, as well as alerting you to any weaknesses in your diet or commitment to self-care.

Exercise helps pregnant women keep in touch with their ever-changing physical status and emotional needs, as well as promoting circulation, elimination, and overall good health. But every mother must be cautioned to immediately desist any activity that causes pain or discomfort. Regardless of prepregnant fitness, her body is different now. If it has been her style to exercise compulsively, she is particularly at risk for ignoring her body's subtle cries of distress. The goal of prenatal exercise is to achieve a sense of balance and harmony, not to reach new heights of performance. Vigorous activity must be moderated within awareness and blended with adequate rest and rejuvenation.

For example, a mother under stress, with baby experiencing a growth spurt, might find her stamina reduced and her appetite increased. These symptoms could alarm her, but if she tunes in to her situation and trusts her body, she will know what to do. Rather than increasing her activity, she needs deep relaxation, extra food for energy, vitamins for stress reduction, time to reflect on both her own and the baby's needs, and plenty of sleep. On the other hand, a woman accustomed to high levels of physical activity who is also able to listen to her body should continue her routine as long as she is comfortable, and then taper off gradually. A sudden drop in activity can cause constipation, circulatory problems, or nervous irritability for the active mother.

Encourage every mother to join a prenatal exercise and support group. These venues help alleviate anxiety and self-consciousness about changing body image, while reassuring participants that their hopes and fears regarding pregnancy are perfectly normal. Yoga is my preference for prenatal exercise, as it inte-

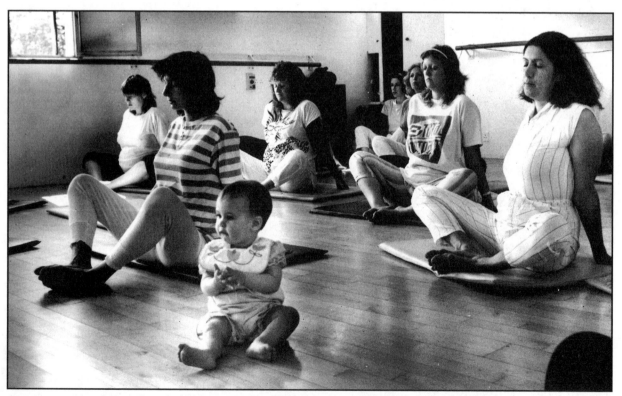

Exercising with others is fun, and helps you relax with your pregnant body.

grates mind and body, movement and rest. At the end of a long day, yoga can dissolve fatigue and boost energy levels in the evening. It helps the body recuperate by stimulating the master glands, which keep hormone levels in balance. This creates harmony throughout the system. Many women also feel that yoga fosters their intuition and creativity.

Mothers who work long hours during pregnancy need special consideration. It is more difficult for them to be spontaneous—to eat when and what they want, to rest when they should, and to be active when they feel like it. Bending the sharp edges of routine can help, but cutting back work hours is better. Pregnancy is a precious time of preparation for birth and motherhood, requiring a somewhat flexible schedule if at all possible.

SCREENING OUT

Ideally, screening out results from a process of decision-making shared by both the mother and the midwife. But sometimes, the midwife must make the final decision. On what basis do you conclude that out-of-hospital birth is not appropriate for a mother, or that you are not the most appropriate care provider?

Beyond preexisting medical problems that contraindicate home birth (as revealed by initial phone screening), other problems, such as contracted or abnormal pelvis, extreme obesity, or essential hypertension, may have become evident at this visit. Psychological contraindications are more complex. An irresponsible attitude, hostility in response to basic suggestions for self-care, or an otherwise rigid belief system should give the midwife pause. A poor diet, particularly if the mother is averse to changing it, may indicate deep-seated indifference, passivity, or lack of self-esteem. Excessive use of drugs, alcohol, or cigarettes has similar implications.

If you sense that you won't be comfortable working with the mother or her partner, suggest they consider other alternatives. This is also appropriate if you sense that she or they were not comfortable with you.

On the other hand, make room for change. I have worked with mothers who smoked or drank in the early weeks, but cleaned themselves up nicely after the initial interview. Provide handouts and suggested reading, make recommendations, and see what happens at the next visit (which should probably be scheduled sooner rather than later to reassess the situation).

For the beginning midwife, a most challenging aspect of screening is determining the relative significance of risk factors. To this end, several state midwifery associations have developed point systems, assigning five points to absolute contraindications such as clotting disorders, lung disease, and so on, and four or fewer points to less serious concerns like borderline anemia, insufficient exercise, having a marginally supportive partner, or partaking in less than optimal nutrition. Under these systems, midwives agree to consult with their peers regarding any situation where women have either a single risk factor of five or *a combination of factors* totaling five points. Apart from absolute contraindications, risk screening is somewhat subjective and, as such, requires a seasoned ability to make judgment calls best learned from training with an experienced midwife.

LAB WORK

If the mother has already had prenatal care elsewhere, she probably has had initial lab work performed. Have her make a written request for release of her records, mailed directly to you.

The **complete blood count** (CBC) or prenatal panel is primarily used to help you determine whether the mother is anemic and, to some extent, what type of anemia she has. Both her **hemoglobin** (HGB) and **hematocrit** (HCT) are critical indicators. HGB is the amount of hemoglobin per red blood cell, and HCT is the percentage of red blood cells per total blood volume. The HGB should be above eleven, and the HCT should be thirty-three or more. Because red blood cells are the oxygen carriers, low HGB or HCT readings mean that mother and baby will suffer some degree of oxygen deprivation. During pregnancy, the mother will be easily fatigued and more prone to infection, and the baby may be growth restricted. If the mother remains anemic at the onset of labor, there is risk of fetal distress, incoordinate or prolonged labor, postpartum hemorrhage (from "tired uterus"), and infection. Even a moderate blood loss can be very serious for an anemic woman because her blood is poorly oxygenated to begin with, predisposing her to shock. (See the discussion on "Anemia" in chapter 3 for more information.)

Blood work also includes **syphilis screening** (VDRL, RPR). Syphilis can cause miscarriage, prematurity, neonatal infection, fetal malformation, or death. Therefore, the desired result on the VDRL/RPR is nonreactive (NR).

Lab work also includes a **Pap smear,** which tests for irregular cells at the cervix. Often performed in conjunction with the initial pelvic exam, a Pap smear is crucial in pregnancy because hormonal changes in pregnancy may precipitate abnormal cell growth. It should be repeated again at six weeks postpartum. The lab will supply slides, cardboard slide holders, and fixative; you will need long-handled, sterile wooden spatulas or cytology sponges, a flashlight, and a speculum (some labs provide supplies in bulk, and some provide individual, all-inclusive kits). You may prefer to use disposable plastic speculums so you won't have to bother with resterilizing; if so, encourage the mother to take her speculum home in case she wants to check her cervix in the future.

To prevent lubricating gel from contaminating test results, do the Pap prior to pelvic assessment. (Plastic speculums are prelubricated, so you won't need gel.) Once the cervix is in view, find the **squamo-columnar junction** (the usual site for abnormality), where red, endocervical cells lining the cervical canal meet the pinker, mucosal cells covering the cervix and vagina (if invisible, it is just inside the cervical os). Take your spatula or cytology sponge and gently rotate at this junc-

ture. It is not necessary to scrape or draw blood, as cells come away freely in cervical secretion, but use just enough pressure so the mother can feel it. Spread your sample on the slide in a lengthwise line, then flip your spatula or sponge and draw another line next to the first (do not press hard or rub back and forth, as this will destroy the cells). Immediately spray the slide with fixative, air dry, and mark with date and mother's name. The lab also provides identification slips and will usually pick up specimens weekly (or you may ship instead).

While screening for abnormal cells, the lab may discover other conditions such as monilia/vaginal yeast, herpesvirus, or **human papilloma virus/HPV.** HPV can manifest as **condyloma accuminata,** that is, visible genital warts or flat lesions difficult to see. HPV is now the most prevalent sexually transmitted disease, and new evidence indicates it may also be possible to contract the virus without sexual contact. Like herpes, it resides in nerve ganglia in the genital area. There is no cure for this virus, only topical treatment for warts or lesions. Certain genotypes of HPV are known to be precursors to abnormal cell growth, dramatically increasing the risk of cervical cancer. Women with HPV are advised to have Pap smears every six months. Venereal warts or lesions are generally painless, may go unnoticed unless clearly visible, and sometimes don't manifest at all, thus a woman can have HPV at the cervix and not know it.

While doing the Pap, inspect the cervix carefully for warts or lesions and for unusual discharge or inflammation. If the latter are evident, the mother may have gonorrhea, chlamydia, or another infection. **Chlamydia** is the second most prevalent sexually transmitted disease in the United States—four times more common than **gonorrhea** (although the two often occur together). Women are rarely symptomatic, but their partners (if male) may have discharge or pain and burning with urination. Perform routine cultures for both gonorrhea and chlamydia, utilizing materials supplied by the lab to take a sample of secretion from the vagina, the cervix, and the anus.

Gonorrhea infection in the mother can lead to chorioamnionitis, premature rupture of the membranes, and preterm labor. It can also cause a blinding eye infection in the baby unless antibiotic drops are administered within the first two hours postpartum. The usual treatment for gonorrhea is a course of Ceftriaxone.

Chlamydia can infect the urinary tract, leading to premature labor. With delivery, the baby has a 70 percent chance of contracting it, resulting in conjunctivitis or life-threatening pneumonia. The usual treatment of tetracycline is contraindicated because it causes discoloration of fetal tooth enamel; erythromycin is nearly as effective and considered safe in pregnancy. For both gonorrhea and chlamydia, the mother's partner must also be treated, and they must use condoms or latex barriers for sexual interaction until additional screens for both confirm the infection to be fully resolved.

Yet another infection that may be sexually transmitted is **hepatitis B (HBV).** Screening is done by blood test, which checks for presence and quantity of surface antigens (HbsAG). HBV is transmitted through blood or blood by-products, saliva, vaginal secretions, or semen. This disease is highly contagious—women who are HbsAG positive have a high risk of transmitting the disease to their newborns, who, if infected, have high risk of becoming carriers and transmitting the disease to their own offspring. Therefore, babies born to infected mothers should be immunized within twelve hours after birth. If this is done, breastfeeding is not contraindicated.

Expectant mothers with active HBV infection (signs are nausea, vomiting, right upper quadrant abdominal pain, chills, and fever) should be hospitalized, and all family members screened. In contrast, HBV carriers are generally asymptomatic, with blood work showing long-term core antibodies (indicating infection contracted at birth). A midwife colleague recently found a client to be a carrier, and noted that although the mother already had several children, neither they nor her husband tested positive, thus no special care was required. Chronic HBV develops in only 15 percent of cases, but can lead to life-threatening conditions such as cirrhosis of the liver and hepatocellular carcinoma.

Hepatitis C (HCV) accounts for about 20 percent of viral hepatitis in the United States. The method of transmission is primarily via blood and blood by-products, but HCV is also sexually transmitted. Signs of active infection are similar to those of HBV, but chronic conditions develop in 85 percent of cases. Perinatal transmission is approximately 5 percent (depending on the amount of virus in the mother's bloodstream), but breast milk is not affected. There is no immunization for HCV.

HIV screening is advisable for all women, particularly if they have ever engaged in high-risk behaviors of unprotected sex or needle sharing. In California, state law requires informing all women of the availability of, and indications for, HIV screening. Testing can and should be done anonymously, either at a testing site or through the mail. The ELISA test is highly sensitive, but has a false positive rate of up to 10 percent. Only if a repeat ELISA proves positive will the more specific Western Blot for HIV Antibodies test be run.

If the mother is seropositive and remains untreated, her baby has a 25 percent chance of contracting the virus. About 5 to 10 percent of this risk is prenatal, 20 percent during labor and birth, and 5 to 15 percent with breastfeeding.[15] Treatment options during pregnancy are ever changing, so get to know the specialists in your community. The mother must be informed of all HIV-related risks and symptoms, and you should consult with backup regarding the advisability of continuing primary care. Note that if the mother is HIV positive, her newborn will likely test positive due to transfer of maternal IgG antibodies during pregnancy. This may persist for six to twelve months, regardless of actual disease status.[16]

As a health worker, you must define your protocol for assisting anyone who has a highly infectious and life-threatening disease. Immunization is available for hepatitis B and may soon be available for HIV. In the meantime, even universal precautions (described fully in chapter 4) cannot offer absolute protection—there is always a marginal risk of a needle-stick or other inadvertent exposure to infectious body fluids. Identify the standard of care within your midwifery community, know your limits, and communicate promptly with your clients should the need arise.

Rubella antibody titre indicates whether or not the mother has immunity to German measles. The test is done by a diluting process that detects the presence of antibodies. For example, a rubella titre of 1:48 means that antibodies can be detected even though the sample has been diluted numerous times. It is proof that the mother has had rubella or has been immunized, even if she cannot remember when. An unusually high reading (greater than 1:64) may indicate recent or current infection. Repeat the titre in this case and consult with backup. If the mother's titre is low (less than 1:10), it means she is susceptible to infection and should be immunized after the current pregnancy and at least three months before the next, to minimize her chances of contracting the disease while pregnant. Were that to occur, her baby would have a 20 percent chance of heart, vision, or hearing defects.

The mother needs her **blood type** too, in case need arises for emergency transfusion. This information is an absolute must for the midwife's records. The four blood types are O, A, AB, and B, with an accompanying **Rh factor** either positive (+) or negative (−).

The Rh factor is an antigen present in the red blood cells. Eighty-three percent of women have this factor and are Rh+; 17 percent do not and are Rh−. If the mother is Rh− and her baby Rh+, and her baby's blood enters her circulation due to intrauterine trauma, premature separation of the placenta, or placenta previa, she will produce antibodies against her baby's red blood cells, rendering it severely anemic. This process is called **isoimmunization.** Isoimmunization is rare with a first baby (as rare as the traumas that can cause it to occur) unless the Rh− mother has had abortions or miscarriages without receiving RhoGAM (an anti-

antigen that blocks the development of antibodies). Because the first-time mother may have had an undetected miscarriage at some point, every Rh− woman is screened for antibodies early in pregnancy, and again at twenty-four, twenty-eight, thirty-two, and thirty-six weeks. If antibodies are found, the baby will be tracked closely and may need a transfusion while still in utero.

It is now standard of care to administer RhoGAM prophylactically during pregnancy at twenty-eight to thirty weeks. This conveys passive immunity, that is, it will not protect subsequent pregnancies. As RhoGAM is commonly formulated with chemicals such as mercury that may be harmful to the fetus, prenatal administration is somewhat controversial.[17] Blood-borne diseases may also be transmitted by RhoGAM, for although blood is routinely screened for HIV and hepatitis, viruses as yet unknown may not be killed by current purification treatments.[18] The mother must make her own informed decision. To this end, I highly recommend the book *Anti-D in Midwifery: Panacea or Paradox?* by British midwife Sara Wickham.

Regarding the need for RhoGAM postpartum, you must take a sample of cord blood immediately at birth to determine the baby's Rh factor. RhoGAM must be administered within seventy-two hours to be effective.

Urinalysis is also standard in prenatal screening. Besides checking for protein and glucose, a complete urinalysis detects the presence of bacteria, with values of +4 or more indicating a **urinary tract infection (UTI),** and necessitating cultures to determine what kind of bacteria are involved. Urine cultures are often accompanied by antibiotic sensitivities to assess which medications are most likely to be effective in eliminating the infection. Whenever values are +2 or +3, repeat the urinalysis before considering treatment.

Because increased progesterone in pregnancy softens and dilates the urethra, women may not notice the usual warning signs of a UTI. An undiagnosed UTI can lead to **kidney infection (pyelonephritis),** which can complicate pregnancy and lead to premature labor. Thus even the slightest symptom is cause for immediate screening, and all women with previous history should be screened periodically to rule out insidious infection.

The **PPD** is used routinely to screen for tuberculosis (TB), an infection linked to crowded urban living among Native American, Asian, Middle Eastern, and military populations. Initial infection is often self-healing, so a woman may remain infected and appear asymptomatic. Her PPD results will be positive, yet she may never develop active disease. Women with inactive TB are at no greater risk for active disease because of pregnancy.

If a mother develops active TB, she may pass the infection to her baby during pregnancy or in the immediate postpartum. She may also readily infect other family members. Any woman who coughs up blood, has difficulty breathing, and suffers weight loss, fever, or fatigue should be immediately referred to a physician for screening. A mother with an active infection during pregnancy should be treated at once, whereas treatment will generally be postponed if the infection is asymptomatic. If a woman reports a previous positive PPD, do not repeat the test but do consult with a physician regarding additional screening and treatment options.

Every mother should be offered **genetic screening.** Depending on her ethnicity (and that of the father), she should be advised of any risk to the baby. If parents are of Greek or Italian descent, the fetus is at risk for B-Thalassemia, or if of Asian or Filipino descent, there is risk for A-Thalassemia, both of which are life-threatening anemias. If parents are of African descent, they may carry the sickle-cell gene that can also cause severe anemia. Ashkenazi Jewish couples may be carriers of Tay-Sachs or Canavan diseases, both of which lead to central nervous system degeneration and death. All northern European populations are at risk for cystic fibrosis, which is characterized by lung disease and limited life span.

Alpha-fetoprotein screening (MsAFP) is the first layer of genetic screening. Offered at fifteen to twenty weeks gestation, this blood test checks for neural tube defects such as anencephaly, microcephaly, hydrocephaly, and spina bifida. It also detects up to 20 percent of Down syndrome cases. Numerous states now require practitioners to inform all mothers of the benefits and risks of alpha-fetoprotein screening. Unfortunately, the test has a 20 percent false positive rate. The **triple screen,** which combines AFP with hCG and unconjugated estrogen levels, is much more accurate, detecting 65 percent of Down syndrome and 80–85 percent of neural tube defects, with a false positive rate of only 5 percent.

If the triple screen is positive, **amniocentesis** is the next step (although some mothers decide against it due to the invasive nature of the procedure and concomitant risk of infection). Amniocentesis is performed by inserting a needle through the abdomen and into the amniotic sac, then withdrawing a sample of fluid. Ultrasound is used simultaneously to visualize the baby. The procedure cannot be performed before fourteen weeks because there is not sufficient fluid; fourteen to sixteen weeks is optimal. It may take several weeks to get results. For perspective, the incidence of Down syndrome at age thirty-five is 1 in 365, equal to the risk of miscarriage or infection caused by the procedure. But by age forty, the incidence of Down syndrome increases to 1 in 100.

Chorionic villus sampling is another option. It can be performed at ten to twelve weeks: an obvious advantage over amniocentesis in case some abnormality is found and the mother decides to terminate the pregnancy. However, the procedure carries greater risks of miscarriage and infection, as the requisite sample of placental tissue must be obtained through the cervix. And because chromosomal construction of placental tissue does not always reflect that of the fetus itself, there are a significant number of false positive and false negative findings. More disturbing are indications (from a recent study at Oxford University) of a possible link between the procedure and subsequent fetal anomalies.[19] Chorionic villus sampling is contraindicated for women with a history of cervical incompetence, miscarriage, or premature labor.

Decisions regarding genetic screening are very personal and often agonizingly difficult. Should a woman decide against it, she will undoubtedly be reminded of her decision repeatedly as friends and family ask if she has had "the test" and whether everything is all right. Amniocentesis has become increasingly routine; in response to the threat of malpractice, some physicians recommend it for every woman over thirty. For any woman uncertain of her risk status, a session with a genetics counselor can help her make a decision. The midwife should be prepared with up-to-date referrals to specialists who are compassionate and willing to spend plenty of time answering questions.

Glucose testing to rule out gestational diabetes is routine from twenty-six to twenty-eight weeks, although it may be performed earlier if there are predisposing factors in the health history. Most common is the glucose screen, for which the mother's blood is drawn one hour after she ingests 50 mg glucose (a thick, syrupy drink). If her blood glucose exceeds 140 mg/dl, further testing is recommended. Many midwives find glucose screening unreliable for their clients, most of whom eat very little sugar and are thus less tolerant to the dosage used in testing. Beyond this, controversy rages as to whether or not gestational diabetes poses a significant risk for women with neither historical nor clinical signs (see chapter 3 for more details).

Another standard screen later in pregnancy is for **group B streptococcus (GBS).** This common bacterium lurks harmlessly in the vagina or rectum of approximately 30 percent of women, but it can have serious consequences for the baby. Although the rate of newborn infection is only 5 percent, 6 percent of infected babies die. The first symptom may be cessation of breathing, with spinal meningitis another common manifestation. Unfortunately, treating strep in pregnancy is almost pointless. Even after a full course of antibiotics in the last trimester, women usually have positive cultures again at term.

Cultures for GBS are standard at thirty-five weeks. If positive, IV antibiotics are advised during labor if it is preterm, if membranes are ruptured for more than eighteen hours, or if the mother develops a fever. And here is where the controversy comes in. One study, which looked at the rates of blood infections in newborns over a six-year period, found that antibiotic treatment in labor reduced the incidence of GBS in newborns but increased the rate of other blood infections.[20] E. coli in particular is on the rise.[21] Some strains of GBS are resistant to all available antibiotics—a study of forty-three newborns with various blood infections (including GBS) found that 88 to 91 percent were resistant to the antibiotics their mothers received in labor.[22, 23] Women unwilling to have antibiotic treatment may therefore wish to waive prenatal screening altogether (see page 242), or may choose to be screened in order to know their status.

To reduce chances of newborn infection, midwives and mothers have devised a number of noninvasive ways to minimize colonization. Midwife Maria Iorillo suggests the following regimen:

Take twice a day, with breakfast and dinner:
2 capsules lactobacillus acidophilus (2 billion per capsule—try Nature's Plus)
1 capsule echinacea, 350 mg
1 capsule garlic, 580 mg
1 capsule or gel vitamin E, 500 mg
Also place one clove peeled, unnicked garlic in vagina every other night, remove in morning.

Here is an alternative, ten-day regimen (to be used near term).

Each day:
6 capsules EHB by NF Formulas (an antibacterial supplement)
Tea tree oil suppositories (soak cotton ball or small cotton tampon with fifty-fifty blend of tea tree oil and olive oil), every four to six waking hours
500 mg vitamin C every four waking hours

For more information, see the excellent article by Christa Novelli, "Treating Group B Strep: Are Antibiotics Necessary?"[24] It also bears mentioning that a vaccine for GBS, administered at thirty to thirty-two weeks, is in the final stages of testing, and thus far results are good.

If a woman comes to her initial visit with no previous lab work and you are unable to do it yourself, send her to a public health facility or women's health center with a full list of requisite tests, including vaginal cultures. But make every effort to acquire these lab skills as soon as possible—your clients will greatly appreciate the continuity of care, and you will enjoy the autonomy of practice.

Fetal Development

The **embryonic period** of fetal development includes the first through the seventh weeks of life postfertilization (or, from the LMP, the third through the ninth week).

The **fetal period** includes all fetal development after the embryonic period and before the time of birth.

Growth and development begin at the moment of fertilization. The **pronucleus** of the sperm and that of the ovum fuse to form a **zygote.** Each pronucleus contains only twenty-three chromosomes (the **haploid** number); when they fuse, the normal forty-six chromosomes (**diploid** number) are restored.

Also determined at the moment of fertilization is the sex of the individual. The pronuclei are carried in the sex cells, or **gametes,** of both sexes. The male gamete carries either and X or a Y chromosome. The female gamete carries only an X. An XX combination is female, an XY, male.

Immediately after fertilization, the zygote undergoes **cleavage** and becomes a **morula.** As the morula develops and fluid enters the mass, it becomes a **blastocyst.** When the blastocyst implants in the uterine lining (on the tenth or eleventh day after fertilization), the embryonic period begins.

Development during the embryonic period, dating from the LMP:

The **heart** starts to beat around the beginning of the sixth week.

The **ears, arms, legs, facial, and neck structures** begin to form at the end of the sixth week.

The **brain and eyes** begin to develop during the seventh week.

The **nose, mouth, and palate** begin to form in the eighth week.

The **neck is established, urogenital development begins,** and all other essential structures are present by the end of the ninth week.

The fetus can **swallow, make respiratory movements, urinate, and open and shut his or her mouth** by the end of the twelfth week.

The embryonic period is a critical one in terms of exposure to teratogens, which may cause congenital malformations or death.

Development during the fetal period, dating from the LMP and taken by lunar months:

Fourth lunar month (thirteen–sixteen weeks): eyelids are fused, body growth accelerates, fingernails develop, reflexes manifest, sex is distinguishable, fetus reaches a weight of about 4 oz.

Fifth lunar month (seventeen–twenty weeks): toenails develop, fetus hiccups, vernix covers the body, fetus reaches average weight of 0.75 lb.

Sixth lunar month (twenty-one–twenty-four weeks): hair growth prominent, fetus covered with fine, downy hair (lanugo), buds of permanent form, fetus makes crying and sucking motions, brown fat (source of heat and energy for the newborn) forms, weight 1.25 lbs.

Seventh lunar month (twenty-five–twenty-eight weeks): eyes begin to open and shut, the fetus grows longer, gains significant weight: average 2.25 lbs.

Eighth lunar month (twenty-nine–thirty-two weeks): fat deposits smooth body contours, thick vernix, rhythmic breathing motions, average 3.75 lbs.

Ninth lunar month (thirty-three–thirty-six weeks): skin smooth, baby looks chubbier, weight 5.5 lbs.

Tenth lunar month (thirty-seven–forty weeks): fetus well proportioned, lanugo disappears, vernix decreases, weight reaches an average of 7.5 lbs. ■

ROUTINE CHECKUPS

The schedule for prenatal visits is fairly standard: up to twenty-eight weeks, every four weeks; from twenty-eight to thirty-four weeks, every two weeks; from thirty-five weeks on, once weekly. The main reason for the increasing frequency of visits is that complications for mother and baby are more likely to arise as pregnancy progresses. It is also important that the midwife have additional personal contact with the mother to foster trust and intimacy as the pregnancy nears completion.

Routine at every visit are urine dipstick for protein and glucose, blood pressure evaluation, fundal height measurement, fetal auscultation, and uterine and fetal palpation. Weight may be checked less frequently, but nutrition and exercise should be discussed each time.

At twenty-eight weeks, certain assessments from early pregnancy should be repeated. Call for another three-day diet report, as needs for protein, calcium, and iron intensify during the last trimester. Check the HCT/HGB again, for if the mother is anemic it may take time to find an effective solution. This is also the cutoff point for initial glucose screening. Otherwise, caregiving during the last trimester should focus on the more personal aspects of helping the mother prepare for labor and impending parenthood.

Throughout the pregnancy there are many appropriate topics for discussion: books and articles read, experiences in childbirth class, partner and family preparation, postpartum support, sexuality, aspects of newborn care, rest and relaxation, work and play. Take your cues from the mother, but avoid the rut of discussing the same subjects over and over. Your task is to expose her and her partner to issues and concerns they may not have considered, in preparation for the multi-faceted experiences of birth and child rearing.

Don't forget to inquire about the mother's general well-being at every visit, as there are a number of physical complaints that may arise from time to time.

And always take good notes. For guidelines, refer to the section on "Medical Records, Charting, Informed Choice, and Client Confidentiality" in chapter 8.

COMMON COMPLAINTS

Ligament pains are experienced as pelvic sensitivity or groin pain when walking; they are caused by stretching of the ligaments that support the uterus as they adjust to its increasing size and weight. Many women do not realize that the uterus is suspended by ligaments, which run from its base to the pelvic bones. The uterus is very movable, more or less a floating organ (see illustration showing the supporting ligaments of the uterus, opposite).

Morning sickness is due primarily to elevated estrogen and human chorionic gonadotropin (HCG) levels. This low-grade, persistent nausea is called morning sickness because it is likely to occur when the stomach is empty, although it also occurs in response to evening cooking odors. Mothers widely acknowledge that psychological upsets contribute to morning sickness, thus emotional support and stress reduction are crucial. Encourage the mother to ask her partner for whatever assistance she may need or for a bit of pampering. Also have her take 50 mg vitamin B-6 at bedtime and again at midday. Other remedies include crackers or plain yogurt upon rising, and ginger or raspberry-leaf tea. Many women report that small meals and nearly continuous eating can help (particularly foods high in protein). This makes sense, as yet another factor in morning sickness is low blood-sugar levels, primarily from fasting during sleep but potentially recurring throughout the day. If the mother is extremely nauseated, Guatemalan midwife Antonia Sanchez recommends that she "feel the vegetable or fruit that she likes most and eat just that."[25]

If nausea progresses to vomiting, recommend ground ginger capsules with meals and maintain daily contact with the mother, at least by phone. Should

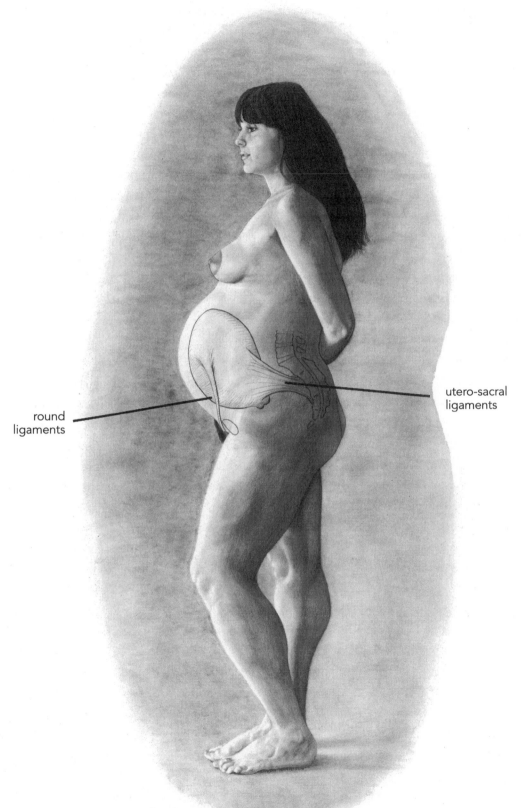

round
ligaments

utero-sacral
ligaments

Supporting Ligaments of the Uterus

hyperemesis gravidarium develop, the mother is at risk for severe dehydration and should be seen by a physician immediately.

Fatigue obviously has a relationship to nutrition and general state of health. But in early pregnancy, fatigue is directly related to physiological adjustments and hormonal changes, and so may serve the positive function of helping the mother tune in to her body's changing needs. If problematic after the first trimester, review the diet. Sometimes mothers get into ruts regarding food and exercise, and may need help breaking away from familiar patterns. A variety of foods, especially fruit and vegetables, provides the range of vitamins and minerals needed to boost vitality. Daily exercise and social interaction can mediate fatigue by stimulating body and mind. Encourage every mother to experiment to find what works best for her. If fatigue is extreme or persistent, screen for anemia.

Indigestion and heartburn result from displacement of the stomach and intestines by the growing uterus, particularly in the last trimester. The best remedy seems to be frequent but small meals, with digestive enzymes (available at many health-food stores) taken as needed. Because digestion slows naturally in pregnancy to increase absorption of essential nutrients, meals should be leisurely. The gall bladder functions less efficiently in pregnancy, reducing fat intake can help. Advise limiting food in the evening, especially right before lying down.

Skin itchiness (pruritis) occurs in 3 to 14 percent of pregnancies. It may be correlated to liver compromise resulting from liver disease, excessive alcohol or recreational drug use, or prolonged use of pharmaceuticals.[26] Dandelion root and yellow dock root tinctures are excellent liver tonics and may bring relief. Liver-cleansing agents like beets, dark greens, lemon juice, and olive oil should be taken freely, along with foods rich in choline like egg yolk, wheat germ, and brewer's yeast. For topical application, plain yogurt rubbed into the skin or oatmeal baths (prepackaged by Aveeno) can help.

If the palms of the hands and soles of the feet are particularly itchy, **intrahepatic cholestasis** may be the cause. Although rare in the general population (0.5 percent), it is quite common in women of Chilean, Mediterranean, or Scandinavian descent.[27] Consult with backup regarding the advisability of a liver profile.

Headaches and other minor pains often respond to relaxing teas such as hops, skullcap, and chamomile. Massage, yoga, and chiropractic care can help. Headaches may also result from dehydration, so stress adequate fluid intake.

If the mother complains of **backache,** see that she is getting sufficient but not overstrenuous exercise, and suggest pelvic rocks to keep the lower spine flexible. These can be performed on hands-and-knees, alternately arching the back like a cat and bringing it back to normal position. She can do these motions standing, sitting, driving in the car, anytime. She should also use her stomach muscles to maintain good posture; suggest she hold her stomach taut periodically throughout the day. Make sure she has plenty of pillow support while sleeping—some women swear by egg-carton foam padding for alleviating back pain. If her abdomen is pendulous, she may benefit from an elastic bellyband, which also provides support for the lower back. Again, chiropractic adjustments can help.

If she indicates that backache is near waist-level, rule out kidney infection by checking for **costovertebral angle tenderness (CVAT).** Do this with the mother in a sitting position, her back fully exposed. Prepare her first, then make a fist and gently strike the area nearest her waist and adjacent her spine, on either side. In order to pound firmly enough to secure your diagnosis, you may wish to place your other hand across the area to cushion your blow. If the mother jumps or otherwise indicates pain, note whether her sensitivity was to the left or right and refer her immediately to a backup physician.

Varicose veins of the legs and vulva are caused by high levels of progesterone relaxing smooth muscle and hindering venous return throughout the body, particularly in the extremities. Hereditary factors also play a part. Standing or sitting with crossed legs for long periods exacerbates the problem, but exercise can help by stimulating circulation, as can elevating the legs and buttocks periodically. Six hundred to 800 units of vitamin E daily may also be beneficial. For best absorption, this fat-soluble vitamin should be taken separately from other supplements and with milk, cheese, or other fatty food sources.

In the absence of hypertension or proteinuria, **swollen ankles** are a normal result of impaired circulation in pregnancy or excessive periods of standing. The diet should be improved with more protein, fresh vegetables, and plenty of fluids, and moderate exercise should be taken regularly. Elevating the feet and legs helps too.

Constipation can be caused by hormones or diet, but plenty of fluids and fibrous foods should remedy this problem. Sometimes women mistake thirst for hunger and must learn to distinguish the two impulses. Regular physical activity is critically important in alleviating constipation.

Vaginal infection, particularly yeast (monilia), is common during pregnancy. Characterized by a white, curd-like discharge, yeast is a naturally occurring vaginal organism that tends to overgrow in pregnancy because of increased vaginal alkalinity, which in turn is caused by elevated progesterone levels. It can be controlled by inserting vaginal sponges (boil first to remove mineral deposits) or cotton tampons soaked in acidophilus culture (available in the cold section of health-food stores). Saturate a sponge or tampon with acidophilus solution, squeeze lightly, insert, and change every three hours. Cotton underwear is essential. Yeast infection at term increases the risk of newborn thrush.

Bacterial vaginosis (BV) (also known as gardnerella or hemophilus) is another common vaginal infection. Although ordinarily benign and transient, it can complicate pregnancy by causing chorioamnionitis, premature rupture of the membranes, and preterm labor. Commonly detected by the mother because of a fishy odor (particularly after lovemaking), bacterial vaginosis produces a thin, gray or white discharge that tends to adhere to vaginal walls. Seldom is there vaginal irritation or itching.

The best way to test for BV without a microscope is by symptoms and odor in combination with the **whiff test.** Touch a cotton swab saturated with discharge to a bit of KOH solution; if it lets off a potent fishy odor (amine), it's bacterial vaginosis. One natural remedy is to insert a peeled, unnicked clove of garlic into the vagina and change three times daily. Follow with five days acidophilus treatment, as just described for monilia. If this does not work, medical treatment is indicated. (It is also important that the woman abstain from intercourse during treatment and that her partner be checked if symptoms persist.)

Trichomonas infection is characterized by a malodorous, highly irritating, yellow-green, frothy discharge. Like BV, it can cause chorioamnionitis, premature rupture of the membranes, and preterm labor. The usual treatment, Flagyl, is contraindicated in the first half of pregnancy. As an alternative, the herbal douche formula outlined in the sidebar on page 46 is effective for both trich and yeast—a bit of trouble to prepare but gentle and nourishing to the mucous membranes (unlike harsh medicinal formulas). Although douching is generally not recommended during pregnancy, it is safe as long as pressure is kept to a minimum (a hand-held squeeze unit is best) with the water warm, not hot. Never insert the nozzle more than a few inches into the vagina. Garlic suppositories also work for trichomonas, particularly if used in combination with the douche.

Keep in mind that trich is sexually transmitted, thus the mother's partner must also be treated. Men may have relatively minor symptoms (such as twinging with urination or slight discharge), but because the organism can be harbored in both the urethra and prostate, they must take oral medication. Condoms and latex barriers must be used for sexual activity until both partners are cured.

All vaginal infections respond positively to the inclusion of dark-green vegetables, high-quality protein, whole grains, citrus, and plenty of fluids in the diet. Unsweetened cranberry juice or concentrate (in capsules) can help increase vaginal acidity (also useful in treating a UTI). Yeast thrives on sugar, so it should be completely eliminated, along with excessive intake of fruit, whether fresh, dried, or juiced. Eating plenty of yogurt with acidophilus can help, as can brewer's yeast.

Herpes simplex virus (1 and 2) is at epidemic proportions and has thus become a common complaint. Small, painful blisters are the prime symptom of this sexually transmitted viral infection. The initial outbreak is usually severe, much like a bad flu. Once the sores disappear, the virus remains in nerve ganglia affecting the genital area, and infection may recur repeatedly. Susceptibility is increased during times of severe stress or exhaustion. Some women have outbreaks every few months; others never have subsequent symptoms, or perhaps not for many years. If a mother reports recurring episodes, inquire as to the number, severity, and usual location of lesions, and note in her chart.

In the event of an outbreak during pregnancy, culture the sores (for a firm diagnosis) and the cervix (to see if the virus is present at this location). Weekly cultures are no longer performed in the last trimester, as visual inspection of the cervix at the onset of labor is considered sufficient to rule out current infection. But if membranes rupture prior to the onset of labor, be sure to screen the cervix within two hours, as the baby may be rapidly affected without the barrier of intact membranes.

Herpes can have a devastating effect on the baby's central nervous system. If an initial outbreak occurs during the first trimester, immediately consult with backup. If lesions are present when labor commences, vaginal delivery is prohibited unless: (1) the outbreak is nonprimary; (2) sores are external; (3) sores are healing; and (4) adhesive surgical film or spray-on bandage is used to prevent contact with the baby.

Treatments for herpes during pregnancy are basically comfort measures. Advise the mother to keep the affected area dry and cool—no nylon underwear, panty hose, or tights. Hot baths tend to aggravate symptoms. Applications of lysine ointment, cold milk, zinc oxide, A&D ointment, ice, and calendula cream (marigold extract) are all reputed to be healing and soothing. Certain dietary changes can also help; one mother reported cutting her usual five-day cycle in half by beginning stress supplements (B-complex) and protein drinks at the first sign of infection. Increased lysine intake is recommended, in supplemental doses of 500 mg daily. Elimination of coffee and black tea, alcohol, and sugar makes a difference, as does getting plenty of rest. Avoid foods containing arginine (an amino acid that supports the herpesvirus), such as nuts and nut products, seeds, and chocolate. Sexual interaction should be discontinued until all sores are completely healed.

Acyclovir (Zovirax) is generally used only for severe or frequent recurrence. This drug is FDA classified as

---

Douche for Vaginal Infections

One part each of:

comfrey root	yarrow
mugwort	rosemary
peppermint	alum

Steep in a nonmetal container using boiled springwater. Allow to cool. Douche with one pint strained solution twice daily for two days. On the third and fourth days, douche as usual in the morning, but for yeast infections add one part acidophilus in the evening, and for trichomonas, one part myrrh in the evening.

Herbs and Homeopathy in Pregnancy

by Shannon Anton, CPM

The following is a list of herbs contraindicated during pregnancy:

Goldenseal, Ephedra, Cotton root bark, Blue cohosh, Pennyroyal, and Birthroot. For more information, refer to *The Natural Pregnancy Book,* by Jill Aviva Romm, CPM, or the *Wise Woman Herbal for the Childbearing Year,* by Susun Weed.

Goldenseal. As Goldenseal has become popular, it has also been overused and overharvested. Once abundant and easily wild crafted, it is now endangered in certain areas. To harvest Goldenseal, you must take the root, thereby eliminating a significant portion of or the entire plant. Goldenseal is also extremely strong medicine; overuse taxes the liver and kidneys. There are only a few conditions for which it is a traditional remedy; other potent and more appropriate remedies abound. Do not use it for cold and flu, as you would Echinacea tincture. There are a few appropriate uses for it postpartum, but do not use it at all during pregnancy. If you must use Goldenseal, preserve its potency and stretch its volume by tincturing it.

Buying Herbs

Dried herbs should hold a deep color and smell strongly of their substance. Faintly colored herbs with little scent have been stored incorrectly or for too long a time, and their potency is questionable.

Herbal tinctures are comprised of either fresh or dried herbs preserved in a liquid form. Herb qualities are extracted using alcohol or glycerin, then the mixture is strained and stored. Tinctures are taken in drops from an eyedropper or by dropperful. When buying tinctures, try to find out how they have been prepared. Tincture from fresh, wild, or organically grown plants is the best. The company Herb Pharm consistently provides quality tinctures prepared with care and respect for the plants.

Working with dried plant material for tinctures is fine. But consider taking a class from an herbalist for an opportunity to observe herbs as they grow and to learn directly from the herbs about their properties and uses.

Using Homeopathy

Although homeopathy is a rich and exact healing tradition, there are beginners' rules that make it easier to work with these marvelous allies. Homeopathic remedies must be properly stored or they are antidoted (negated). Store homeopathics out of sunlight, protect them from heat and extreme cold, and never keep them near strong aromatic substances like herbs, camphor, peppermint, toothpaste, perfumed products, and so on. Avoid storing them in your medicine cabinet or in your birth bag near your herbal tinctures.

If possible, one must avoid eating or drinking for fifteen minutes prior to taking a remedy (in labor, this cannot always be achieved).

The strong potencies listed in this sidebar are not for everyday use; birth is exceptional in its requirements. Potencies of 6x or 30C are applied in most other situations. Unless you are sure of your expertise, never treat issues outside of birth with these stronger potencies.

In critical situations, as when resuscitating an infant or dealing with maternal hemorrhage, dosing and then dosing quickly again is appropriate. Once relief is experienced or a shift is noted, discontinue the remedy. If symptoms return, apply the remedy again.

I urge you to read *Homeopathic Medicines for Pregnancy and Childbirth,* by Richard Moskowitz, MD, to better understand the nature of homeopathic medicines and to further research the following remedies.

Herbs for Pregnancy Support

The most basic and well-known nutritional herbs are also beneficial for pregnancy. Herbal infusions are a simple and delicious way to take herbal nourishment. To make an herbal infusion, use one ounce of fresh or dried herb (a good handful) per one quart boiling water (removed from heat).

continued →

Steep at least four hours in a covered, nonmetal container. You can mix two herbs per quart water, or double the batch and mix three or four. You may also want to add honey or lemon. If you like, brew peppermint tea separately and add it to your infusion for taste.

Nettle leaf provides excellent support for kidneys and is rich in vitamins A, C, D, and K, as well as calcium, potassium, phosphorus, iron, and sulfur. It prevents leg cramps and postpartum hemorrhage, eases postpartum afterpains, nourishes the circulatory system to reduce hemorrhoids, and encourages abundant breast milk.

Dandelion leaf is nature's special gift to nourish and revitalize the liver and also provides great kidney support. It is rich in calcium, potassium, and iron as well as vitamins A, B complex, C, and D. It is also essential in the prevention and treatment of preeclampsia and is a reliable digestive aid.

Red Raspberry leaf is the classic uterine toner and pregnancy tonic. It prepares the uterus to function at its best. The leaf can ease morning sickness and gently aid digestion.

Red Clover leaves and blossoms greatly nourish the whole reproductive system as well as nourish and balance the endocrine system. They are rich in calcium, magnesium, and trace minerals.

Lemon juice and water safely detoxify the liver during pregnancy (or at any time of stress). It is best to drink it in the early part of the day.

Remedies in Pregnancy

NAUSEA

Nausea can be greatly relieved with **Ginger** tea. Pour one cup boiling water over three to five slices of fresh ginger root. Let steep five minutes and sip slowly. Homeopathic remedies can be extremely effective for easing morning sickness. The remedies are specific to symptoms. Research **Pulsitilla, Sepia, Nux Vomica,** and **Ipecacuanha.** Additional remedies to consider include **Antimonium Tartrate, Argentum Nitricum, Petroleum, Sulfur,** and **Tabacum.** Good references are *Homeopathic Medicine for Women,* by Trevor Smith, MD, and the already mentioned *Homeopathic Medicines for Pregnancy and Childbirth,* by Moskowitz.

ANEMIA

Anemia is often diagnosed in pregnancy. Herbal and green sources of iron include **Dandelion, Nettles, Kelp,** and **Parsley. Yellow Dock root** improves absorption. **Floradix Herbs plus Iron,** a concentrated herbal and food compound, is an excellent tonic.

HEARTBURN

Slippery Elm lozenges greatly relieve the worst heartburn. Also try chewing raw **almonds,** raw **papaya,** or papaya enzyme tablets.

SLEEP DIFFICULTIES

Apart from deep relaxation and exercise during the day, a silky eye pillow filled with flax seed and lavender has proven to be my own best remedy for sleeplessness. Stronger remedies include: half a dropperful of **Skullcap** tincture or **Valerian** tincture. Or, during the last trimester, half a dropperful of **Hops** tincture. Some women are awakened by anxiety or worry that keeps them from getting back to sleep. Homeopathic **Aconite** 30C is very effective to calm and quiet nervous tension and fears. Use this remedy only during anxious episodes.

BACK PAIN, SCIATICA, OR CARPAL TUNNEL SYNDROME

Chiropractic care can be crucial: joints softened by pregnancy may become misaligned, and if readjusted, other remedies can be more helpful. Even if you are unfamiliar with chiropractic care, don't hesitate to try it in pregnancy.

Saint John's Wort (hypericum) oil is the best remedy I've found for nerve or muscle pain. Apply it directly over the sore area, as well as a bit above and below. Especially if used before sleeping, Saint John's Wort brings amazing relief. Depending on the severity of pain, use it straight from the bottle or dilute one ounce in six ounces of almond or olive oil. Arnica oil can also be beneficial, though it is Saint John's Wort oil that earned the reputation of "miracle cure" during the middle ages. For nerve pain, **Saint John's Wort** tincture may be taken orally, half a dropperful tincture every few hours. Homeopathic remedies include **Hypericum** 30C, taken every two hours during painful episodes, and topical application of a gel compound, **Arniflora.**

HEMORRHOIDS

Red Clover and **Nettle** infusion nourishes the circulatory system and prevents or improves hemorrhoids, especially if taken routinely. Grated raw **potato** may be used as a compress directly on hemorrhoids, or a thin slice of raw potato may be inserted into the rectum to shrink and relieve painful swelling. The classic standby, **Witch Hazel extract,** is very effective. Apply directly on hemorrhoids or use compresses. It may also be taken orally as homeopathic **Hamamelis** 30C when hemorrhoids flare up.

CONSTIPATION

Hydration is of utmost importance when dealing with constipation. Plenty of vegetables and whole foods offer sufficient bulk to avoid constipation. For additional bulk, **psyllium seed** (the main ingredient in Metamucil) can be added to oatmeal or taken in capsules; take lots of water with it. **Prune** juice is the faithful elixir our grandparents knew and loved; it works great.

DIARRHEA

Even pregnant women get the stomach flu. The biggest concern is keeping enough fluid down to prevent dehydration. Often, plain water is abrasive to the system. Add **honey** or **maple syrup** to warm or room temperature water and sip slowly. To stop diarrhea, here are two proven remedies:

> **Rice water.** Cook white rice with a four to one ratio of water to rice. Cook only until rice is tender, then pour off excess water and drink it.

> **Tea x3.** Using black tea and boiling water, brew one cup of tea. Save the tea bag, dump the tea. Use the same tea bag and brew a second cup, then dump. Brew a third time and drink.

Both of these remedies are complemented by **polarity** therapy. To practice this, the woman and her partner face each other and fully relax. The partner places one hand on the woman's right shoulder and one hand on her left hip. Waiting until both hands feel even or seem to pulse together, the partner then gives the woman warning that a change is coming and shifts hand positions to hold the woman's left shoulder and right hip. When the energy in both hands feels even again, the partner slowly removes both hands. **Rescue Remedy.** A Bach Flower Remedy, is helpful in any case of physical or physiological upset.

BREECH BABIES

Besides the usual postural exercises for turning a breech baby, two additional remedies have proven effective. Homeopathic **Pulsitilla** 30C taken several times a day can also encourage the breech to rotate. Even more reliable is **moxa** treatment. Moxa is a roll of tightly compacted **Mugwort,** used in traditional Chinese medicine. When lit, moxa looks rather like a cigar. The ash of burning moxa is extremely hot, so care must be taken in handling. Place the burning end near the outer, lower corner of the pinky toenail; heat at this "point" facilitates rotation of the breech. Treat the toes on both feet two or three times daily until a change occurs—and don't worry, women know how hot is hot enough! Moxa treatment is most effective done on a slant board.

PRETERM LABOR

The sooner preterm labor symptoms are addressed, the better your chance of getting them to stop. In times of threatened preterm labor, good hydration is critical. In addition, **magnesium** supplements have proven invaluable in preventing preterm labor in any woman with predisposing factors, or forestalling it if it occurs. Too much magnesium causes diarrhea; reduce intake as necessary, and space doses throughout the day. Follow this routine until thirty-seven weeks. If preterm labor begins, extra doses of magnesium and plenty of fluids should be taken at once, along with a deep, warm soak in the tub.

Homeopathic **Mag Phos** 30C is also useful. Using a nonmetal cup, put seven pellets in half a cup of hot (not boiling) water and stir with a nonmetal stick a hundred times. Slowly and continuously sip little sips of this remedy until it is gone. Contractions should slow or stop within an hour. Continue to monitor for preterm labor symptoms: if labor is not slowing or is accelerating, or if cervical change is occurring, consult a physician.

POSTDATES

In addition to the famed **Evening Primrose Oil** remedy, the cervix may be softened with homeopathic **Cimicifuga** 30C, taken once an hour for eight hours. Follow with homeopathic **Caulophyllum** 30C, taken as above. If the cervix is already soft, go right to Caulophyllum. Often, one dose of Caulophyllum 200C before bed will result in labor during the night. ∎

C-category, that is, risk cannot be ruled out because human studies are lacking or animal studies have shown adverse effects. The newer drugs Valaclovir and Famciclovir are FDA classified as B-category, wherein no evidence of risk has been shown in animals but insufficient information is available on humans.

COMMON FEARS AND COUNSELING TECHNIQUES

Certain fears regarding pregnancy and birth are universal and deeply rooted in survival, such as fear of the unknown, fear of death, fear of separation, and fear of change. These fears serve to alert the mother to the needs of her developing baby and help prepare her for parenting. Almost every mother wonders if her baby will be normal. Most women have some fear of labor, wondering if they will be able to tolerate it. These worries are often alleviated simply by explaining how commonly they occur.

Besides these universal fears, there are concerns unique to our times and culture. Working mothers may fear losing career-related identity and being buried in domesticity. Others struggle with changes in primary relationships, fearing losses of intimacy and freedom. Some worry deeply about being able to parent effectively. These concerns are specialized according to the mother's background, her role in society, and the nature of her relationship with her partner. When these fears arise, you may need to do a bit of counseling. Focus the mother on her own problem-solving capabilities, but take pains to sympathize with her distress. (See chapter 3 for specific psychological issues and configurations.)

Validating the hormonally enhanced sensitivities of a concerned mother is most effective if spiced with humor and a bit of personal disclosure. In the midwifery model of care, counseling is an expression of friendship and reassurance. What are some basic techniques? By receiving impressions and reflecting them back without judgment or distortion, you **mirror** the mother. You can also try **pacing** the mother's rhythms, **matching** her speed and style of self-expression as a means of making a connection. **Active listening** requires that you use all of yourself—not just your ears, but your heart and soul—to fully receive what the mother is trying to communicate. When the mother has moments of truth or reckoning, give her **positive reinforcement** for her revelations.

Contrary to the medical model's premium on clinical detachment, personal involvement is integral to the midwife/client relationship. By committing yourself to help the mother work through her problems, you inspire her commitment in return. And by letting your own character shine through, strengths and weaknesses alike, you help the mother feel courageous enough to accept newly revealed truths about herself. When the mother embraces her realizations and begins to make them manifest, the ultimate aim of counseling—**eliciting responsibility**—is achieved.

Truth be told, midwives need to be needed. Healers in a traditional sense, we have strong maternal instincts nourished by giving. On the other hand, our desire for intimacy must at all times be tempered by respect for client privacy and pacing. We must avoid the codependence of projecting personal needs and concerns into our caregiving relationships. Working in partnership with other midwives can keep us from going overboard in this respect, and help us maintain the necessary balance between personal involvement and objectivity.

PARTNER PARTICIPATION

The mother's partner has his or her own vital role to play in the experience. Some need time to warm up to the idea of playing a significant role, while others want to be very involved and hands-on. Some plan to catch the baby, and there is no reason this can't happen, barring unforeseen complications. For many women, the thought of easing the baby into their partner's loving hands is the ultimate dream. Your job is to provide reading material with clear, reasonably detailed information, at the same time describing the sensual aspects of birth, like how the baby's head will look and feel as it emerges. Then schedule a practice session a few weeks before the birth, perhaps at the home visit, using a model pelvis and doll to demonstrate.

Some fathers see "making the catch" as a virility test. Explain the need for sensitivity to the mother in the moment, and how anyone assisting must at all times follow her lead. Ideally, partner preparation is mostly personal, an extension of the couple's intimacy. Here is Frank's story:

> I wanted to share the birth process with my mate and felt that my involvement was necessary and my right as a father. Practicing exercises and massaging Bridget almost every night put me in tune with her body and spirit. By participating in this way I believed that my mind and body would appreciate the mystical aspects of birth when the time came.
>
> My participation was not limited to prenatal classes, exercises, and reading material. This was our second pregnancy and once again my goal was to catch the baby and cut the cord. I had performed this mighty ritual during our first birth. That labor was only three hours; Bridget went immediately into hard labor-transition. Even though it was hard to absorb this rapid labor, I still made the catch. Lydia was small, yet perfect to the touch. I caught her and held her close to my joyful, tired body.
>
> I did not catch our second child. His shoulders were stuck and we needed assistance. His birth was twelve hours long, which let Bridget and me absorb ourselves at every stage. We touched, massaged, showered, and supported each other in every way. This made up for not catching Paul.
>
> During this second birth I felt fully in touch with Bridget sexually and spiritually. I noticed that my

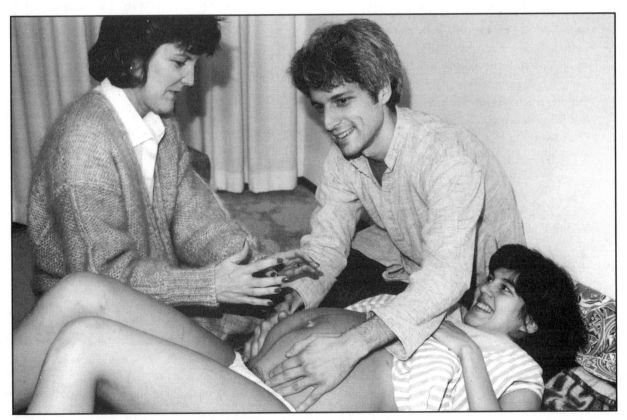

This father is discovering how to feel his baby's head.

sensitivity was greater than before, and my love for Bridget and my family grew with every phase of the encounter. Patience, listening, and empathy were at their peak. I felt then that I truly understood both birth and Bridget.

Here is the joint perspective from Watta and her partner Kenna (herself a midwife):

We both always knew that we wanted to be moms, but somehow each of us had always pictured herself as "the" mom. Learning how to fill the role of non-biological mother has been a challenge for both of us, but a challenge with great rewards. We have the two most beautiful boys in the world, each one born to a different mother. But they both "belong" to each of us. Here are our stories of learning to be there for each other:

Kenna:

Watta was incredibly beautiful when she was pregnant. I adored rubbing her belly and putting my ear against it to hear the baby's heartbeat. I also struggled a lot with jealousy, as I had been wanting to be pregnant for a long time. Our journey to this pregnancy was a difficult one, and many plans had fallen through along the way. I wanted to be there for Watta as a perfectly supportive partner, but trying to suppress my less-than-perfect feelings didn't work very well. It was very hard at times, but in the end, I knew that the most important things held true: I loved Watta, I was completely in love with the baby who was growing in her belly, and together we were a family.

Watching her give birth was one of the great privileges of my life. She was so graceful, even in the midst of all that pain. She was so strong that it made me want to cry. She labored all night with me at her side offering up soft words of encouragement, drinks of Recharge, a bowl to throw up in, and my complete and utter faith that her body knew what to do. Not long after sunrise, she pushed our son Rio out into the water of the birth tub and into my hands. I was, and still am, completely in awe of her.

Watta:

Even though I gave birth first, I wanted Kenna to feel special and as if she was having the first child. As the birth progressed, it was so hard and so long that I got really scared. I was scared for Kenna and I was scared for the baby. I wanted her to have an easy birth, but that's not what she got. I felt really helpless. It was very intense in that I knew what she was going through, but at the same time I didn't know what she was going through.

After twenty-four hours I was ready for it to be over. I reached a level of exhaustion where, if it wasn't for the midwife, I don't know if I could have kept my faith in the process. It had gone on for so long with no change. Watching her get through it was . . . like she was superhuman, not real in some way. She finally told me to go to sleep. I didn't want to go to sleep until the baby was born; I felt like I needed to be around. But when she told me to go I did—for two hours. That was hard for me, although she did the best part of her work when she was alone.

When we got to the end and the head was coming out, I was right in position to catch the baby. I hadn't planned on that, but the midwife said, "Catch your baby," and took her hands away, so someone had to catch the baby and it was me! That was such a surprise and such an honor and so great. In that moment of holding the baby, I realized that it was all about Kenna's transformation into motherhood. In the end, the experience was about Kenna and her work.

Here is another account, with comments from the father, Eugene, and the mother, Pamela.

Eugene:

Every man should catch his own baby. I didn't realize that, when my daughter was born eight years ago. We had her at home, I cut the cord, and it was the high point of my life. Yet it would have been even better if I had caught her.

I didn't because I was ignorant. I didn't know how easy it was, and nobody told me that I could or should. But when my son was born, I found out that catching your baby is the next best thing to having it. I urge all fathers to do it, to insist on it.

I enjoyed being down there between Pamela's legs. At my daughter's birth I was at her mother's side and didn't have the intimate perspective. This time I could see what was going on.

Pamela:

I was not sure where I wanted Eugene to be—at my side or at my feet. But as our cycle was near completion, I realized that this was the only time we, the three of us, would be connected in that intense moment of birth. Watching Eugene's concentration, his hands and the message of love that they carried, and seeing my baby's head in the mirror helped me to stay focused. Soon I was feeling those irresistible urges to push and feeling my baby's body moving through the passage. First the head then swoosh the body into the hands of the man I love. A beautiful baby boy was born so right. The connection is made and is never lost.

Eugene:

When Lenny slithered into my hands I immediately felt bonded to him. I was the first one able to see that he was a boy. That was a special thrill. Though Pamela carried Lenny and gave him up like ripe fruit; I was his first contact with the world as a whole person. In this first, total contact I knew he could feel my protective, loving feelings. And when I gave him to Pamela, completing the cycle, I felt truly satisfied.

SIBLING PARTICIPATION

Children who will be at the birth need preparation too. Have picture books available to lend for this purpose. Many parents worry that the sights and sounds of birth will frighten their children. Usually, these fears are unwarranted. As my midwife Ann Govan said regarding the presence of my son, then two, at his sister's birth, "They take it like an apple falling off a tree." Still,

you may wish to lend out birth videos to help with preparation. Mothers can also make "birth noises" with small children, helping them be better prepared for the intensity of the event. And it is a good idea to encourage the mother to invite an adult companion especially for the child, someone who can take her or him out of the room if she or he becomes upset during the birth and decides she or he wants to leave.

I recall one mother who planned to have her two-year-old at the birth but changed her mind in light of how ultra-sensitive her daughter had recently become (crying if anyone around her was hurt and responding intensely to her mother's every mood). Each mother must make the best decision for her child.

If a child is to be included, the atmosphere at prenatal visits is of utmost importance. Here's one mother's experience of preparing her three-year-old daughter:

From the beginning of our second pregnancy, we wanted to include Lydia in the birth. We felt that this would ease the transition from being an only child and lessen any jealousy that might arise. A home birth would enable her to comfortably share this joyous family occasion. Although some friends and relatives thought she was too young to participate, our

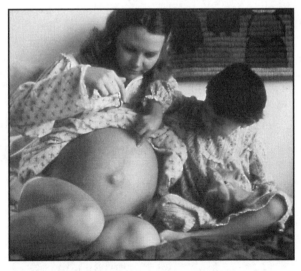

Mother encourages her daughter to touch and enjoy.

midwife and other friends invited to the birth supported the idea.

Our preparation started with prenatal exams in the home of our midwife, Elizabeth. Lydia accompanied us on all of these visits, and with each one became more interested in the proceedings. We tried to explain each step to her and encouraged her to take part by imitating Elizabeth. The relaxed atmosphere and obvious enthusiasm of everyone in the room made her more comfortable.

In preparation for the actual birth, we asked a friend who is close to Liddy to look after her during labor and to try to gauge whether she wanted to be in the room while the baby was born. We were happy that she slept through most of my labor because this reduced the chance that she would become bored, plus Frank and I were better able to concentrate on each other and the birth.

Liddy entered the room in the arms of a friend just as I was pushing the baby out. She was very calm, putting to rest our fears that the intensity of pushing might upset her. Even after the birth, much of my attention went out to Lydia, who seemed a bit shy at first. But a few hours later when the four of us were alone, she warmed up considerably and has continued to show a deep affection for her little brother. We feel that bringing her to clinic and letting her attend the birth has a lot to do with her present warmth and tolerance.

THE LAST SIX WEEKS

The emphasis of caregiving shifts dramatically during this final phase of pregnancy. The birth is imminent, and that is the focus. Parents have last-minute preparations to consider and more questions than before, while the midwife attends more assiduously to assessing the readiness of both mother and baby. She carefully palpates the baby for position, size, and growth, and also checks for descent, flexion, and engagement. These additional assessments can be done abdominally and by internal exam.

Lack of flexion can be corrected if the head is not too far into the pelvis; in fact, the deflexed head can

and should be flexed before it engages. The maneuver is simple—facing the mother's feet, press the occiput (back of the baby's head) down into the pelvis while pulling the sinciput (forehead) toward you, thus tucking the baby's chin to its chest (see illustration "Checking for Engagement and Securing Flexion" on the opposite page).

Internal exams are not mandatory but may help satisfy everyone's curiosity regarding the mother's readiness for labor. When examining near term you should: (1) check the cervix for dilation and effacement, (2) note the station (level of descent) of the baby's head, and (3) note any increase in vaginal lubrication or softening of the musculature common when birth is imminent. If a first pregnancy, the cervix may remain somewhat closed until labor begins, with perhaps a centimeter of **dilation,** whereas a woman who has had children before may be 2 or 3 cm dilated at term. **Effacement,** or the softening and shortening of the cervix, depends largely on how far the baby has descended and how much pressure it is exerting on lower uterine tissues. If the baby's head is still high and the cervix posterior, it is rare to find much effacement or dilation.

The degree of effacement is recorded in terms of percentage. An uneffaced cervix feels thick, firm, and about an inch long. A cervix 50 percent effaced feels softer, "mushier," with a less distinguishable neck, just half an inch or so in length. Sometimes the cervix is almost fully effaced but the os feels ringlike, with a clearly defined and somewhat rigid edge. Or the cervix may efface unevenly if the baby's head comes down at an angle (asynclitism) and puts pressure on either the anterior or posterior aspect. It is fairly common to find 60–80 percent effacement in the final weeks. Rarely, the cervix is **100** percent effaced at term (paper-thin and smooth against the baby's head) with little or no dilation but great propensity to open precipitously in labor. Some women dilate to 5 or 6 cm weeks before labor begins; these labors are also apt to be quick.

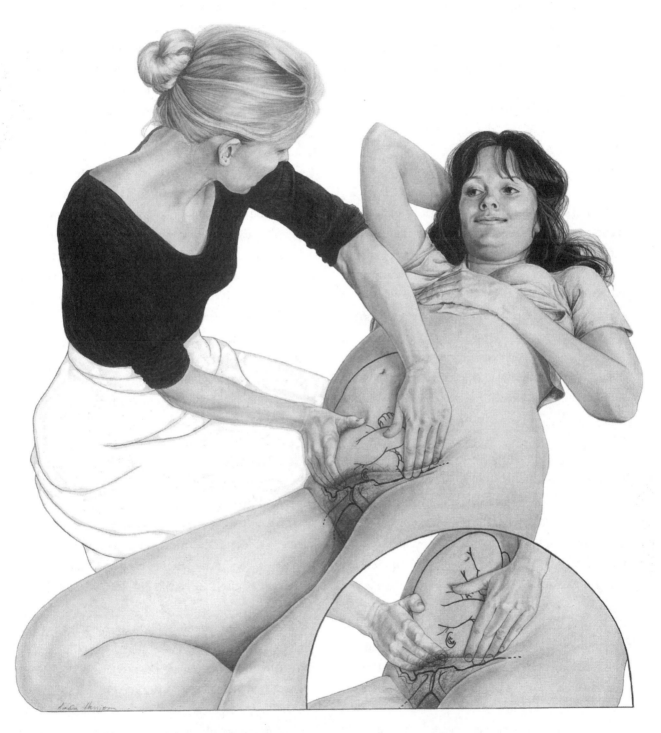

Checking for Engagement and Securing Flexion

If you find the cervical opening to be rigid and taut, or you know the mother to have scar tissue there from previous infection or surgery, have her do self-massage with evening primrose oil (available at most health-food stores). This will soften tissues and break up adhesions, preparing the cervix for dilation.[28] This can also be done in early labor, in case it is prolonged. Help the mother find her cervix in case she has never felt it before, and direct her to massage twice daily for several minutes. (This is contraindicated for any woman with a history of premature labor until she is at least thirty-seven weeks.)

The phenomenon of **false labor** commonly occurring in the final weeks of pregnancy is characterized by irregular contractions. Instead of increasing in duration and frequency, they eventually just taper off and stop. Little or no dilation takes place because uterine action is **incoordinate.** The uterus is comprised of three layers: the external, longitudinal layer, the internal, circular layer, and the middle, connective layer. In incoordinate labor, only certain long muscle segments contract, but all must work together harmoniously in order to pull open circular muscles of the cervix. Still, the term "false" is both discouraging and somewhat misleading, as these contractions often facilitate the baby's descent and engagement and may accomplish some effacement.

Descent is measured according to the relationship between the level of the presenting part and that of the ischial spines (which mark the midpoint of the pelvis). If the head is one centimeter above spine level, the station is termed –1. The head can be as high as –2, –3, or –4 and still be felt internally. If the top of the head is exactly level with the spines, it is at 0 station and considered to be **engaged.** If the head is a centimeter or two below spine level, it is at +1 or +2 station. Rarely will the presenting part be lower than +2 before labor begins.

Checking for station is difficult for beginners. It is essential to have some experience with pelvimetry to be certain you can find the spines. With the mother reclining, insert two fingers, bend the middle one and place it on the spine, then extend the index finger to find the presenting part. Your reading will only be accurate if you keep both fingers on a horizontal plane. If you must move your index finger up to touch the presenting part, the station is negative. With a positive station, your finger will move below the spine until the head is too low for the spine to be felt. At this point, assessment of the station is based primarily on a qualitative sense of how much the head (or butt) fills the pelvis. With practice, this ceases to be such a mysterious and painstaking procedure.

If you have not done so already, teach the mother **vaginal muscle awareness and control** to help her avoid vaginal and perineal tears. If she can learn the difference between contracted and relaxed states of her vagina and perineum, she will be able to create either at will. Encourage her to do some exploring; have her place her fingers inside and attempt to contract her muscles around them. Being able to stop the flow of urine (one way vaginal muscle awareness is taught) does not indicate a full range of control and may actually lead to urinary retention and infection.

The classic vaginal exercise is the "elevator." To do this, imagine pulling your pelvic floor muscles up, like an elevator ascending to the first floor (pause), second floor (pause), third floor (pause), fourth floor (pause), and fifth floor. Hold for thirty seconds, then descend slowly to the fourth floor (pause), third floor (pause), second floor (pause), first floor (pause), the basement (pause), and finally the subbasement (from which we give birth). Yet another exercise that imparts control of the muscle most likely to tear at birth (the bulbocavernosus) is to make quick, snapping movements lower in the vagina, near the introitus. These exercises also help to restore vaginal tone and speed tissue healing postpartum.

A new, physiologic approach to pelvic floor exercise was developed by midwifery instructor Verena

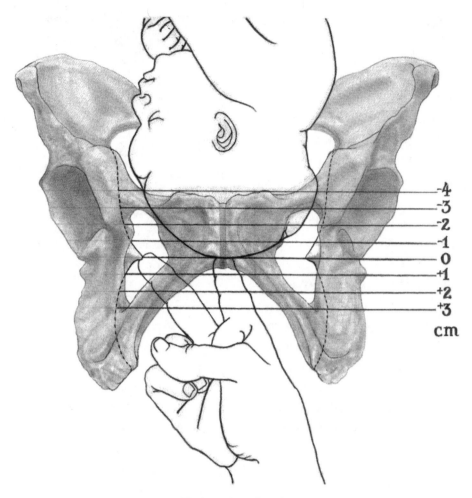

-4
-3
-2
-1
0
+1
+2
+3
cm

Estimating Station

Schmid. She suggests that contractions be performed in layers, beginning with the bulbocavernosus muscle. To activate this muscle, gently draw pubic bone and coccyx together. Next, add the transverse perineal muscle by pulling the ischial tuberosities (sitz bones) together. Now draw the entire vaginal canal together (it helps to tip the coccyx forward as you do this). Finally, activate the wide bands of levator ani running between the pubic bone and sacrum by contracting the pelvis in the opposite direction (coccyx back). Hold all four layers tightly, then release one by one.[29]

Vaginal/perineal massage is optional but can serve to make tissues supple and liable to stretch by increasing circulation. Have the mother use olive oil, and with clean hands, place her thumb against the floor of the vagina, running back and forth in a half circle with increasing pressure. Deep breathing helps facilitate this process. Some women feel awkward about massaging themselves and prefer to involve their partner.

Sometime in the last few weeks of pregnancy, it may be wise to carefully examine the mother's external genitals so if tearing occurs, you have some idea of how she looked previously and can more easily approximate tissues. Many women have **caruncles**—hymeneal skin tags irregular in shape—which can confuse suturing efforts. And check for scar tissue from previous repair that might require extra attention or support during perineal distension.

HOME VISITS

Home visits are obviously a critical part of home birth preparation. In fact, a number of midwives provide care exclusively by home visit. A minimum of two is essential: one early in pregnancy to see the mother and her supporters in their own element, and another around thirty-five weeks to be sure that supplies are ready and last-minute concerns are fully addressed. Extra home visits are definitely called for if a mother complains of family problems, reports feeling unsettled in her environment, or her partner hasn't come to prenatal visits for a while, whatever the reason.

The last home visit should be scheduled around thirty-five weeks and should include a review of prepared childbirth techniques (especially if the mother and her partner have not taken classes). Schoolage children can be included in dinner discussions, then afterward can feel mom's belly and listen to the baby's heartbeat. The entire birth team should be present at this gathering so that roles can be clearly delineated in advance.

Use this visit to appraise the home for order and cleanliness and see that a tabletop or some other protected area will be available for laying out supplies. A most crucial assessment is for **adequate heat in the birth room;** newborns quickly lose body heat and are almost impossible to resuscitate if cold. Also appraise the sleeping arrangements for baby—beware of the crib or cradle in a separate part of the house. Emphasize the importance of skin-to-skin contact in the early weeks, and debunk fears about bringing the baby to bed. You might want to come prepared with handouts or other reading material should your discussion progress to baby care or other postpartum concerns.

If the mother has felt shy or awkward with vaginal exams at your office, perhaps her own bed will be better. If she agrees, her children might be allowed to watch so they will be less likely to be alarmed at intimate procedures during the birth.

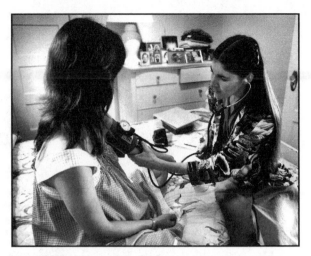

Combining a prenatal check-up with a home visit.

This is a perfect time to discuss any unresolved concerns the mother or her partner may be harboring with regard to the birth. Because this is a leisurely visit and the mother is in her own environment, she may become more vulnerable than ever before and reveal her deepest fears. However long it takes, consider this time well spent, as the birth may be shorter and smoother because of it. The main purpose of this visit is to affirm home as the birthplace and to inspire confidence and intimacy among the entire support team.

PREPARATION FOR WATER BIRTH

If the mother intends to have a water birth, she will need an ample sized tub (now widely available for rent). The tub should be scrubbed with iodine and rinsed thoroughly before it is filled with water. It is generally agreed that a mild saline solution can help discourage the growth of microorganisms and keep the birth environment similar to that which the baby has known in utero. The mother and her partner should shower before entering the tub. Be aware that it can be difficult to utilize universal precautions when assisting water birth.

Parents' most common concern regarding water birth is for their baby's safety: What if it tries to breathe while still under water? This fear is unfounded, as the baby will not be stimulated to breathe until its body is exposed to air, due to the **dive reflex** that keeps the glottis closed when the baby is submerged. Still, it is wise to bring the baby out of the water as soon as it is born.

Benefits of water birth include increased relaxation and comfort for the mother, greater intimacy for the couple, and an easier transition for the baby. Water birth can greatly ease a painful or tumultuous labor. German expert Cornelia Enning claims it lowers blood pressure in cases of borderline hypertension and is ideal for breech and posterior babies, as well as for women having a VBAC.[30]

The temperature of the water is very important; it must stay between 86 and 95 degrees F. Ideally, it should be between 92 and 94 degrees F for late labor, 86 degrees F for placental delivery, and then warmed back up to the low 90s for breastfeeding. Under these circumstances, the following benefits accrue:

1. Neurotransmission of pain is reduced.

2. Oxygen uptake via uterine vessels is increased.

3. Muscle tone is normalized.

4. Glucose metabolism is improved.

5. Levels of stress hormones are lowered,

6. Placental separation is facilitated.[31]

The mother must be in the water for at least thirty minutes before maximum effects are realized. After two to three hours, benefits as per hormone stimulation diminish.[32] Advise her to stay flexible, and see how she feels about being in the water as labor progresses. Never put a cold cloth on her forehead to cool her—if she gets hot, cool the water down or have her come out. If she gets claustrophobic in the tub, or feels like she cannot get enough leverage to bear down, she should get out immediately.

Auscultate fetal heart tones using a Doppler with a waterproof probe. If there is fetal distress, meconium, or blood loss during labor, the mother should get out of the water. If she is at risk for postpartum hemorrhage, or the baby may be slow to start, have her leave the tub as transition ends. Once she leaves the water, it can take between thirty minutes and an hour and a half for her metabolism to return to normal. Therefore, she should stay out of the tub for at least an hour before reentering.[33]

It is best to avoid touching the baby as it is born. If the mother is undisturbed, she will touch the head herself, and the baby will spiral out (literally pushing itself out with its feet) and turn to face her. It may expel fluid from its lungs (seen jetting into the water), and may reach one arm toward her with the other bent, as if swimming (the asymmetric tonic reflex). Mom and baby will then make eye contact, and she and her partner can lift it and bring it to her chest.

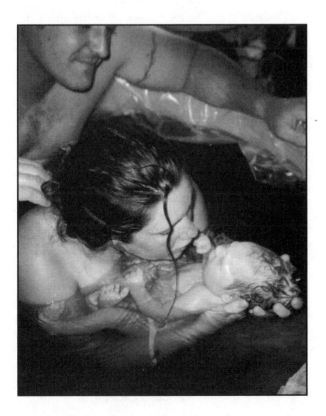

LAST-MINUTE CLIENTS

What about mothers calling for help just weeks before their due date? In general, the last-minute scramble to obtain all essential information and develop intimacy in short order will challenge even the most experienced midwife. If the mother has been receiving care and her records are available, your task is less daunting. Without prenatal records, you have no maternal or fetal baselines from which to extrapolate norms during labor. And if her dates are at all uncertain, you have no point of reference regarding the baby's maturity except its current size. You also have very little time to assess the mother's needs and expectations of you, or to assert your own needs and expectations of her. All this increases your liability, and you must decide if the additional effort and risk can be justified.

Your decision to assist must be based on a strong sense of rapport, and the conviction that the mother and her supporters are utterly committed to home birth. If they are coming to you from another midwife's care, explore their reasons carefully to make sure they are not just chasing rainbows. Get right down to it: What do they want from you? Make a home visit as soon as possible, and schedule longer or extra appointments. You must still cover all the essential information on emergency care, the mechanics of labor, and birthing techniques. Some last-minute clients expect a major discount; explain that providing care in these short-order circumstances requires a challenging condensation of your services.

Tina, a midwife practicing in rural Hawaii, shared this tale of assisting a true last-minute client. Her account also exemplifies how the midwife's work can overflow into her personal, home, and family life:

> This lady-in-waiting called me two days after her due date—I'd met her before, and I said sure, I'd find time to see her. But I made no promises, as I'm wary of "last-minute goodies." She had no support, no man, not even a place to call home. She'd seen a doc-

tor three times, but didn't feel comfortable or prepared for the hospital situation.

> There she was on my doorstep; I had just returned from one of my huge food shopping expeditions. So I put the groceries away, made some tea, sat down with the woman and felt out the situation. She looked pretty tense, had been having contractions all night but didn't want to go to the hospital. She didn't even know if she wanted to keep the child. Very much alone, she felt she had other things to do with her life besides mothering. But she did have enough incentive to give the baby a good beginning with natural birth and breast milk. She also was willing to give herself some time to feel out motherhood.

> It was early afternoon, and I got the feeling that she was definitely in labor and would have her baby that night. But I didn't even know this woman, didn't even know if I liked her! All I knew was that she was confused, and I wanted to help her. She couldn't have her baby at my place—too much traffic with five children. So I told her I'd go to the hospital to ease the doctor confrontation and serve as her support person and coach. She seemed relieved at this decision. She took a walk outside in the banana patch for about an hour and came back a different woman: resigned, courageous, strong. She began squatting for most of her now regular contractions. I suggested that she lie down and rest in the loft where it was quiet and where Adrian (my one-year-old) was sleeping. The older children came in from playing and we gathered around the table for dinner.

> No sooner were the dishes cleared than we heard some serious "Oh-oh-ohs" from the loft. I dropped everything and got ready to examine her, but she was already on her way down the ladder saying she had to go to the bathroom. She came back out to kneel on the living room floor and her water bag broke. "Can I check you?" said I. "No, no, no, oh, oh, oh," said she, "I've got to go to the bathroom again." Then she really began complaining, she said she wasn't comfortable at all, couldn't see any point in all this discomfort, wanted to go to the hospital and get drugged out. She got off the toilet and leaned on the sink, but was still . . . pushing!

Uh, oh . . . what's this? Oh god, quick, wash those hands, catch that baby, plop, flop, she's out, gorgeous! Her mother was stunned but finally uttered something, and the baby gave a cry back. Relief, release. I wrapped the babe in a towel, set another towel on the floor so they could lie down, and waited for the placenta. I opened the bathroom door and there were some little faces eager to greet the baby; the children all heard that first cry. Haydon (nine-and-a-half years old) announced that it happened at two minutes to eight. Chana (eight years old) got a blanket for the baby. Nara (six years old) got my birth kit so I could clamp the cord, and also a bowl for the placenta. Then I announced bedtime but of course I wasn't heeded; the excitement was too much.

I assisted the mother with baby-holding and bonding and the placenta came out fine. "Now," I thought, "if I can just get them up off this floor and onto a bed in the living room to check for tears . . . hmm, well, she was standing and there was no support." So after a good nursing session I suggested she go to the hospital to be sutured and stay for a few days. She would rest better there and wouldn't have to think about her personal care for a while.

They came to stay with us for several weeks before finally leaving the island. We really fell in love with the baby—it was quite an experience for all of us.

Notes

1. Robert Briffault, *The Mothers* (New York: Atheneum, 1977).

2. Verena Schmid, Midwifery Today conference notes.

3. Schmid, Midwifery Today conference notes, London, June 2003.

4. Verena Schmid, "Birth Centres in Italy," in *Birth Centers: A Social Model for Maternity Care*, ed. Mavis Kirkham (UK: Butterworth Heinemann, 2003).

5. M. Plaut, M. Schwartz, and S. Lubarsky, "Uterine rupture associated with the use of misoprostol in the gravid patient with a previous cesarean section," *American Journal of Obstetrics and Gynecology* 180 (1999): 1,535–42.

6. Ina May Gaskin, *Ina May's Guide to Childbirth* (New York: Bantam Dell, 2003), p. 300.

7. F. M. Cowan and P. Munday, "Guidelines for the management of herpes simplex virus infection in pregnancy," *Sexually Transmitted Infections* 74 (2): 93–94, 1998.

8. Peggy McIntosh, "White Privilege: Unpacking the Invisible Knapsack," from Working Paper 189, "White Privilege and Male Privilege: A Personal Account of Coming to See Correspondences through Work in Women's Studies," Wellesley, College Center for Research on Women, Wellesley, Mass., 1988.

9. R. Mittendorf and others, "The length of uncomplicated human gestation," *OB/GYN* 75 (6): 929–32, 1990.

10. Carol Wood Nichols, "Postdate Pregnancy, Part II: Clinical Implications," *Journal of Nurse Midwifery* 30 (5): 259–68, 1985.

11. B. G. Ewigman, J. P. Crane, D. Fredric, F. D. Frigoletto, M. L. Le Fevre, R. P. Bain, D. McNellis, and the RADIUS study group, "Effect of prenatal ultrasound screening on perinatal outcome," *New England Journal of Medicine* 329 (12): 821–27.

12. J. Newnham, S. F. Evans, C. A. Michael, F. J. Stanley, and L. I. Landau, "Effects of frequent ultrasound during pregnancy: a randomized controlled trial," *Lancet* 342 (1993): 887–91.

13. J. M. Jiminez, J. E. Tyson, and J. S. Reisch, "Clinical Measures of Gestational Age in Normal Pregnancies," *Obstetrics and Gynecology* 61 (1983): 483.

14. American College of Obstetricians and Gynecologists, "Fetal Heart Rate Patterns: Monitoring, Interpretation, and Management," *ACOG Technical Bulletin* 207, July 1995.

15. K. M. De Cock, M. G. Fowler, E. Mercier, and others, "Prevention of Mother-to-Child HIV Transmission in Resource-Poor Countries: Translating Research into Policy and Practice," *Journal of the American Medical Association* 238 (9): 1,175–82.

16. Anne Frye, *Understanding Diagnostic Tests in the Childbearing Year*, 6th ed. (Portland, Oreg.: Labrys Press, 1997), 422.

17. Sara Wickham, *Anti-D in Midwifery: Panacea or Paradox?* (Oxford, England: Butterworth-Heinemann, 2001), 7.

18. Wickham, *Anti-D in Midwifery*, 7.

19. Frye, *Understanding Diagnostic Tests*, 726.

20. E. M. Levine and others, "Intrapartum Antibiotic Prophylaxis Increases the Incidence of Gram Negative Neonatal Sepsis," *Infectious Disease Obstetrics Gynecology* 7 (4): 210–13.

21. M. Dabrowska-Szponar and J. Galinski, "Drug resistance of Group B Streptococci," *Pol Merkuriusz Lek* 10 (60): 442–44.

22. C. V. Towers and G. G. Briggs, "Antepartum Use of Antibiotics and Early-Onset Neonatal Sepsis: The

Next Four Years," *American Journal of Obstetric Gynecology* 187 (2): 495–500.

23. C. J. Baker, M. A. Rench, and P. McInnes, "Immunization of Pregnant Women with Group B Streptococcal Type III Capsular Polysaccharide-Tetanus Toxoid Conjugate Vaccine," *Vaccine* (Netherlands) 21 (24): 3468–72.

24. Christa Novelli, "Treating Group B Strep: Are Antibiotics Necessary?" *Mothering*, November 2003.

25. Antonia Sanchez, Midwifery Today conference notes, Oaxaca, Mexico, October 2003.

26. Frye, *Understanding Diagnostic Tests,* 288.

27. Stephen G. Gabbe, Jennifer R. Neibyl, and Joe Leigh Simpson, *Obstetrics: Normal and Problem Pregnancies,* 4th ed. (New York: Churchill Livingstone, 2002), 1286.

28. Frye, *Understanding Diagnostic Tests,* 249.

29. Schmid, Midwifery Today conference notes.

30. Cornelia Enning, Midwifery Today conference, lecture notes.

31. Enning, Midwifery Today conference, lecture notes.

32. Enning, Midwifery Today conference, lecture notes.

33. Enning, Midwifery Today conference, lecture notes.

For Parents: Self-Care in Pregnancy

Prenatal care is more than just the checkups you receive from your practitioner every few weeks—it is the care you *give yourself* each and every day. Here are some of the main components of self-care in pregnancy, with a rating system to help you see how well you are doing. Enter one of the following with each category:

4: Do this automatically, naturally

3: Do this consistently but with definite effort

2: Do this occasionally, with some resistance

1: Just can't seem to do this or haven't thus far

Nutrition

_____ Eat from the four basic food groups daily

_____ Take supplements that I know I need

_____ Drink at least two quarts of water, juice, and so on per day

_____ Pay attention to my inner voice of hunger and respond accordingly

_____ Treat myself to something I know is especially good for the baby and me

_____ Indulge myself in favorite foods (that are also healthful) for pure pleasure

Exercise and Relaxation

_____ Take fresh air and (if available) sunshine daily

_____ Do something to work up a sweat each day

_____ Stretch out my back, legs, shoulders, and neck daily

_____ Do exercises specific to pregnancy several times a week

_____ Dance, move rhythmically and freely with music

_____ Do vaginal toning and relaxation exercises daily

_____ Completely let go at least once every day

_____ Practice progressive relaxation at least twice a week

_____ Have my partner (or someone else) massage me at least once weekly

_____ Dress in clothing that allows freedom of movement and is comfortable

_____ Deliberately release areas where I know I hold tension, several times daily

_____ Allow myself the necessary comforts to curl up and take it easy before bed

Emotional Well-Being

_____ Let myself cry whenever I feel like it

_____ Ask for support, acknowledgement, touch, and sex from my partner whenever I need it (if applicable)

_____ Vent my frustrations before they become explosive

_____ Feel free to be loving and tender with my partner (if applicable) day by day

_____ Feel loving and tender with myself at least once each day

_____ Give myself time alone and find new ways to enjoy it

Intellectual Preparation

_____ Read something on pregnancy at least once a week

_____ Formulate and ask questions of my care provider

_____ Take stock of my status in pregnancy by reviewing my daily or weekly activities and looking for areas that need improvement

_____ Discuss technical aspects of pregnancy, birth, and parenting with my partner and/or supporters on a regular basis

continued →

_____ Work on developing my birth plan by noting ideas and preferences as they arise

_____ Attend information sessions or film series on birth whenever possible

Social Preparation

_____ Meet with other pregnant women at least once a week

_____ Talk to mothers of infants or pregnant women in public places

_____ Observe infant behavior and family interaction whenever possible

_____ Ask for concrete support from friends and relatives for needs in pregnancy and postpartum

_____ Think about the changes having a baby will bring and formulate ways to adapt

_____ Support my partner (if applicable) in talking to other new parents, reading about parenting, or discussing the baby with me

There are several different ways to score this exercise. First add up your total score in each section; this will give you a general idea of areas where you are strong and those where you could use improvement. Your overall score can be viewed as follows:

110–44: Yes, you are enjoying being pregnant and are taking good care of yourself.

80–109: You are doing well enough, but could stand to focus a bit more on the pregnancy. Look carefully at your areas of resistance, and see what you can do to discipline or motivate yourself more.

36–79: Well, perhaps you are very busy with other things, but you definitely need to give your pregnancy some attention. Try combining an activity where you scored low with one where you scored high; for example, if you get outside every day but can't seem to take your vitamins, make it a prerequisite before leaving the house (like locking the door, turning off the lights, etc.).

You'll feel much better if you care for yourself regularly. ■

Chapter 3

PROBLEMS IN PREGNANCY

The challenge in caring for problem pregnancies is to differentiate psychological and physical factors, for they often overlap. One must be wary of oversimplifying physical complications with a psychosomatic view; on the other hand, psychological disequilibrium for an extended period of time can definitely cause physical illness or jeopardy. The hallmark of a competent midwife is her ability to enlist the mother in unraveling any emotional aspects of her condition, while promptly securing medical consultation or assistance if indicated.

Physical problems still in incipient stages call upon the midwife to utilize her insight and expertise to formulate, with the mother's assistance, a remedy as holistic as possible, one combining health-giving physical treatments with self-awareness practices. Safe leeway for finding the most effective remedy always depends on close and continued surveillance of the mother's condition. Under these circumstances, prenatal visits should be scheduled more frequently—perhaps as often as every few days, with phone contact in the interim. And don't hesitate to consult with another experienced midwife or another expert within your network of health-care providers.

Physical Complications

The following section on physical complications will not address every pathological condition of pregnancy, but will focus on those pertinent to low-risk women already established as good candidates for home birth. For more information, consult a medical textbook or your backup physician.

ANEMIA

Nutritional anemia is common in pregnancy, due partly to dietary quirks and partly to the normal physiology of pregnancy. **Iron deficiency anemia** accounts for 95 percent of nutritional anemias; however, supplemental iron is seldom enough to remedy the problem. Adequate protein is necessary to build new red blood cells, and folic acid must be available to maintain the integrity of cell membranes. Vitamin C is crucial for iron absorption. If stress is a lifestyle factor, vitamin C, B-complex, and trace minerals may also be depleted, thus increased intake is advisable. The best approach to dealing with anemia is to dramatically revamp and improve the entire diet by adding more fresh fruit and vegetables, high-quality protein, whole grains, mineral-rich seeds and nuts, and nourishing herbal teas.

Take care with iron supplements, as they are toxic in large quantities. I recommend ferrous peptonate or gluconate, in low doses (25–50 mg) spread throughout the day, and no more than 100 mg total. Supplemental iron is difficult to assimilate; often, no more than a third is absorbed. The unused portion can irritate the kidneys and intestines and cause indigestion, constipation, and black stools. This is particularly true of ferrous sulfate. Note that supplemental calcium and dairy products virtually block absorption. If the mother is vegan, she can try one of several brands of iron that contain no animal products.

If a woman is anemic in early pregnancy, meaning hematocrit (HCT) at or below 33 or hemoglobin (HGB) at or below 11, suggest 100 mg iron daily, taken with 500 mg vitamin C. Repeat blood work in three to four weeks. An extremely anemic woman may benefit from higher doses of vitamin C and iron, but emphasize dietary changes too. Good food sources for iron include prune juice, molasses, pumpkin seeds, sesame seeds, sunflower seeds, beans, raisins, dark greens, and organic beef liver. An herbal elixir called Floradix Iron Plus Herbs (or Floradix Floravital Iron Plus Herbs for vegans) is concentrated and easily absorbed by many women.

Around twenty-eight weeks, HCT/HGB readings often dip due to **hemodilution,** that is, an increase in blood volume that temporarily decreases the percentage of red blood cells. This condition is known as **physiologic anemia.** Check for this at the onset of the last trimester, and if need be, advise the mother on how to bring the HCT/HGB to optimal levels by the time of the birth. Keep in mind that it takes several weeks to build red cells, and an effective therapy for one woman may do nothing for the next.

Anemia creates numerous problems for the mother. Fatigue and diminished vitality affect her appetite, her resistance to infection, and her general enjoyment of the pregnancy. She is susceptible to premature labor, but even if she goes to term, labor may be prolonged by incoordinate contractions, and she is at risk for maternal exhaustion. Her uterus is less likely to contract efficiently after birth, placing her at risk for postpartum hemorrhage. And with less oxygen-carrying cells in her bloodstream, she may go into shock more rapidly than usual. Anemia in the postpartum period can be devastating too, as it renders the new mother more susceptible to infection, poor healing, difficulties with establishing a milk supply, and postpartum depression.

The baby of an anemic mother may be growth restricted, lacking sufficient body fat for insulation and stress resistance during the early weeks. Normally, it will store enough iron in the last six weeks of pregnancy for the first six months of life, but if the mother's intake is inadequate, she may have to begin feeding solids before she or the baby is ready. During labor, decreased oxygen levels in the maternal bloodstream can lead to fetal distress, a cesarean, or the need for neonatal resuscitation. For all of these reasons, a woman wanting a home birth should strive to maintain an HCT of 34 or an HGB of 11.5 throughout most of her pregnancy.

Before treating the mother for iron-deficiency anemia, double-check her lab work to rule out a 5 percent chance of anemia caused by a deficiency of either folic acid or vitamin B-12. How do you identify this? Look at the prenatal panel and notice the figures given in the **mean corpuscular volume (MCV)** and **mean corpuscular hemoglobin (MCH)** categories. The **MCV** indicates the average size of her blood cells. The **MCH** indicates the average amount of hemoglobin per cell. In iron-deficiency anemia, the MCV is normal but the MCH is lower than usual; this type of anemia is called **microcytic** (small cell) anemia. In B-12 and folic acid anemias, the MCV is elevated but the MCH is normal; these anemias are **macrocytic** or **megaloblastic** (large cell) anemias.

If it appears the mother suffers from a macrocytic or megaloblastic anemia, more testing will be necessary to determine whether a deficiency of folic acid or B-12 is at fault. In the meantime, carefully reassess the diet. Sources of folic acid include egg yolks, orange juice, melons, strawberries, and dark greens like spinach, chard, kale, and collard greens—the darker the green, the better. Although food comes first, four large servings of the above per day would barely remedy a minor deficiency during pregnancy. So advise the mother to combine food sources with supplemental folic acid, about 2,400 mcg daily.

B-12 is found almost exclusively in dairy foods and animal products and will therefore be lacking in a vegan diet unless a supplement is taken. B-12 deficiency can cause central nervous system damage in the newborn, and should deficiency persist into childhood, there will be slow, insidious, and irreversible brain damage. Thus all vegan mothers must be sure of their intake. Purported vegetable sources such as fermented soy products, seaweed, shiitake mushrooms, or spirulina actually contain analogs of the vitamin that can block absorption of the active form. Have the mother look for sublingual tablets containing cyanocobalamin or hydroxocobalamin. Soy products or fresh juices fortified with cyanocobalamin or hydroxocobalamin are also good sources. In severe cases, intramuscular injections are the only remedy.

There are certain types of hereditary, microcytic anemias such as thalassemia or sickle-cell anemia that may also render MCV values unusually low. If the MCV is below 80, and the woman is of African, Asian, or Mediterranean descent, consider ordering a hemoglobin electrophoresis (test for normal hemoglobin).

PROBLEMS WITH WEIGHT GAIN

Determining whether weight gain during pregnancy is inadequate or excessive depends partly on prepregnant weight. The average weight gain in pregnancy is about a pound per week, although underweight women may gain more and overweight women may gain less. In either case, extensive nutritional counseling may be necessary to assure that adequate nutrients and calories are being taken. As a rule of thumb, the expectant mother should gain at least ten pounds by twenty weeks and about a pound a week thereafter.

What causes weight gain in pregnancy? There is increased water retention due to hormones, increased fatty insulation deposited over the belly and backside, increased weight in the breasts, increased blood volume, plus the obvious weight of the enlarged uterus including amniotic fluid, placenta, and fetus. Most women lose an average of fifteen pounds with the birth or a few days thereafter, and the remaining weight is used for sustenance during the first few months postpartum. Making breast milk, getting up several times a night to nurse, and dealing with the stress of a new baby definitely burn up the fat reserves!

If a mother seems to be gaining weight more rapidly than usual, check for a fetal growth spurt. It is not unusual to see a gain of five pounds in two weeks linked to a corresponding increase of three or four centimeters in fundal height. Sometimes a mother gains weight *just before* a growth spurt, so wait a couple weeks before jumping to conclusions. Double-check her diet to see if she's made any deleterious changes (perhaps because of something she has read or heard). If so, reiterate nutritional basics and remind her to heed her instinctive voice of hunger. Excess sugar intake may signal a need for more protein. Suggest she have vegetable snacks instead of high caloric fruits and juices; see which fruits appeal to her and find vegetables with equivalent vitamin and mineral content. Also recommend low-fat protein sources like cottage cheese, fish, or chicken breast in place of high-fat sources like ice cream, hard cheese, or cream cheese. Be sensitive to the mother's response to your ideas, and try to work positively around her attachment to certain foods.

Mothers with a history of eating disorders may require care from a specialist. Anorexic women often have difficulty conceiving and may have serious problems maintaining a pregnancy. Even when the pregnancy is well established, increased appetite combined

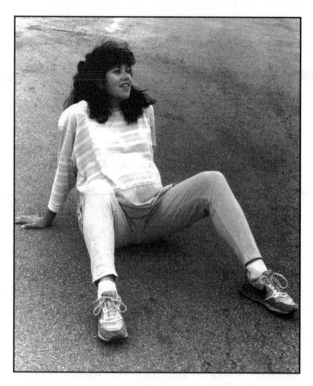

active, used to running around constantly, more or less "living on air." Help her slow down enough to tune into her pregnant body, particularly if she has nervous symptoms of insomnia, dizziness, or fainting. Your slender client may adore fresh squeezed juices, raw vegetables, and tofu, but unless she gets enough calories each day she will not look and feel her best. Thin women often complain of feeling bloated, heavy, or "clogged-up" with more food, especially carbohydrates. If so, suggest smaller meals, with an snack extra at bedtime. Better yet, encourage continuous snacking throughout the day, with baggies of goodies ever available. Explain to the mother that her body makes nourishing the baby a priority, so if she is underweight, there may be little left for her own needs. This puts her at risk for anemia, preeclampsia, premature labor, prolonged labor, postpartum hemorrhage, poor recovery, and postpartum depression. With her cooperation, set a goal of around twenty-five pounds of weight gain.

The mother's partner must also understand her liability with inadequate food intake; see that he or she understands the nutritional demands of pregnancy and is fully supportive. Make sure the mother is not dieting or trying to control her weight in order to please her partner. Emphasize the positive physical changes of pregnancy, such as the mother's rosier complexion, her fuller, more sensitive breasts, that warm pregnant glow, and for many, an increased sexual appetite.

with changing body image may reactivate eating disorders. Mothers with a history of bulimia are particularly at risk for hyperemesis gravidarium, and those who have been anorexic, for malnutrition. Schedule prenatal visits more often if necessary, and plan to see the mother in her home (where you can share meals together) as much as possible.

In fact, any mother who claims she must "watch her weight" should be taken seriously. If she defines eating as an out-of-control, emotionally based activity, she may never learn to trust her instincts for nourishing herself and her child. She may have strong feelings of guilt associated with eating, linked to years of criticism from family or friends regarding her appearance. Do take history in this regard, but avoid dwelling on the negative aspects. Encourage her to bring variety to her diet, honor cravings for treats from time to time, and find some type of physical activity she can embrace. Brisk walking is a good beginning; prenatal exercise classes are ideal.

How about the underweight woman who gains very slowly in pregnancy? She may be somewhat hyper-

MISCARRIAGE (ABORTION)

The proper technical term for miscarriage occurring before twenty weeks is **spontaneous abortion;** beyond this point, it becomes **fetal demise.** In the vast majority of cases, the cause of spontaneous abortion is abnormal development of the fetus or placenta due to chromosomal abnormalities. Less commonly, a mother may miscarry due to viral infection, severe malnutrition, substance abuse, or an antibody effect toward the father's sperm.

Threatened abortion is presumed whenever the mother has vaginal bleeding in the first half of pregnancy, particularly if combined with cramping or persistent backache. Remember, though, that one in four women experience bleeding in the first trimester, while only half of these actually miscarry.[1] With threatened abortion, bright-red blood loss may be either dramatic or slight but continuous for days or weeks. **Inevitable abortion** ensues if the membranes rupture or if the cervix dilates.

Is there any intervention that can keep a threatened miscarriage from becoming inevitable? Probably not, but certain measures may be worth a try. If symptoms are acute, recommend bedrest and complete cessation of all sexual activity. If there is cramping without bleeding, a glass of wine may halt uterine activity and forestall miscarriage. But if it does become inevitable, console the mother as best you can and focus on helping her safely through the physical aspects of the process.

If she wants to go through her miscarriage at home, be certain she is not anemic and keep close watch for possible hemorrhage. *Two cups of blood is the maximum safe blood loss.* If the miscarriage extends for more than a day or two, she is at risk for infection and must take her temperature every four hours. If bleeding or pain persists, she should see a physician to determine whether everything has been shed—that is, that the abortion is complete. She may also wish to save the remnants of her miscarriage (insensitively referred to as "products of conception") and either have them tested for possible causative factors or handled in some ceremonial way.

Occasionally, women have light bleeding (brownish in color) for many weeks, with no distinct episode of resolution. This may be due to **missed abortion,** that is, the fetus has died but is retained in utero. The mother may notice that her breasts have returned to their normal size, or that she has lost several pounds. Upon examination, her uterus may seem small for dates. The most conclusive sign of missed abortion is lack of fetal heart tones.

In case of suspected missed abortion, it is important to make a determination with ultrasound as soon as possible. Although rare before twenty weeks, a coagulation disorder known as **disseminated intravascular coagulation (DIC)** may result from retained products of conception, leading to catastrophic bleeding when the pregnancy is terminated. The incidence of DIC increases exponentially the longer the mother has been pregnant and the longer the fetus is retained after it dies. If a mother with signs of missed abortion notes excessive bleeding from the gums, nose, or minor injury sites, she is extremely high risk. Have her seen by a backup physician immediately.

I have had only one case of missed abortion in my practice. The mother came for her first visit at eighteen weeks, reporting brown spotting for the last week or so. She had a history of previous miscarriage, although she had also had a baby at term (whose birth I assisted several years earlier). Her uterus felt normal for dates. I couldn't hear the baby with the fetascope but was not concerned, as she was not yet twenty weeks. Two weeks later she came in again, reporting what she thought was fetal movement, but the brown discharge had been continuous since her last visit. This time I was alarmed at not finding the fetal heart and sent her for an ultrasound. She called to report a missed abortion; it was unclear exactly when the fetus had died, but development appeared to have arrested at twelve weeks. She was screened for DIC and was negative, but immediately scheduled a therapeutic abortion because she couldn't stand the agony of waiting.

With any type of miscarriage, emotional support is critical at every phase of the process. Studies show that women grieve as deeply with miscarriage as they do with fetal demise, stillbirth, and neonatal death.[2] Feelings of guilt, shame, anger, and frustration are common and must be validated and worked through. Support groups for women who have miscarried may also be found through a local birth resource center or online.

In addition, most women worry about their future prospects for carrying to term. Occasionally, miscarriage becomes **habitual**—that is, it occurs more than three times, in which case genetic or other factors may be at fault. Refer a woman (or couple) with this problem for consultation with a specialist.

ECTOPIC PREGNANCY

Ectopic pregnancy refers to implantation occurring outside the uterine cavity. The blastocyst implants in one of the fallopian tubes 95 percent of the time. Depending on the portion of the tube in which implantation occurs, the fetus may either be expelled into the abdominal cavity as it grows too large or may cause the tube to rupture, usually between ten and thirteen weeks. This is a serious, life-threatening complication. With tubal rupture, the mother will lose the baby and is at risk for severe internal hemorrhage, which may lead to shock or even death. Tubal pregnancy or rupture may be misdiagnosed as pelvic inflammatory disease, severe gastrointestinal upset, or appendicitis, particularly if the woman does not know she is pregnant.

The primary cause of tubal pregnancy is pelvic inflammatory disease, which leaves behind scar tissue that may partially occlude the tube and cause reduced cilliation or the formation of blind pockets. Ectopic pregnancies have risen fivefold in the last decade due to the prevalence of sexually transmitted diseases, trauma from intrauterine devices, progesterone-based contraception, and infection following abortion.[3] Prior ectopic rupture and reconstructive surgery (tuboplasty) also predispose a woman to ectopic pregnancy. One of my colleagues, whose practice has had more than its share of ectopic pregnancies, now routinely does bimanual exam on any woman with first trimester bleeding to rule out any luteal pelvic masses.

Symptoms of tubal pregnancy include pelvic pain (consistent and more intense than cramping) and often, spot bleeding, sometimes brown. Pain becomes quite severe with actual rupture and may be referred to the shoulder area. A definite sign that the mother is suffering from tubal rupture (as opposed to miscarriage) is that the degree of shock far exceeds what would normally be expected for the amount of blood loss. If an expectant mother calls to report symptoms that lead you to suspect tubal pregnancy or rupture, contact your backup physician *immediately* and have her call an ambulance for transport. Even if per an initial phone consultation, avoid sending her to the emergency room, as the wait may be life jeopardizing.

Treatment of tubal pregnancy (if not ruptured) involves one of two options: surgical removal of the pregnancy or use of the drug methotrexate to dissolve the pregnancy. At first glance, the latter seems preferable; it can spare the loss of the tube and is the only reasonable choice if the other tube is ruptured. But keep in mind that methotrexate is a potent chemotherapy drug, a folic acid antagonist and teratogen.[4] Do your best to assure your client informed choice regarding her treatment.

Emotional recovery from ectopic pregnancy is complex. The woman has come close to losing her life, and has lost a child that may have been long-awaited. Her future fertility may be affected. Her partner may struggle as well, with multiple shocks of nearly losing her plus the disappointment of losing the baby. See to it that both are offered counseling and support.

HYDATIDIFORM MOLE

This extremely rare complication occurs in 1 per 1,500–2,000 pregnancies. The hydatidiform (pronounced "high-duh-tid-ah-form") mole results from abnormal development of the chorionic villi, which ordinarily form the membranes and placenta but in this case, become a mass of clear, grape-like vesicles filling the uterus. In 95 percent of cases, a hydatidiform mole is thought to be caused by an abnormal sperm inactivating the chromosomes of the ovum. This is called a **complete mole;** there is no fetus. In the remaining 5 percent of cases there is fetal tissue present, though chromosomes from sperm and ovum are abnormal in number and the fetus almost never survives. This is called a **partial mole.** Molar pregnancy is more common in women over forty.

Light brown bleeding is the most outstanding symptom, persisting for weeks or months (though rarely past the first trimester). What distinguishes the hydatidiform mole from other complications correlated to light brown bleeding, such as missed abortion or ectopic pregnancy, is that the uterus is typically large for dates and feels woody hard or doughy to the touch. The overgrowth of chorionic villi also leads to abnormally high hCG levels, which are subnormal with missed abortion and ectopic pregnancy.

Elevated hCG levels tax the liver, giving rise to secondary symptoms of hypertension and proteinuria. Hyperemesis occurs in 25 to 30 percent of all cases but tends to develop later than usual in pregnancy, generally at the onset of the second trimester. The mole almost always aborts spontaneously but occasionally must be surgically removed. Approximately 20 percent of molar pregnancies progress to invasive cancer, thus follow-up examination and testing are necessary for at least a year.[5] (A former student of mine related that during her training as a nurse-midwife, she took care of a woman who had metastasis to her brain from cancer originating in molar pregnancy!) If you suspect a hydatidiform mole, refer to a physician promptly.

As with ectopic pregnancy, attend to the mother's emotional recovery or any need for additional psychological support.

BLEEDING LATE IN PREGNANCY

Occasionally, vaginal bleeding a bit heavier than spotting occurs after intercourse in the second or third trimester. The cervix has increased vascularity during pregnancy and is often quite friable, that is, easily abraded with friction. Or if the mother has a vaginal infection, the mucosa will be irritable and more prone to bleeding during and after sex.

Another possible source of bleeding is a **ruptured cervical polyp.** Polyps are small, tonguelike protrusions at the cervical os, visible by speculum exam. Bleeding from a ruptured polyp is sudden and somewhat dramatic but tends to resolve quickly and completely. If blood loss is significant and persistent in the second or third trimester, it is probably due to placental abruption or placenta previa.

Placental abruption refers to premature separation of the placenta. It may be caused by cord entanglement, physical trauma, or hypertension, but often the cause is unknown. There are several types of abruption. **Marginal abruption** refers to separation at the edge of the placenta only, causing blood to flow from the vagina. **Concealed abruption** refers to separation of the central portion of the placenta while margins remain attached, so bleeding is concealed. **Complete abruption** refers to total separation of the placenta. These are all rare, particularly the last—and fortunately so, because abruption may prove fatal for the baby and sometimes for the mother. If abruption occurs during labor and delivery is imminent, the baby will probably survive and the mother will be fine. But if it occurs late in pregnancy or early in labor, even an emergency cesarean may not be quick enough to save the baby, and depending on the degree of abruption, the mother's life may also be in jeopardy.

Symptoms of abruption vary depending on degree. With concealed abruption, bleeding is not evident but there is acute abdominal pain, distinct from uterine contractions in its persistence and location. The uterus is woody hard and exceedingly tender to the touch. With marginal abruption, bright-red bleeding is apparent but abdominal pain may be less intense (and less noticeable in hard labor). In either case, the mother should be rushed to the hospital unless she is in labor and about to give birth. Administer oxygen and **treat** her for shock with feet elevated, head down, and body warmed with blankets.

Repeated episodes of light bleeding or heavy spotting with no report of abdominal pain may indicate **placenta previa,** that is, placenta implanted low in the uterus. It is believed that the blastocyst seeks unscarred tissue in which to imbed, thus most risk factors for this condition are associated with uterine scarring. They include (1) previous uterine surgeries (including more than three D+Cs), (2) endometritus (uterine infection) with a previous pregnancy, (3) multiparity, (4) pregnancies with short intervals between, and (5) maternal age over thirty-five. Placenta previa is also correlated to an unusually large placenta—for example, with a multiple pregnancy.

Why does blood loss occur with this condition? In late pregnancy, the lower uterine segment begins to distend and thin as the presenting part of the baby enters the pelvis and presses downward; if the placenta is imbedded in this area, small portions will detach wherever underlying uterine tissues stretch. There are varying degrees of placenta previa: **total previa,** in which the placenta completely covers the cervical os; **partial previa,** in which the os is partially covered; **marginal previa,** in which the edge of the placenta is at the edge of the os; and **low-lying placenta,** in which the placenta is close to the os but does not actually reach it.

Prospects for vaginal birth depend on the location of the placenta at the onset of labor. Total and partial previa necessitate cesarean delivery. A marginal previa will inevitably separate as the cervix dilates, and depending on the degree of maternal blood loss, may also require a cesarean. Vaginal delivery is more likely with a low-lying placenta, but maternal blood loss must be carefully monitored. Placenta previa is also associated with an increased risk of third-stage hemorrhage (see chapter 5) due to poor contractibility of the lower uterine segment.

Placenta previa may manifest as early as twenty-four weeks. If so, the placenta will appear to migrate upward as the lower uterine segment stretches downward with advancing pregnancy. I had one case like this in my practice; I could barely believe my client's bleeding was due to placenta previa because it occurred so early. The mother was put at bedrest for a number of weeks until an ultrasound showed the placenta to be out of the way, and she had a perfectly normal vaginal birth.

Diagnosis of placenta previa must always be done by ultrasound. As *Williams Obstetrics* admonishes, "Examination of the cervix is never permissible unless the woman is in the operating room with all the preparations for immediate cesarean section, since even the gentlest examination of this sort can cause torrential hemorrhage."[6] *Never, ever do a vaginal exam when there is bleeding in late pregnancy!* And have the mother suspend all sexual activity until a diagnosis is made.

GESTATIONAL DIABETES

This term for decreased glucose tolerance during pregnancy was coined in 1979, when blood glucose levels for pregnant women (as distinct from the general population) were first established. The validity of these levels remains controversial, as the study on which they were based included women at high risk and in poor health, as well as prediagnosed diabetics.[7] Subsequent studies utilized management protocols such as starvation diets, early induction, and withholding nourishment from the newborn.[8] The data do show a correlation between elevated blood glucose levels in pregnancy and the tendency to develop diabetes later in life, but no correlation to increased risk for the fetus or other prenatal/intrapartal complications.[9] (The purported correlation between high glucose levels in pregnancy and stillbirth was merely extrapolated from risks for babies of mothers with Type I or Type II diabetes).

The midwife's greatest concern is that if a mother in her care has an abnormally high glucose screen, conservative medical protocol may define this woman as high risk and no longer suitable for home birth, or, at best, will funnel her into a regimen of risk screening that may negatively affect her experience of pregnancy and ability to labor with confidence.

Because so many women are falsely diagnosed, it is difficult to estimate the incidence of true diabetes unmasked by pregnancy. Predisposing factors are family history of the disease, marked obesity, age over thirty-five, or previous delivery of a baby weighing nine pounds or more. **Macrosomia** (large baby) does in fact correlate to increased risks of prolonged labor, shoulder dystocia, and birth injury. Common sense dictates that women with any of the above risk factors should receive glucose screening, and the earlier, the better.

This is a moot point, though, as far as the medicine is concerned—the standard of care is to screen *every* woman at twenty-four to twenty-eight weeks. The test most commonly used is the **glucose challenge test (GCT),** for which the mother ingests 50 mg liquid glucose/orange pop, with a blood draw an hour later. As the liquid concoction is somewhat revolting, alternatives of apple juice (about three-quarters cup; the exact amount depends on the brand) or eighteen full-sized jelly beans may be used instead.[10] It is also recommended that the mother carbo-load for three days prior to the test, and that it be performed at twenty-four weeks, as insulin resistance continues to increase as pregnancy advances.

If her glucose level exceeds 140 mg/dl, the mother is referred for an **oral glucose tolerance test (OGTT).** For this, she should once again carbo-load for three days before the test. She must fast overnight and then have blood drawn to establish baseline glucose levels before ingesting 100 mg glucose. Blood draws are repeated at one, two, and three hours. During this time, she cannot eat but should exercise lightly, which may be challenging as many women suffer nausea, vomiting, headache, bloating, or profuse sweating in response to glucose syrup. Maximum sugar levels in whole blood are (1) fasting, above 90 mg/dl; (2) one

hour, above 165 mg/dl; (3) two hours, above 145 mg/dl; and (4) three hours, above 125 mg/dl. Note that both the GCT and the OGTT have extremely high false positive rates. Although the OGTT is considered the gold standard by most physicians, 75 percent of asymptomatic women with positive results never develop diabetes, rendering the test only 25 percent accurate.[11] If a woman in your practice chooses not to be screened, she will need to sign a waiver indicating her informed decision.

If backup is amenable, many midwives prefer to use the **fasting glucose screen.** This is done first thing in the morning without any special dietary preparation. Using a lancet to prick the mother's finger, measure her blood sugar levels with either a glucosometer or a Visidex testing strip; levels should not exceed 120.

If this test is positive, a **two-hour postprandial whole blood test** is preferable to the OGTT. The mother should eat a high-carb diet for three days prior to testing. She then fasts for twelve hours, after which a blood sample is drawn for a baseline. Next, she eats a high-carb meal, such as whole grain pancakes with butter and syrup, eggs or some kind of meat, and a large glass of orange juice, and her blood is drawn two hours later. Readings will be more accurate if she exercises lightly after eating. Normal levels are 120–40 mg/dl. If results are borderline, ask about her diet in the days preceding the test and also check to see if she has been under stress, as excess adrenaline blocks insulin. If there is any question, repeat the test in a few days.

What if the mother is truly diabetic? Because glucose readily crosses the placental barrier, elevated maternal blood sugar can cause a significant rise in the baby. The fetal pancreas reacts by greatly increasing production of insulin, which leads to an increase in growth. Besides complications associated with macrosomia, the baby may experience respiratory distress (production of surfactant in the lungs can be interrupted by increased levels of insulin). The mother has a four times greater chance of developing preeclampsia, ten times greater incidence of polyhydramnios, and a high risk of postpartum hemorrhage. The newborn may have severe problems with **hypoglycemia** (low blood sugar) or **hypocalcaemia** (low calcium levels) after the birth.

Treatment for diabetes in pregnancy depends on the degree. Nutrition is central—a diet high in protein and complex carbohydrates, with limited simple sugars, is strongly recommended. Regular, aerobic exercise is also encouraged. Monitoring of the fetus via nonstress testing and kick counts should begin no later than thirty-six weeks (see the section on "Postdatism" in this chapter for more information). In severe cases, insulin therapy is recommended and the woman will be risked out for home birth.

HYPERTENSION

Hypertension (high blood pressure) may manifest in several ways during pregnancy. **Essential hypertension** is a preexisting condition indicated by initial and subsequent readings of 140/90 or more. When high readings first occur in the latter part of pregnancy, we call the condition **gestational hypertension.** These two types can be hard to differentiate if a mother begins care in her last trimester and presents with hypertension. In this case, you must obtain records of previous care, either during the pregnancy or before. Home birth is contraindicated for women with essential hypertension and may be contraindicated with gestational hypertension, depending on the degree. *Note: I have deliberately avoided the use of the more common term for gestational hypertension—pregnancy-induced hypertension (PIH)—because in most texts it is synonymous with preeclampsia. Gestational hypertension, independent of other clinical signs of preeclampsia, can be considered low risk and may be treated by the midwife.*

Keep in mind that blood pressure fluctuates dramatically with emotional upheaval and tension. In *Holistic Midwifery (Volume I)*, Anne Frye mentions a study done by Kevin Dalton at Cambridge University, showing fluctuations as great as 40 points systolic and 22 points diastolic in ten-minute intervals.[12] Therefore, no conclusions should be drawn unless blood pressure is high on at least two occasions a full six hours apart. It helps to do repeat readings with the woman on her left side, as this position induces optimal circulation and is thought to render the greatest accuracy.

Severe and prolonged hypertension may cause intrauterine growth restriction, as the resulting vasoconstriction affects the flow of oxygen (and nutrients) to the baby. For the same reason, elevated blood pressure during labor can cause fetal distress. If readings rise to 160/100, medical intervention will be necessary to prevent severe vascular damage from occurring. Therefore, any woman showing a consistent rise in blood pressure during pregnancy, no matter how slight, should be treated to prevent the problem from progressing. Here are some suggestions:

1. **Exercise is critical** whenever blood pressure is just starting to rise, and as long as it is no more than moderately elevated. Exercise increases circulation and forces blood vessels to stretch and dilate, which reduces the pressure inside them. Most effective are aerobic activities such as brisk walking, hiking, or swimming. Have the mother start out slowly, depending on what she is used to. One midwife colleague advises all her clients to work up a sweat every day, as a preventive measure. If blood pressure goes above 140/90, rest takes precedence over conditioning. The mother should lie on her left side for extended periods to allow optimal uptake of oxygen.

2. **Deep relaxation** goes hand in hand with exercise. Women who live in a state of chronic tension may have little experience of complete release for days at a time, even while sleeping. Relaxation practice can help relieve tension in the voluntary muscles, which in turn reduces tension in the involuntary system. A calm state of being also contributes to emotional stability, which helps prevent overreaction to challenging situations.

3. **No stimulants whatsoever.** These include coffee, black tea, some carbonated beverages, chocolate, nicotine, and cocaine. The last two stimulants in particular have been proven to cause vasoconstriction and low birth weight. Strong spices like mustard, black pepper, ginger, and nutmeg should also be avoided.

4. **Good diet and healing herbs** help immensely when used in combination with the above measures. Improper eating and abnormal weight gain place stress on the system; encourage the mother to eat plenty of high-quality protein, whole grains, and lots of mineral-rich fresh fruits and vegetables. Watermelon, cucumber, parsley, and onion specifically reduce blood pressure, and garlic is a must. Contrary to popular opinion, salt is a necessary nutrient and should be used according to taste. (See Gail and Tom Brewer's excellent book, *What Every Pregnant Woman Should Know.*)

    Herbs like hops, skullcap, passionflower, hawthorn, and chamomile (listed in order of potency) can be used to induce relaxation; these are perfect for the mother with elevated systolic pressure who mostly needs to calm down. On the other hand, a woman with elevated diastolic pressure can benefit from cayenne pepper, which replicates the effects of aerobic exercise by causing vasodilation and stimulating the heart (take in capsules with meals). Chinese herbs and acupuncture may also be helpful. Increased fluids are crucial, as is increased intake of calcium, potassium, and magnesium. In a 1996 analysis of nearly 2,500 women, those who took 1,500 to 2,000 mg of calcium a day were 70 percent less likely to have hypertension in pregnancy than those who did not.[13] A subsequent study disputed these findings, but recent data indicate that calcium does in fact reduce the risk of hypertension in pregnancy.[14]

5. **Counseling** may be the first step if you are working with a woman so tense and distracted she can hardly take responsibility for herself. Assist her in getting to the roots of her anxiety, which may help her release tension and find new enjoyment in the pregnancy. If she is enabled to work through whatever is troubling her and can feel good about herself and her situation, attending to messages from her body will not seem so difficult or overwhelming.

I have seen two cases of gestational hypertension that bear repeating. In the first, the mother made immediate changes to her diet and began exercising daily. Relaxation was difficult for her as she had a very active work schedule that couldn't be altered. But she tried to moderate her activities with a more relaxed attitude and periodic meditation. In a matter of weeks, her blood pressure was down from a high of 150/86 to 120/70. Pride in this accomplishment motivated her to continue her new routine. Toward the end of pregnancy her blood pressure rose again to 136/80; she was experiencing much emotional tension on the job. She began to use relaxant herbs daily, and by her next visit her blood pressure was back to baseline. Throughout labor, it was steady at 120/70.

In the second case, the mother showed a rise in blood pressure at about thirty weeks to 130/86. We gave her suggestions on diet, relaxation, and exercise to nip the problem in the bud, but she was decidedly indifferent. Her diet was not the best: she ate a lot of red meat and refined foods, and was already thirty-five pounds overweight when pregnancy began. Her blood pressure was 140/90 at her next visit, and she grew angry and defiant in response to ideas of how she might lower it. A few days later, readings of 140/100 prompted us to recommend that she see a physician. At this, she burst into tears, releasing a flood of anger toward her partner for working too much and neglecting her needs. They asked for more time and went home seriously resolved to work on their situation. Two days later, her blood pressure was still 140/90 and continued to rise for the next few exams, so we referred her for hospital birth. She was given intravenous magnesium sulfate (standard treatment for hypertension) during labor and gave birth without further complications.

Occasionally you will have a mother who manifests a sudden rise in blood pressure just two or three weeks before term, with no other clinical problems. If she is well hydrated and not unduly stressed, this is probably a message that her body has reached its limit regarding circulatory volume, and the matter will resolve as soon as labor begins. If she is sure of her dates, her cervix is ripe (partly effaced), the baby is term (by size and recent growth pattern), and the head is well down in the pelvis, suggest acupuncture, herbs, or other nonpharmaceutical means to get labor going. When contractions begin, check frequently to see that her blood pressure is stable and within normal range.

It is not uncommon for previously normal blood pressure to jump as high as 140/90 with the most rigorous transition contractions. But a steady rise during labor may herald preeclampsia or lead to vascular damage, and the mother should be transported (see chapter 4 for more details).

PREECLAMPSIA

One of the main reasons for routine prenatal care is to screen for preeclampsia. The exact cause of preeclampsia may be subject to debate, but this dangerous disease poses a threat to the lives of both mother and baby. Generally occurring after twenty-six weeks, early signs include hemoconcentration, hypertension, generalized edema, sudden and excessive weight gain, and protein in the urine.

There is ample empirical evidence that preeclampsia directly results from protein deficiency and malnutrition. Inadequate albumin in the bloodstream causes fluid to leak from cells, resulting in reduced blood volume hemoconcentrations, and generalized edema. Blood flow to the kidneys is then reduced, which triggers a compensatory rise in blood pressure. Blood flow to the uterus is also reduced, leading to fetal growth restriction (and possible fetal distress in labor). If hypertension becomes severe, vasospasm and irritation of cell

walls cause microthrombi (tiny clots) to form. These microthrombi stretch the filtering slits in the kidneys so that large protein molecules begin to slip through, leading to proteinuria. Microthrombi can do significant harm to other parts of the body; they can impair circulation to the liver leading to epigastric pain and liver damage, or in severe cases, can lead to DIC as the body exhausts its clotting factors.

Nutritional guidelines for preventing preeclampsia include a minimum of 80 g protein daily, combined with ample calories, complex carbohydrates, as well as fresh fruits and vegetables. High-fiber foods are recommended, and adequate fluid intake is absolutely crucial.

Genetic research also indicates that a protein made by the placenta, sFlt1, may play a significant role in the disease. This protein halts growth and is normally released when the placenta reaches its full size. But evidence shows that in women who develop preeclampsia, this protein is made too soon, which stunts placental growth and reduces circulation to the baby. Interestingly enough, pregnant rats injected with sFlt1 develop preeclampsia. These findings may account for the occasional client who eats well, gets plenty of rest, and has good support but nonetheless develops the disease.[15]

Hemoconcentration may be the earliest indicator of preeclampsia, revealed by an abnormally high hematocrit indicating reduced blood volume. This is in sharp contrast to the usual dip in hematocrit readings with hemodilution at this stage of pregnancy. *Preeclampsia is diagnosed when hypertension and an additional sign (see below) are present on two occasions at least six hours apart.*

Check **for edema** by observing the mother's hands and face—her features will look coarse, the hands and fingers will be puffy and inflexible, and all rings will usually have been removed. Ankle edema is physiologic and therefore not significant, but edema of the upper shins, breastbone, or sacrum is definitive. Assess the degree of edema by checking for **pitting,** that is, press a fingertip into the skin and see whether or not a depression remains. The rating system is as follows: 2mm depression equals +1, 4mm equals +2, 6mm equals +3, and 8mm equals +4. Pitting of +2 or greater is a sign of preeclampsia.

When checking for **proteinuria,** the mother should take a clean catch to prevent vaginal discharge from affecting results. This is done by washing the labia with a towelette, and then allowing a bit of urine to flow before collecting the sample. Anything over a trace of protein is significant.

Hyperreflexia is a transitional sign, indicating that preeclampsia has progressed to a more serious stage. Check for hyperreflexia by checking for **clonus.** Have the mother sit in a straight-backed chair, lift and support her calf with one hand, then dorsiflex her foot (bend toes toward her knee). Maintain this hold for a moment, then release. Ordinarily the foot will fall back to its natural position with no extraneous movement; if you notice jerking while it is dorsiflexed, or oscillation as it falls, the test is positive. (It is wise to check all reflexes at some point in early pregnancy to establish baselines.)

The preeclamptic mother should immediately rest in bed on her left side, while the backup physician is contacted. If he or she is willing, you may be able to comanage care. The mother should be seen twice weekly and should be advised to report any of the following indications that her condition has worsened: (1) severe headache, (2) epigastric pain (pain in upper abdomen), (3) visual disturbances, (4) decreased output of urine, (5) extreme nervous irritability, or (6) decrease in fetal movement.

One of my clients became preeclamptic at thirty-seven weeks. I knew it as soon as she walked into my office; her face had that coarse look I had so often read about. We had made a home visit once in early pregnancy, at which time her diet was clearly excellent. However, just a week ago we had gone to her home again and had been served a vegetable dinner with no protein whatsoever. I was concerned and intended to bring it up at this visit but was obviously too late.

Remarkable in this case was the mother's blood pressure; it never went higher than 120/76. However, her baseline was 98/56, and some texts cite a diastolic rise of more than 15 points or systolic rise of more than 30 as indicative of hypertension. We referred her immediately to backup, and alternated visits twice weekly with her physician. Her condition remained borderline: periodic facial edema with blood pressure high but stationary, proteinuria from a trace to +2. She took bedrest as much as possible, and we transported as soon as labor was established.

What are the dangers of preeclampsia? As mentioned earlier, reduced uterine blood flow may lead to intrauterine growth restriction and fetal distress in labor. There is also a higher incidence of placental abruption (about 8 percent), which can lead to fetal death or jeopardize the mother's life. If preeclampsia progresses to eclampsia, convulsions in labor may threaten the lives of both mother and baby. A grim picture indeed, but not entirely hopeless if dietary changes are made at once and the mother is kept under close surveillance by her midwife and backup.

POLYHYDRAMNIOS/ HYDRAMNIOS

This is a term referring to excess amniotic fluid. It occurs in fewer than 1 percent of all pregnancies, often in conjunction with multiple pregnancy (8 percent), Rh incompatibility (11 percent), or diabetes (5–25 percent). It is also associated with fetal anomalies (18–39 percent), particularly with atresia of the esophagus, hydrocephaly, anencephaly, or spina bifida.[16]

Polyhydramnios may occur suddenly and acutely, but this is rare. It is more common to notice a slight elevation in fundal height around twenty-eight weeks, with a steady increase in the weeks that follow. This is called **chronic polyhydramnios.** Typically, there is difficulty palpating the baby at a time when it should be filling the uterus. It is possible to confuse a thick uterine wall with excess fluid; in both cases, heart tones will be difficult to hear and the baby, challenging to feel. Check for the classic sign of polyhydramnios, **fluid thrill,** by placing a hand on each side of the uterus, and if a tap from one sends a vibration to the other, the test is positive.

A woman with noticeable polyhydramnios should be seen again in several days regardless of gestation. If you find an additional increase in fluid, send her for an ultrasound to try to determine the cause. Polyhydramnios can lead to premature labor, thus hospital birth is likely unless the condition is borderline. It can also result in serious complications during labor, such as uterine dysfunction, placental abruption, and postpartum hemorrhage, all from overdistension of the uterus. Fetal malpresentation and cord prolapse are not uncommon.

I recall referring a mother for ultrasound whom I assessed to have a considerable degree of excess fluid, only to be told that everything was fine. Nonetheless, her fundal height was above normal from twenty-eight weeks, reaching 42 cm at term (with head in the pelvis). Early labor was characterized by spastic and painful incoordinate contractions. We transported, and imagine my frustration when membranes ruptured in a quantity sufficient to bring the entire labor and delivery staff to have a look! At this point, the uterus began to work more efficiently, and labor progressed normally. However, the mother sustained a fairly severe postpartum hemorrhage.

Another mother developed polyhydramnios before I had any idea she was carrying twins. The extra fluid really alarmed me; her fundal height at twenty-five weeks was 29 cm—a rise of 6 cm in just three weeks, with an accompanying weight gain of eight pounds. In less than a week, her fundal height increased three more centimeters, she gained three more pounds and was almost impossible to palpate. I made no mention of twins, but she brought up the possibility. Sure enough, ultrasound showed two babies, plus extra fluid within normal range for multiple pregnancy. Two weeks later

she went into labor, and no wonder, with a fundal height of 39 cm at only twenty-eight weeks!

Adequate rest (feet elevated) can help mediate common side effects of polyhydramnios, such as severe ankle edema and varicosities of the legs and vulva. Heartburn remedies, such as smaller meals and digestive enzymes, are essential. If you are comanaging the care of a woman with polyhydramnios, check her cervix weekly to look for changes that might portend premature labor.

OLIGOHYDRAMNIOS

Oligohydramnios is an abnormally small amount of amniotic fluid. It is associated with a marked increase in fetal mortality, due to underlying conditions such as intrauterine growth restriction, postmaturity syndrome, and congenital anomalies. Reduced amniotic fluid renders the fetus susceptible to cord compression and fetal distress/hypoxia during labor. Although amniotic fluid volume varies considerably from mother to mother, oligohydramnios is readily detected when the fetus is tightly compacted in the uterus and fundal height is lagging. Continuity of care enables the midwife to notice small fluctuations in amniotic fluid volume without having to resort to serial ultrasound.

Studies have shown that amniotic fluid can be increased by adequate hydration: the more fluid the mother drinks, the more amniotic fluid she produces.[17] However, as oligohydramnios rarely occurs in the course of a healthy pregnancy, consider it a sign of something amiss that must quickly be identified. (See the sections on "Small for Gestational Age and Intrauterine Growth Restriction" and "Postdatism" later in this chapter.)

MULTIPLE PREGNANCY

A fundal measurement greater than gestational age in weeks should immediately lead you to consider twins. But first, rule out other possible causes of a uterus large for dates (see the section on "Large Gestational Age" later in this chapter). Consider your clinical findings: Have you noticed an abundance of small parts when palpating? Does the head feel somewhat small relative to fundal height? Twins are sometimes missed if one is tucked behind the other's body.

Unless a woman has had serial ultrasounds, twins are not usually detected until twenty-eight to thirty weeks, with clinical confirmation through the auscultation of two heartbeats. But take care—what appears to be two heartbeats may be just one, audible over a wide range. If you note a ten to fifteen point difference in rhythms with distinct patterns of variability, you have almost certainly identified twins. When in doubt, schedule an ultrasound.

There are two types of twinning. **Identical, or monozygotic,** twins result from the union of one egg, one sperm, with the fertilized ovum separating into two. **Fraternal, or dizygotic,** twins represent two eggs, two sperm, thus two separate pregnancies occurring simultaneously. Dizygotic twins have separate placentas and separate amniotic sacs, whereas monozygotic twins share a placenta and may also share an amniotic sac, although usually there are two separate sacs. Sixty-six to 75 percent of twins are dizygotic. Monozygotic twins occur at a rate of approximately 1 per 250 births, whereas dizygotic twinning varies dramatically according to maternal race and age. With in vitro fertilization or embryo transfer, the rate of multiple pregnancy is as high as 22 percent.[18]

Although these stats are relatively up-to-date, the past few years of routine serial ultrasound have shown twinning to be even more common. I know of several women who, at about twelve weeks, had such heavy bleeding that they were sure they had lost the pregnancy, only to find they were still pregnant. Twins were diagnosed only after one was lost.

It is important to identify twins as soon as suspected, as there are increased risks in pregnancy for mother and babies. Anemia is common with twin preg-

nancy, and the incidence of premature birth is greatly increased (guidelines for recognizing and reporting signs of premature labor should be immediately provided). Mothers with twins need expert nutritional counseling, and recommendations for moderating daily activity with adequate rest (feet up for twenty minutes, twice a day). Rarely, **twin to twin transfusion syndrome (TTTS)** (identical twins only) will cause blood to be shunted from one twin to the other, putting the "donor" baby at risk for growth restriction and other complications.

The risks with twin birth are numerous. Cord prolapse can occur if the first baby is footling or kneeling breech. The second baby is at even greater risk, especially if it remains high in the uterus after the first has been born. It may also become hypoxic, as reduced uterine volume can cause constriction of placental vessels. For the same reason, there is risk of placental abruption. Finally, there is considerable risk of postpartum hemorrhage from an overdistended and tired uterus.

In the area where I practice, assisting twins at home is out of the question. However, I have diagnosed twins a number of times and have continued to provide prenatal care in conjunction with a physician (including catching babies in the hospital). Even if the midwife is no longer the primary provider, she can still provide critical assistance by focusing on the emotional and practical aspects of caring for two babies. And, if the mother is helped to maintain her pregnancy to at least thirty-seven weeks, hospital management may be relatively noninterventive. That is—if vaginal birth is permitted. Increasingly, physicians insist that all twins be delivered by cesarean. Some still assist vaginal twin births, but usually both babies must be vertex. This trend is due to fear of malpractice litigation, lack of exposure to vaginal twin births, and lack of training in vaginal breech birth. Beyond the skills and the inclination of the physician, much depends on hospital policy. For myself, having witnessed many vaginal twin births before the standard changed (a number of them

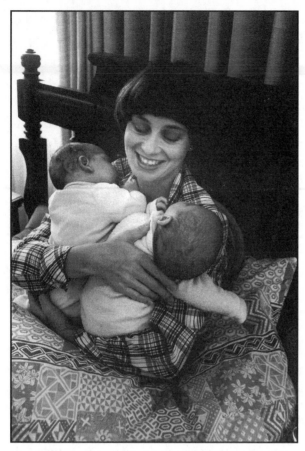

Twice the work, but twice the joy and fulfillment.

breech, and all spontaneous and uncomplicated), I find it outrageous that women are being funneled into cesarean birth without a choice, regardless of their health status.

On one occasion, I seriously considered assisting twins at home. The mother was in excellent health, sensitive and cooperative, her partner was fully supportive, and both babies were head down. Amniotic fluid was within normal range, and she was at 37 weeks. We jointly considered her situation. My hesitation was mostly political; if transport became necessary, I knew I could lose my backup. And because she too had fears, she opted for vaginal birth in the hospital. Had her only option been cesarean, she might have felt differently—and I might have assisted her at home.

If the birth will be in hospital, be certain the mother and her partner know what to expect from the experience. Even if the birth is to be vaginal, there will be many attendants besides the obstetrician, including the full neonatal team. Emphasize the emotional aspects of the experience, and the support you will provide before, during, and after.

BREECH PRESENTATION AND TRANSVERSE LIE

Because of the backup situation in my area, I have not been free to assist breech births at home. If I had a choice, I would do so (but very selectively). It is more than unfortunate that we treat breech birth as a life-threatening complication simply because medical schools have stopped teaching physicians the skills to assist breech vaginally.

The greatest risk with breech birth is cephalopelvic disproportion (CPD). In vertex positions, the head has hours to negotiate the pelvis, but in breech positions, it must be born quickly as exposure of the body and cord to air prompts respiration. In other words, if the body is born but the head proves too large for the pelvis and is stuck behind the brim, fetal hypoxia and death will likely result. Cord prolapse is another risk, particularly with footling or kneeling presentations, as there is nothing to prevent the cord from slipping past the body when the water breaks.

What are wise criteria for breech birth at home? The mother should have an ample gynecoid pelvis and an average-sized baby. If she has already given birth without a problem, the risks diminish. However, the baby should either be frank breech (legs extended up over the chest) or complete breech (legs crossed over the abdomen), in either anterior or transverse position, and with head well flexed so it can readily negotiate the pelvis. In order to make certain of these factors, ultrasound must be used.

Even so, complications may arise that require special expertise. An arm impacted behind the head must be deftly and quickly manipulated; a head deflexed during labor must be repositioned without delay. These maneuvers are beyond the scope of this text. Suffice to say, it is not advisable to attend breech birth without the assistance of someone experienced in both basic and advanced midwifery techniques (including neonatal resuscitation).

Before presenting breech, the baby may assume a **transverse lie.** This is common up to twenty-six weeks, at which point the baby generally finds greater comfort in lying longitudinally. If the baby remains transverse after twenty-seven weeks and is high in the uterus, listen in the lower portion of the mother's abdomen for placenta sounds (swishing sounds at the same rate as the mother's pulse). Do this to rule out placental previa, which could be preventing the baby from presenting either breech or vertex. If the baby remains transverse past thirty weeks, an ultrasound is necessary to locate the placenta precisely.

Rarely, the breech rotates to vertex in the final weeks of pregnancy or right before labor. Rather than wait and see, have the mother try to turn the baby with **postural tilting** if it remains breech beyond thirty weeks. To do this, she must empty her bladder and lie down comfortably, hips elevated about twelve inches on pillows, three times daily for twenty minutes. Suggest she do deep relaxation while in this position, and visualize the baby turning while asking it to do so. If she feels major movement, have her come in right away to be checked.

Other ways she can encourage the baby to turn include:

1. Doing somersaults or handstands in a pool.

2. Doing elephant walking (on her hands and feet).

3. Placing headphones low on the uterus and playing music (baby may turn toward the sound).

4. Shining a flashlight low in the uterus or between her legs (baby may turn toward the light).

5. Placing a bag of frozen vegetables on the backside of the baby's head (baby may turn away from the cold).

6. Partner talking to baby low on her belly, asking the baby to turn.

Another possibility is to use the **rebozo** to turn the baby. A rebozo is a long shawl used by midwives in Mexico for numerous remedial purposes throughout the childbearing cycle. To rotate a breech, the mother should be on knees and elbows with swayed back (belly sagging toward the floor). Place the center of the rebozo where her buttocks meet her thighs, and then stand at her head with one end in each hand pulled taught. Pull firmly on one end and then the other to establish a brisk, rocking motion: 1, 2, 3, 4, 5 (pause) 1, 2, 3, 4, 5 (pause) and so forth, for several minutes. Repeat daily.[19]

If the baby has not rotated after several weeks and is beginning to feel rather snugly encased, **external version** is another option. This is a tricky maneuver for all but the most experienced midwife, as it requires great expertise in fetal palpation and a highly refined sense of touch. There is also some risk of cord entanglement or compression, so the fetal heart must be monitored continuously by another experienced practitioner.

Have the mother drink a beer or glass of wine to promote uterine relaxation, and make sure her bladder is empty before you begin. Position her in a tilt, and then *gently* attempt to reposition the baby. Be sure to keep the head flexed, and rotate the baby in the direction it is facing. If any resistance is felt or changes in the fetal heart rate are noted, the version should be stopped and the baby returned to its original position. Because of the risks involved in this procedure, informed consent is essential and must be added to the chart.

Some mothers report massaging their babies into vertex position all by themselves. But if, despite all efforts, the baby has not rotated by thirty-six weeks, you might ask your backup physician to give version a try. Most physicians wait until thirty-seven weeks to perform external version, for fear of causing premature labor. However, they generally employ a much more forceful technique than do midwives, due to the use of terbutaline or other uterine tocolytic (relaxant) in conjunction with the procedure. If all attempts at version fail, prepare the mother for hospital birth and most likely a cesarean. (Refer also to "Surprise Breech" in chapter 5.)

PREMATURITY

The medical standard of care defines prematurity as birth prior to thirty-seven weeks, although this limit is somewhat arbitrary. The chief concern is that the baby's lungs may not be mature, yet the lungs are almost always mature by thirty-four weeks. The thirty-seven-week cutoff simply includes a margin of error in calculating the EDD.

If the baby's lungs are not fully developed, it will struggle to get enough oxygen and **respiratory distress syndrome (RDS)** will result. Signs of RDS include **cyanosis** (blue color), **tachypnea** (rapid respirations), **grunting** (with expiration), **retractions** (skin between the ribs sucks in each time baby inhales), and **nasal flaring.** These signs are caused by inadequate **surfactant,** a lubricant that permits the alveoli to inflate.

Causes of preterm labor include vaginal or urinary tract infection leading to chorioamnionitis and premature rupture of the membranes, incompetent cervix, polyhydramnios, multiple pregnancy, uterine anomalies, faulty implantation of the placenta, substance abuse, short interval between pregnancies, malnutrition, fetal death, and extreme or chronic stress. The latter is little acknowledged in the literature, but there is evidence that maternal stress may cause up to one-third of premature births by activating the fetal hypothalamic-pituitary-adrenal axis.[20] There is also an association between preterm birth and stressful working conditions, such as those involving prolonged standing or strenuous physical activity.[21] Mothers with chronic gum disease in the second trimester are at three to eight times greater risk, due to an increase in prostaglandins.[22] Maternal dehydration can also lead to prematurity.[23]

Any mother with a history of miscarriage or previous premature birth is automatically at risk. Make sure she is well hydrated, and that her diet is excellent. She should eat fatty fish—for example, salmon, mackerel, sardines, or trout—once weekly, or take a supplement of fish oil daily, as women who do so have only a 1.9 percent prematurity rate as compared with 7.1 percent for women who don't.[24] Monitor her carefully from twenty-four weeks on; schedule visits every two weeks, and perform gentle cervical examination each time. Suggest that she reduce her workload, both in and out of the home. Screen at the first sign of vaginal infection, and recommend the use of condoms (if applicable) to reduce the risks of sexually transmitted diseases and exposure to prostaglandins in seminal fluid that can soften the cervix. If her cervix begins to efface, have her curtail sexual activity, make sure she knows how to distinguish contractions from fetal movement, and see her weekly thereafter. If regular contractions occur or the cervix begins to dilate, immediately contact a physician.

Medications commonly used for stopping labor include magnesium sulfate, ritodrine, and terbutaline; these generally do the job but cause nervous irritability and nausea. They are also quite toxic and should be used no more than several days. If you find the cervix only minimally changed, contractions are mild, and the mother has no history of alcoholism, suggest she take a couple of stiff drinks. Alcohol inhibits oxytocin and relaxes the uterus. (Before labor-stopping, tocolytic drugs were developed, alcohol was given intravenously for premature labor.)

One of my clients began premature labor at thirty-five weeks. Her cervix was quite effaced and about 2 cm dilated (this was her second baby). She took two shots of vodka in grapefruit juice, stayed in bed, and was fine until the following morning. Her contractions resumed upon arising, so she repeated the previous routine. This went on for almost a week, during which I checked her daily and in spite of regular uterine activity, found her cervix to be stable. Contractions then stopped completely. She carried her baby to forty-one weeks and birthed at home, but not without some difficulty. Severe shoulder dystocia, partial separation of the placenta necessitating manual removal, and postpartum hemorrhage made for an interesting trade-off of complications.

Another of my clients carrying twins had a fundal height of 38 cm at thirty weeks, with slight polyhydramnios. She began premature labor and was given ritodrine, which did little to stop her contractions. However, as a student of yoga, she discovered that postural tilting several times daily definitely stopped uterine activity, probably by taking pressure off her cervix. The obstetrician was so impressed that he called in the staff to observe her innovation. Ritodrine was discontinued, and she carried her babies to term.

If a mother in your care gives birth prematurely, she may have to deal with long periods of separation from her baby and disrupted breastfeeding, although much depends on the gestational age of the baby and hospital policy. Fortunately, a number of intensive care nurseries now incorporate the practice of **kangaroo care** in stabilizing the premature infant. Much as it sounds, kangaroo care involves continuous skin-to-skin contact—the baby wears only a diaper and is held between the mother's breasts with a blanket or a sling. Developed by doctors in South America, where intensive care facilities were not adequate to treat a growing number of premies, kangaroo care reduced infant mortality from 70 to 30 percent.[25] It has been shown to stabilize the newborn's heart rate, temperature, and breathing, as well as boosting growth and brain development. Mothers who use kangaroo care report increased confidence, better postpartum recovery, and greater success with breastfeeding. The mother's partner is encouraged to participate too.

Do all you can to prevent premature labor, but learn all you can about support organizations for parents with premies. And know that apart from worries about the baby, the mother may grieve the loss of her home birth dream and have no one else with whom to process this loss but you.

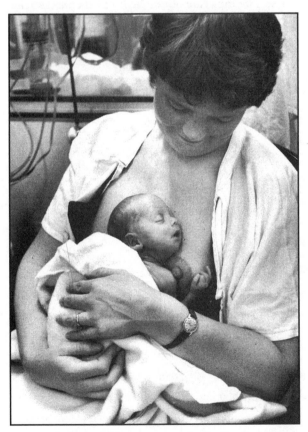

When a baby needs intensive care, the family must be creative as well as assertive in finding ways to stay close to the baby.

SMALL FOR GESTATIONAL AGE AND INTRAUTERINE GROWTH RESTRICTION

With regard to uterine size, causes of **small for gestational age (SGA)** include miscalculated dates, fetus transverse or low-lying, hereditary predisposition to small babies, and **intrauterine growth restriction (IUGR)**. The first three are fairly easy to rule out, but the last is a complication requiring special attention.

Although babies grow in spurts, normal growth results in an average fundal height increase of about one centimeter per week. IUGR is suspected when fundal height has been normal to twenty-four weeks and then begins to fall behind this average. We can differentiate the baby genetically destined to weigh six pounds and one truly growth restricted in that the former will have consistent, but slightly less than normal increments of growth, whereas the latter will have *steadily decreasing increments of growth*. In other words, with IUGR the growth curve flattens out.

The causes of IUGR are numerous, including malnutrition, anemia, chronic hypertension, substance abuse, fetal malformation or infection, abnormalities of the placenta and cord, and prolonged pregnancy. Chronic stress and overwork are also implicated: an analysis of studies involving 160,988 women showed that neonates born to women who work at physically demanding jobs weigh less at birth.[26]

Here is an interesting case history. This mother started care at twenty-seven weeks with a fundal height of 23 cm, certain of her dates. Her nutrition was poor and she smoked half a pack of cigarettes daily, but she made a commitment to improve her diet and cut back her intake of nicotine. Her baby began to grow in spurts over the next few weeks, and steadily thereafter. Total maternal weight gain was about twenty pounds. Ultrasounds at thirty-one and thirty-five weeks determined a normal rate of fetal growth, but a baby so small for gestational age that a month was added to the EDD. This seemed arbitrary to say the least, considering that neither the menstrual history nor the couple's sexual history corroborated this. Nevertheless, if "sonogram says," we had best believe it!

Her final checkup revealed her cervix to be slightly dilated and 60 percent effaced. At thirty-eight weeks by original dates, thirty-four weeks by revised EDD, labor commenced with ruptured membranes. What to do? Was the baby premature, or simply small for gestational age? And what about the impact of earlier IUGR? We estimated the baby to be about five pounds and so decided on hospital birth. This was a real disappointment to the parents, who had never accepted the revised dates anyway. After six hours of labor, the mother gave birth to a healthy, vigorous girl

of five pounds, estimated to be about thirty-eight weeks gestational age. No respiratory distress; the lungs were fully mature. There was some indication of fetal compromise in that the placenta was spongy, shredding, and full of calcifications. But the baby showed no other signs of growth restriction; it was neither wizened or emaciated, and had Apgars of 9/10.

In retrospect, this birth could have taken place at home. But if a baby is SGA, and care begins later in pregnancy when accuracy of dates is more difficult to determine, hospital birth is more or less by default. Premature babies face significant risks at delivery, whereas complications linked to a minor degree of IUGR are more easily managed until a pediatrician is contacted. These include **hypoglycemia** (low blood sugar) and **hypothermia** (difficulty maintaining body temperature), both of which are due to insufficient body fat. These conditions are not immediately life threatening and can be dealt with initially by the midwife; still, it is wise to have the baby seen by a pediatrician within the first few hours after the birth.

If significant IUGR persists throughout pregnancy despite every attempt to remedy the situation, hospital birth is advisable. Even with minor degrees of IUGR, it is wise to do nonstress testing, assess amniotic fluid volume, and have the mother start fetal kick-counts at thirty-four weeks (for more on these procedures, see section on "Postdatism" in this chapter), because some studies show a correlation between IUGR and stillbirth.

If you are preparing to assist the birth of a small baby who has grown well in the latter part of pregnancy and whom you believe to be term, have oven-warmed flannel blankets and an aluminum outer wrapper (space blanket) ready as insulation. Place the baby skin-to-skin on the mother's body, then wrap in three flannels with aluminum blanket over all. It is crucial to keep the head covered at all times; use a stockinet cap so that the mother will not have to fuss with the blankets and instead can focus fully on the baby. Take the baby's axillary temperature several times an hour until you are certain it has stabilized. Also check the baby's blood sugar level by doing a **dextrostix** (heel prick with test strip). If the level is below 45, contact the pediatrician at once. If it is just slightly below normal, encourage the mother to nurse, and afterward give eyedroppersful of sterile water and molasses, one teaspoon per cup (never use honey, due to risk of infant botulism). Repeat the dextrostix every two hours to assess whether feedings are raising the blood sugar level. Be sure to chart each time fluid is given, how much, and how well the baby tolerated it. If the baby vomits, intravenous feeding may be necessary, so contact the pediatrician without delay.

Even a minor degree of IUGR puts the baby at risk for **polycythemia** (an excess of red blood cells), which predisposes to severe jaundice. If the baby looks ruddy at birth, do a hematocrit, and if elevated, immediately consult the pediatrician. Once the baby is fully stable, make certain that parents understand how critical it is to keep the baby warm and dry, and to call you immediately if the baby gets irritable or lethargic. Ask them to report back after seeing the pediatrician, and plan to do postpartum checks daily for the first four days, minimum.

LARGE FOR GESTATIONAL AGE

Causes of large for gestational age (LGA) have already been presented in other sections of this chapter; they include miscalculated dates, hydatidiform mole, gestational diabetes, twins, polyhydramnios, maternal obesity, hereditary predisposition for big babies, fetal anomalies, baby high in fundus due to placenta previa or abdominal muscle tone, fibroids (internal or external) displacing the baby upward or positioned atop the fundus, and postmaturity.

Whenever a mother measures large for dates, each of these possibilities must be considered and ruled out. I recall a woman who came to me at twenty-eight weeks with fundal height of 32 cm, wide abdominal girth (but not overweight), and +4 glucose in her urine. On palpating her I felt a good-sized head entering the pelvis, butt in the fundus, and small parts everywhere (posterior position, I assumed). I sent her immediately for a glucose screen, and it was negative. Next week, there was no glucosuria but two heartbeats were audible; a sonogram soon confirmed that she had twins!

A big baby is of concern only if the mother's pelvis is not ample. To assuage this fear, check for engagement, assessing not only the station of the head but how well it fits into the pelvis. If the baby is still high, **check for ability to engage** by grasping the head externally and pressing it toward the sacral promontory, then down into the inlet. If the head feels movable and enters the pelvis readily, things are fine so far. Another way to check is to place your hand above the pubic bone with the mom in a semi-sit position, and then have her sit up completely. If the head bulges into your hand instead of slipping into the pelvis, it will have difficulty clearing the inlet.

I have had only one obvious case of cephalopelvic disproportion (CPD) in my practice. This was a first pregnancy, the mother was certain of her menstrual history but the baby was consistently large for dates. She had a small pelvis with adequate inlet, but android characteristics of close-set ischial spines and a slightly flattened sacrum. She was about 5 feet 3 inches tall, and the father, 6 feet tall. I remember feeling alarmed at 37 weeks by the size of the baby's head, particularly in that it overrode the pubic bone and bulged into my hand. Upon discovering this condition of **fetal overlap**, I encouraged her to give birth as soon as she was ready (her cervix was soft, about 60 percent effaced). She started labor at 40 weeks, dilated completely (with the help of pitocin—we transported for arrest at 6 cm) but pushed for two hours without the head engaging and ended up with a cesarean. Her dates proved correct, as the baby showed no evidence of postmaturity— he simply grew too large for her pelvic dimensions.

If a similar situation arose again where we were certain of dates, I might suggest home-based induction as early as thirty-seven weeks. Successful induction largely depends on the condition of the cervix—it must be ripe (soft and partially effaced) before attempting to stimulate contractions. If the mother's partner is male, sexual intercourse can ripen the cervix via prostaglandins in seminal fluid (and may also stimulate contractions via the release of oxytocin). An alternative is cervical massage with evening primrose oil. The tried-and-true method of **castor oil induction** is hardly pleasant, but the resulting diarrhea triggers the release of prostaglandins. Have the mother take two tablespoons initially with orange juice, followed by another tablespoon a half hour later, and a final tablespoon in another hour.

Ways to get (or keep) contractions going include acupuncture techniques, herbal formulas (blue cohosh tincture, a dropperful every few hours), and periodic nipple stimulation. Or have the mother wear one of her partner's shirts (saturated with his or her scent) to get the oxytocin flowing.

There are certain risks attendant to LGA deliveries. The uterus is typically overdistended and less able to contract efficiently, resulting in prolonged labor, arrested progress, or postpartum hemorrhage. If the mother becomes clinically exhausted, the baby is at risk for hypoxia and may require resuscitation at birth. There may also be shoulder dystocia. Be prepared for these possibilities.

POSTDATISM

The standard definition of postdatism is pregnancy progressing past forty-two weeks (based on Naegele's Rule). However, it is estimated that up to 19 percent of pregnancies reach this marker.[27] This is hardly surprising, considering the findings of the Mittendorf study (see page 21).

Sometimes there is hereditary predisposition for longer-term pregnancy—for example, the mother reports that she herself was born three weeks late, as were all her siblings. Commonly, there is no obvious physical cause. Perhaps some babies simply need to gestate longer than others—the fruit on our trees doesn't ripen at exactly the same rate, so why should our babies?

Occasionally, emotional factors may cause a mother to go beyond term. Perhaps this is to be her last pregnancy, and she is hesitant to give it up. If this is her first baby, she may be wary of the responsibilities of parenting and loathe to surrender the special attention she has enjoyed while pregnant. Or, if she has been obliged or otherwise compelled to work until her due date, she may take extra time to enjoy being pregnant and wind down in preparation for labor. If her partner has uncertainty about his or her changing role, this too can prolong pregnancy. When exploring these possibilities (which can be done simply by asking the mother if she feels ready to give birth), make sure she does not feel judged or accused, as this may exacerbate any tension she is already feeling. Encourage her to make her own observations, draw her own conclusions. Such a difficult time, these postdate weeks of waiting!

The risks of postdatism are twofold. If all is well in utero and the fetus continues to grow, cephalopelvic disproportion or shoulder dystocia may result. If, on the other hand, the mother ceases to eat and drink sufficiently (perhaps for fear of having a large baby), the fetus may suffer weight loss, cord compression due to oligohydramnios, fetal distress, or even stillbirth. We used to think these risks were linked to the condition of the placenta, that it was a "timed organ" set to expire with advanced gestation, but research has shown this not to be true. We do know that maternal malnutrition and chronic dehydration can lead to reduced blood volume and oligohydramnios, which in turn can cause cord compression and fetal compromise. This is known as **fetal postmaturity syndrome.**

But if a mother is simply postdates, and is well nourished, well hydrated, well rested, and (based on pelvimetry and estimated fetal weight) has plenty of room to birth her baby, why is there cause for concern? According to the classic text, *Human Labor and Birth:* "While prolongation of pregnancy beyond 42 weeks may have an adverse effect on neonatal outcome in some cases, fetal death is rare. Induction of labor does not improve results. What the latter practice does achieve is an increase in the rate of cesarean section because of failed induction. An uncomplicated postdates pregnancy is not an indication for induction of labor. Early delivery is necessary only when tests of fetal health show that deterioration is taking place."[28]

There are several assessments that help determine fetal well-being in the postdates period. Have the mother do **fetal kick-counts** every day for an hour after her largest meal: she should notice about eight to ten movements in this time period. (Although routine for postdate pregnancies, some practitioners recommend that all women begin counting fetal movements at least once daily from thirty-four weeks on.)

Another common assessment of fetal well-being is **nonstress testing (NST),** which evaluates fluctuations in the baby's heart rate in response to its own movements. The desired or positive response is moderate acceleration. The NST can be performed in hospital by external monitor, or the midwife can simply listen with her fetascope for twenty minutes and look for heart rate changes with fetal activity. In recent years, the validity of the NST has been called into question as no definitive correlation has been shown between negative findings with this test and fetal outcome; nevertheless, it remains standard of care for postdatism.

Reduced **amniotic fluid volume** is much more significant. This can be assessed by serial ultrasound commencing at forty-one weeks, or by careful uterine palpation performed week to week by the same care provider. Assessment of amniotic fluid volume in combination with nonstress testing has less than a 15 percent margin of error—the two taken together

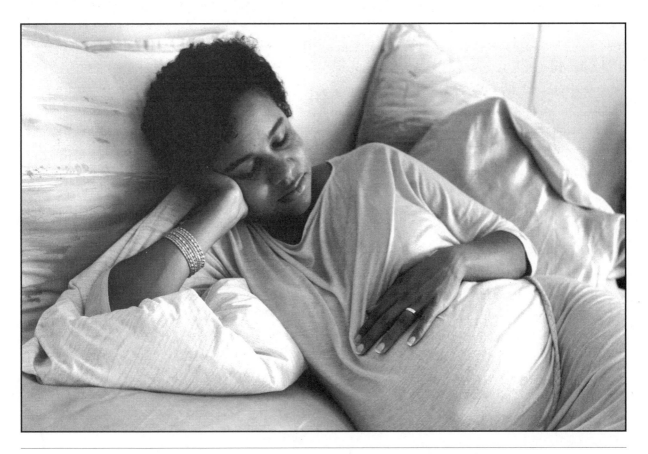

dramatically reduce the chance of being either falsely reassured or unnecessarily alarmed by individual results of these procedures.[29]

Current medical protocol for postdatism combines the aforementioned assessments with a few more obtained by ultrasound. Fetal muscle tone and breathing movements are evaluated and are combined with NST results, fetal movement counts, and amniotic fluid volume assessment to form the **biophysical profile (BPP).** With a scoring method similar to the Apgar system, zero to two points are given for the five categories cited above, with ten the highest possible score. A total score of less than seven is considered an indication for induction. BPP screening generally begins at forty-one weeks and is performed twice weekly.

Can the midwife's assessments as cited earlier provide enough information to substitute for the biophysical profile? In my opinion, the answer is yes. Although fetal breathing movements cannot be assessed directly, these may be presumed to be adequate on the basis of normal muscle tone, as demonstrated by kick-counts. NST is readily accomplished with a standard fetascope. And to reiterate, even the subtlest changes in amniotic fluid volume are easily noted with continuity of care.

Depending on the results of your assessments, consult with backup, leave well enough alone, or, assuming the head is well into the pelvis, recommend home-based induction (see the previous section, "Large for Gestational Age"). Induction might also be wise if the baby is getting a bit large for the mother's dimensions. Check carefully for fetal overlap, and beware of the previously engaged head rising up in the pelvis.

For the truly postmature fetus, the most stressful time in labor is the onset. Uterine contractions are much stronger than are Braxton-Hicks, thus any degree of fetal compromise will show up almost immediately. Plan to attend the postdates labor from the very beginning, and take heart tones more frequently than usual.

Psychological Issues and Complications

The vast majority of emotional upsets in pregnancy result from hormonal changes: complaints forgotten by the next visit are typically hormone induced. If emotional problems become chronic, ask for more background. You may uncover issues in the mother's relationships, environment, or health unknown to you before. Rarely, a client becomes increasingly imbalanced as pregnancy progresses, and you may find yourself unable to continue primary care (see "Psychological Screening Out," at the end of this chapter).

On the other hand, midwives know that pregnancy is a tempestuous time and encourage mothers to use the volatile energy of this period to take personal inventory and forge new modes of self-expression. After many years of practice, I have come to believe that the best way to promote a pregnant woman's well-being is to help her see weak or neglected aspects of herself in a positive light, so she will feel good about doing some work in these areas. Self-reliance and self-love are the cornerstones of wellness in pregnancy, birth, and parenting.

If some aspect of ourselves is weak or neglected, another is probably overstrong in compensation. For example, a mother who is extremely physical in nature may become anxious over normal changes as pregnancy ensues. If highly athletic—for example, used to competitive sports or marathon running—she may find fatigue, nausea, and loss of muscle tone to be extremely frustrating, even frightening. She runs the risk of pushing past physical imperatives for rest and relaxation and is therefore more susceptible to infection, hypertension, and premature labor.

I had one such client, a black belt in karate and a marathon runner, who broke down and cried at about twelve weeks, "My body just doesn't work anymore!" I explained that her body was actually working hard, making critical adjustments in metabolic rate and circulatory volume. I reassured her that her fatigue would abate, and that the softening of her muscles and ligaments would make the birth and her recovery easier. I encouraged her to trust her body's wisdom and intelligence in adapting to pregnancy and growing the baby. I suggested that she hold on to her strength, but experiment with pacing herself. She went on to enjoy her pregnancy. In labor, she found the dilation phase to be challenging, but really reached a peak with pushing. Afterward, she viewed the entire experience as positive and became a fiercely proud mother.

A more emotionally based woman will usually savor the changes of early pregnancy, particularly the dreamy quality of her heightened sensitivities. She may drive her partner a little crazy with her mood swings and forget to eat or get regular physical activity. She is at risk for anemia, dehydration, and prolonged labor. Encourage her to read for factual information, and help her develop a nutrition and exercise plan. She might also keep a diary, in which she can make observations on how changes in diet and activity affect her feelings. In labor, emotionally oriented women tend to dilate without much trouble, but may dislike the intensity of pushing. Help mothers who are somewhat ethereal in nature prepare for the physicality of second stage with activities requiring endurance, such as aerobic dance, hiking, lap swimming, and so on.

The mentally oriented woman generally chooses the particulars of her birth plan methodically. She is extremely well read and tends to practice what she has learned regarding diet and exercise, but may repress her emotions. If you ask her how she is feeling, she will probably answer with just a word or two, "Fine" or "I'm okay." (In contrast, an emotionally based woman can talk for twenty minutes on every nuance of her sentiments.) Massage or other bodywork can help her find both physical and emotional release. Nevertheless, it may be difficult to forge a close connection with the self-contained intellectual woman until labor. She is at risk for hypertension, postdatism, and postpartum depression.

I had one such client whose mother arrived a few days before her due date. Days and then weeks went by, and the expectant mother continued to report that her relationship with Mom was "just great." The day after her mother left, she went into labor. True to her mental nature, she labored with remarkable control; she didn't want to be touched or assisted by anyone (including her husband). Caring for the baby was her biggest challenge; she kept trying to get him on a schedule.

Few women are as extreme as these examples. But many women have one aspect of themselves (whether physical, emotional, or mental) noticeably less developed than the others. If you can help a mother identify and activate this latent part of herself, she can find skills for birthing and parenting that otherwise might not have occurred to her.

Expectant mothers may also benefit from awareness of the four elements that comprise our physical nature and all existence: earth, air, fire, and water. Midwife Verena Schmid has devised a method of prenatal care and therapy in which mothers experiment with movement that expresses each of these elements, discovering what feels easy and what feels challenging.[30]

But movement is just one way to get in touch with the elements. Fire is passion, so a mother might explore her relationship to feeling and expressing herself passionately. Air is cool intellect, the ability to take the overview, so a mother might explore her ease at being calm in her truth. Water is emotion, deep feelings of love and tenderness, so a mother might explore the depths of her openness to letting go. Earth is solid, ground of being, so a mother might explore her ability to stand firm, be strong, and believe in herself.

And yet, beyond any formula lies the Mystery of Birth, in which ease or difficulty with dilation, fast or slow pushing, liking one phase of labor, hating another are all in the cards for women, and may vary for the same mother from labor to labor. As midwife Janice Kalman has said:

> Sometimes birth is energetic, sometimes emotional, sometimes challenging depending on aspects of relationship, or the mother's physical or psychological state that day . . . it's always Mr. Toad's wild ride as to how these aspects create the warp and weave of the story of labor. The trick during pregnancy is for the midwife to recognize red flags of fear, anger, anxiety, discord at home or about who will be at the birth, and then, facilitate open communication around these issues and help a woman come to her truth, no matter what the outcome.

That is what counseling in pregnancy is all about—helping women come to their truth, no matter what. Beyond this, certain circumstances in life pose special challenges to women in pregnancy. The following sections explore these circumstances in depth.

CHALLENGES FACING SINGLE MOTHERS

It has become increasingly common in our society for women to choose to parent alone. Some reach an age when they decide, "It's now or never," selecting the baby's father quite deliberately and then absolving him of any further emotional and financial entanglement. Women who become pregnant accidentally with men they barely know or with whom they cannot hope to establish a lasting relationship have other adjustments to make. And the mother estranged from but still emotionally attached to her baby's father has yet another psychological set.

Particularly if the mother is recently separated, pregnancy can be a time of unprecedented apprehension and loneliness. Alone at night, with the baby kicking and disturbing her sleep, she wonders how she will ever handle her impending responsibilities with everything in her hands, her keeping. No matter what their circumstances, single mothers feel vulnerable because they have no intrinsic support. They may choose home birth out of fear of being abandoned in the hospital situation—a topic worth exploring, to make certain that the responsibilities of birthing at home are well understood. And although most single mothers need extra nurturing from the midwife, they must be encouraged to meet other expectant mothers for lasting friendship and long-term support.

How can you help the single mother with this task? First, make sure she has good self-esteem. Encourage her to talk through concerns she may have about her ability to parent, while stressing her positive traits, aptitudes, and accomplishments. Be on the lookout for signs of depression—see whether she gets out socially, and how she spends her free time. Just be careful not to assume sole responsibility as confidant, because after the birth she will have a whole new set of emotional

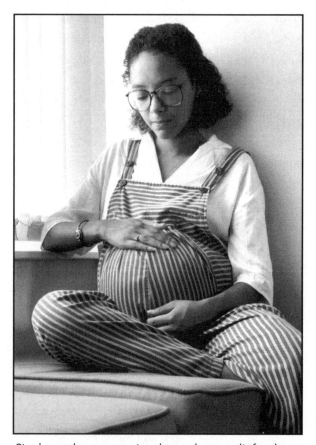

Single mothers must give themselves credit for the courage and strength it takes to go it alone.

needs, and you will have other expectant mothers counting on you. Don't make the beginner's mistake of engendering the single mother's dependency.

When it comes to parenting, most single mothers worry about whether they will have the emotional and physical stamina to do the job. In contrast, if your client chooses to keep the prospect of motherhood veiled, floating through pregnancy with little thought to what lies ahead, initiate a practical discussion of the postpartum period. Ask her how she plans to cope with her own needs in the first few weeks, and how prepared she is to care for the baby. Does she have an adequate supply of baby clothes, furniture, and accessories? Has she ever diapered or bathed a baby before? With little time to prepare food or get to the store, how will she feed herself? And if an emergency should arise (whether physical or emotional), whom can she call for help? These are useful checkpoints for any expectant mother, but for one who is single, this line of inquiry is especially critical.

What about fears concerning the actual birth? Fears of being overwhelmed and losing control are universal, but the single mother is especially susceptible for lack of an intimate partner. Who will stand by her if she falls apart? Besides you, she should have a woman friend, a female relative, or a doula for support during the birth (not to mention before and after).

The sexual dimension of birth may also give a single mother pause, especially if she is celibate. Broach the subject with details on the physiology of labor, explaining how hormones affect pelvic circulation and how the vagina adapts to the baby's contours. Discuss the role of vaginal awareness in the final stages of labor, and teach the mother pelvic floor exercises. Reassure her that masturbation and orgasm are beneficial in pregnancy and help prepare for the birth. Explain the sensations of labor as vividly as you can, and encourage her to feel free to make noise and move uninhibitedly when the time comes.

This brings up a major concern of the single mother: the prospects for love after birth. Are women with babies desirable as sexual partners? Let her know that there are plenty of single parents out there looking for companionship. Some single mothers report being pleasantly surprised by a new lover's relief at being spared the pressure to start a family. Enable the single mother to feel confident about her chances for a loving relationship, and she will approach her birth with confidence and enthusiasm.

DIFFICULTIES OF WORKING MOTHERS

"Every Mother Is a Working Mother," the popular bumper sticker reminds us. If expectant and juggling the demands of a busy career with domestic engineering, a woman may find herself more than overwhelmed. If her life is centered almost entirely on her work, she may need help focusing on pregnancy and her developing baby. Encourage her to stay tuned to her feelings and connected to her body throughout the course of each workday.

Here are some questions for a hard-working mother to help her assess whether her career is negatively affecting her pregnancy. Does she have problems sleeping? During her free hours, is she preoccupied with concerns stemming from work? How is her sex life? Does she make time for deep relaxation every day? Does she get exercise on a regular basis? Her answers to these questions will shed light on how well she is supported, whether or not she is able to unwind, and whether she is making time for the introspection and surrender essential in preparing for labor.

The most common problem of working mothers is chronic stress. Stress tends to manifest in aches and pains at night, or insomnia, and may be mediated by increased vitamins B and C, trace minerals, calcium, and protein. Herbal tinctures of hawthorn, passionflower, or hops can help induce sleep. Chiropractic adjustments may be appropriate, and massage can make a big difference. Meditation and deep relaxation also help, along with regular aerobic exercise. Any woman dealing with stress needs an excellent diet and regular means of emotional and physical release.

If income from employment is so essential that a mother must continue working even when physical and emotional signals say it is time to quit, suggest that she lie down and relax as soon as she gets home, and keep weekends completely free. Discuss this plan with her partner and significant others so they will be able to support it fully. Regardless of their situation, I urge all expectant mothers to quit work at least a week or two before the EDD. Particularly if stressed, women who work to term are frequently overdue, as if making up for lost time.

If the mother plans to return to work soon after the birth, emphasize the importance of taking as much time off as she possibly can to (1) get to know the baby, (2) establish a good milk supply, and (3) develop a workable routine at home. None of this can be done without adequate rest and recuperation. Recommend that she line up a woman relative to assist her full time with everything but baby care, or hire a postpartum doula. Also help her find a support group: cogent discussion with other new moms can reassure the career woman that she is not alone. Do your best to explain how critical the early days and weeks are in establishing intimacy, and how a few months of undivided attention to the baby make parenting more pleasurable and fulfilling in the long run.

If the mother plans to work and breastfeed, make sure she contacts her local chapter of La Leche League. This magnificent organization offers cost-free phone counseling and referrals to nursing mothers' groups. Without support, a busy mother may unconsciously begin limiting nursing periods, which leads to a reduced milk supply and early weaning.

The working mothers category also includes pregnant students, who can accumulate tremendous physical tension from sitting still and concentrating over long periods. Help the pregnant student assess her best times for effective, relaxed study, and then commit to using these and no others. Also help her take a realistic view of continuing her studies after the birth, for even if she limits in-class hours, she may be so preoccupied with subject matter that she may find it hard to give her baby (and herself) sufficient attention.

CHALLENGES FOR ADOPTIVE MOTHERS

Begin by looking closely at any biases you have regarding mothers who give their babies up for adoption. If in your heart of hearts you consider adoption to be child abandonment or, at best, an evasion of responsibility, you must refer the mother to another care provider. The decision to let go of a baby is a painful one—never an easy choice, in the best of circumstances.

The first home birth I attended took place in a milk shed in rural Oregon; I was twenty-one years old and just five months pregnant with my first child. There was no midwife to be found in our community, but the mother had already given birth twice before at home and felt comfortable with the responsibility of birthing on her own. This was in 1971, when humanistic care was virtually nonexistent in hospital.

This experience was remarkable in many ways, but especially in that the mother did not intend to keep the baby—she would give it up for adoption to a couple (her friends) who could not have children and would be at the birth to receive it. Besides the astounding energy of birth and the mother's remarkable power, what I recall most vividly was her restraint at the time of delivery. For the hands that caught the baby were the adoptive mother's, and it was she who first took the baby to breast. The women remained friends, and the child continued to have contact with the birth mother.

This account is an example of **open, private adoption,** which seems preferable in most cases to **closed, agency adoption,** where the identity of the birth parents is concealed from both the adoptive parent(s) and the child (although the mother may be able to sign a waiver allowing the child to seek her out upon reaching legal adulthood). With agency adoption, a facilitator meets with adoptive parents and birth parents alike, to assess appropriate placement. If your client prefers an agency adoption, advise her to contact the Child Welfare League of America, or the Family Service Association. Private adoptions increasingly result from the efforts of an intermediary, such as a lawyer or an independent adoption facilitator, who works for the adoptive parents and charges a substantial fee. It is crucial that the birth mother hire her own legal counsel to protect her rights, and make sure the intermediary is above board. Concerned United Parents (800-822-2777) counsels birth parents and provides referrals to local social service agencies.

Suzanne Arms, author of *Adoption: A Handful of Hope,* suggests that two midwives are needed in the adoption process: one for the birth mother, and one for the adoptive mother.[31] In caring for the birth mother, Frye has observed that grieving usually begins during pregnancy, and having the baby is a major loss, like a death. Thus the birth mother may want to name the baby, take photos when it is born, snip a lock of hair, take hand- or footprints, or save a baby shirt or blanket from the birth.[32] And unlike my experience in the milk shed, she may want and need to nurse the baby, in order to bond sufficiently to make peace with her decision. She may also ask your assistance in developing a ritual or ceremony to formalize her act of letting go, with the witness of family and friends.

Adoptive mothers and parents have their own anxieties, especially postpartum. Whatever will they do if the birth mother changes her mind? How on earth will they cope, especially if the baby has been in their care for a while? State regulations vary regarding the number of days that must elapse after the birth before consents can be signed, as well as time limits for withdrawal. Even after papers are signed, there is a probationary period lasting an average of six months, depending on locale.

In some states, the biological father must also sign his consent. Know the regulations in your area—and if you feel ill equipped to handle the emotional issues, make an appropriate and timely referral.

ISSUES FOR WOMEN WHO DELAY CHILDBEARING

It used to be that any woman having a first baby after age thirty-five was termed an elderly primigravida and considered at risk. The main concern was that labor might be complicated by deteriorating health or inhibited by age-induced rigidity of pelvic bones or muscle tissue. But the standard has changed: as increasing numbers of women delay childbearing and maintain their health and fitness throughout the years, age has proven to be a nonissue.

As for stamina, the older woman who knows herself and clearly wants her baby can manifest phenomenal endurance, more than enough to see her through the longest labor. She has the obvious benefit of life experience, and often, a high degree of self-assurance linked to worldly success. With adolescence far behind her, she is less apt to project maturation issues onto the experience of mothering than a younger woman might be. She knows how to care for herself; she knows what works for her.

On the other hand, psychological rigidity may occur with aging. This can cause problems in labor; for example, if a mother thinks she is doing everything right and still feels out of control, her frustration can greatly hinder progress. When a woman has focused primarily on her own development, honing and finetuning her likes and dislikes, the surrender of established routines to meet a newborn's needs can be more than a little disconcerting. And if conception has been by default—that is, the biological clock is running out—disrupted schedules, unwashed dishes, and hurried meals postpartum may make an older mother feel panicked or even depressed.

You can help by emphasizing that emotional maturity is the key to good parenting. Let her know that the best mothering techniques depend on integrity and forthright communication: attributes she has probably long since refined. Urge her to form friendships with other mothers, especially if her social circle is comprised mostly of childless women and couples. Her greatest asset may be a well-seasoned sense of humor; appeal to this with anecdotes that illustrate how levity can mediate the toughest trials of parenthood. A woman of experience is quick to appreciate what it takes the younger, less mature mother much longer to comprehend—that her child is his or her own person, right from the start.

Attitudes have also changed regarding the grand multipara—the woman who has given birth five times or more. Long considered at risk for fetal malpresentation, prolonged labor, and postpartum hemorrhage due to lax muscle tone, research has shown no risks based on multiparity alone. With attention to nutrition, exercise, and rest during pregnancy, a woman's physical condition and birth experience can be optimal regardless of age or previous childbearing.

PROBLEMS OF ESTRANGED COUPLES

Working with estranged partners is complex: you strive to help them reconcile their differences, at the same time supporting the mother in finding autonomy should reconciliation prove to be impossible. The latter is important regardless of what transpires during pregnancy. Help the mother articulate her core needs and identify those not being met in the relationship. Reaffirm her ability to single-parent if she must, while encouraging her to communicate assertively with her partner.

There are many variations on the theme of estrangement in pregnancy. Perhaps the couple has been together for a while but has not stabilized, with parties vacillating on whether to marry or otherwise define their relationship as long-term. Be prepared for tearful prenatal sessions and continued repetition of problems. Your own counsel may begin to repeat itself too, and you may decide to refer the couple to a specialist who can work with them more intensively.

How best to deal with the mother's partner? Seldom does an estranged partner request advice or assistance; more often than not, he or she simply drops out of the picture. On a few occasions, I have been beeped in the middle of the night by drunken, distraught fathers. These contacts were unproductive and more than a little disturbing. Should this happen to you, tell the father that you will speak to him during normal business hours *only*, unless his partner has a physical emergency. Take care to be professional in your tone of voice and manner of speaking—men can read strange meaning into the midwife's sensitivity and compassion. Refer the couple to counseling, and reassert your role as care provider for the mother.

Hopefully, there will come a time well before labor when the couple in distress decides whether they will stay together. If they remain undecided late in pregnancy, it is important to advise them of the difficulties emotional ambivalence can create during the birth. If they cannot work out their differences, suggest that the mother prepare to labor without her partner. Explain that she must feel fully at ease and supported in order to give birth safely. Contemplation of this fact may make partners decide to reconcile or cause them to see that it is impossible. If separation seems inevitable, have the mother take a close friend to classes or contact a doula. As soon as possible, begin to broach the same topics of discussion as you would with a single mother.

If the couple does reunite for the birth, go out of your way to facilitate partner involvement. Encourage him or her to support the mother in difficult stages, to provide massage and loving contact, and to feel the baby's head as it emerges. Partner participation is intrinsic to bonding and can make a tremendous difference for the tentative couple.

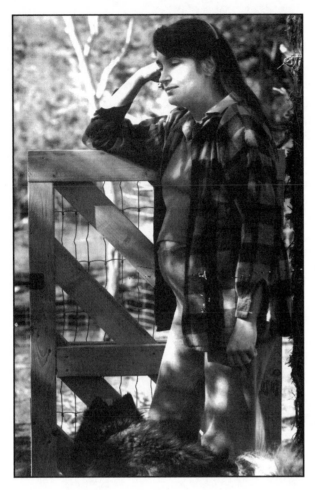

Yet another situation you may encounter is a mother with a new love interested in sharing the pregnancy. The newcomer may be very excited about witnessing the birth, but quite let down postpartum. Passionate, fledgling couples approaching parenthood must be briefed on the difficulties of the early weeks, and you must persist through their joking affection to get at the thorniest issues. Have they discussed their respective roles after the birth? Are they prepared to deal with sleepless nights, hours of baby-crying, loss of privacy, and so on? Do they understand how emotionally volatile the postpartum period can be, and how lack of privacy and breastfeeding may temper sexual activity for quite some time? At some point, see the mother alone in order to broach the subject of single parenting. Ask her how she would cope if she and her new love grew apart after the birth, and whether or not she has any

backup plan for physical assistance or financial support. Remind her of her former self-reliance, and suggest she not lose sight of it if the relationship flounders.

CHALLENGES FACING LESBIAN MOTHERS

In the past, lesbian women openly contemplating motherhood met with ridicule or hostility. Now that same-sex couples are more positively portrayed in the media, these antiquated reactions are falling away. The notion that lesbians are unfit to parent is being replaced with an understanding of how much their children benefit from being carefully prepared for and very much wanted. Nevertheless, lesbian couples need the same guidance and support for handling the stresses of pregnancy and early parenting as do heterosexual partners.

If consultative visits or transport become necessary, make sure you understand how the expectant mother and her partner want their relationship presented to the backup physician and medical staff. Some of your lesbian clients may want to be closeted, while others are definitely "out."

Help with artificial insemination is increasingly available through midwives. Sperm is obtained from sperm banks for 94 percent of inseminations. Otherwise, fresh sperm is secured from known or unknown donors, after careful screening for HIV and other diseases. (Sperm banks also screen donors for HIV, which is critical since the virus can survive freezing.) Rarely, the donor may want some knowledge of the child or may wish to co-parent. But the relationship between mother and donor is usually tentative, thus legal contracts are advisable to delineate these agreements and prevent future custody battles. In numerous states, the donor surrenders all claim to the child if insemination is done through a physician.

The actual insemination process often takes many months. The success rate quoted by most sperm banks is only about 19 percent. It takes an average of six to nine months to conceive, and with two inseminations performed each month, the process can be quite costly. Again, this points to the fact that lesbian women desiring motherhood must be thoroughly committed to their decision.

The birth certificate poses a special problem. If the mother indicates that she was artificially inseminated, the state may try to track the father if she later applies for aid. Better to leave the space for father's name blank or write "unknown." With few exceptions (Vermont, for example), only the birth mother can be registered as legal guardian. In most states, her partner cannot adopt the child either. And if anything were to happen to the mother during the birth (or after) that rendered her disabled or incompetent, her partner would have no authority unless she established power of attorney in advance (in which case she would be treated as next of kin).

Encourage lesbian mothers to find others in their community for support. It is a sobering fact that some lesbian mothers do not tell their midwives the truth, but pose as single mothers. Check yourself for homophobia, and if you personally feel you cannot serve lesbian mothers lovingly and well, refer them to midwives who can.

ISSUES IN FAMILY RELATIONSHIPS

The family in Western society has undergone a major transformation. More often than not, blood relatives live at great distances from one another and communicate infrequently. Thus, most first-time mothers think little of how their family relationships might affect their experience of childbearing and may be surprised to find memories of childhood surfacing as pregnancy progresses. Whether they delve into these memories or not, many feel the urge to talk with their mothers about birth and baby care.

This desire to reanimate family ties links to the power of bonding, which may remain unconscious until maternal (or paternal) surges turn the wheel and complete the cycle of biological relatedness. Particularly with a first pregnancy, the mother and her partner may express negativity about how they were raised and resolve to do a better job than their own parents did. This process of individuation requires letting go of anger and resentment—reactions of attachment—toward their parents and the past, while culling the best techniques and greatest wisdom from their upbringing.

Help expectant partners to fully explore their feelings in this regard, at the same time encouraging them to find forgiveness if at all possible. This may require counseling, particularly if there is history of abuse. Those in their early twenties may confuse bitter memories of adolescence with an otherwise happy childhood—help them recollect the good times. The most difficult (and profound) aspect of first-time parenting is reckoning our ideals with our limitations. Stress that parenting is about process, not perfection; about receptivity, not mastery; about flexibility, not control.

Also, expectant partners may have very different ideas about childrearing. One may have many preconceptions of what is best, while the other maintains a "wait and see" approach. Along these lines, any disagreements arising in your presence are best treated lightly, as ultimately, time will tell. Just be aware that partners with rigid ideals about parenting may likewise fanatic in their expectations of birth and may need to broaden their perspective. Those with decidedly unhappy childhood experiences may confide that they do not really like children and wonder how they will ever survive parenting. Those blessed with happy memories may nonetheless lack exposure to infants and worry that their enthusiasm is much less than it should be. The hardest thing for prospective parents to grasp is that their baby will be *kin,* not just some abstract, alien little infant like everyone else has.

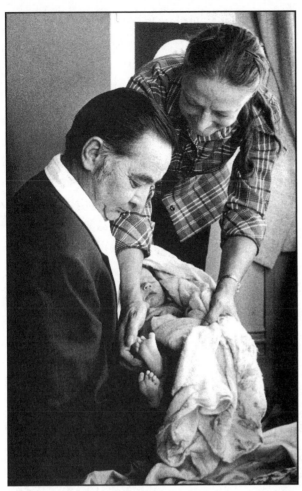
Grandparents thrill to the miracle of birth.

Fear of becoming a parent may be linked to the fear of perpetuating a negative role model. If a first-time father remembers Dad as rigid and unfeeling, or harried and stressed, he may unconsciously believe that becoming a parent means behaving this way. Thus, instead of being cause for celebration, pregnancy is viewed as a sobering event concomitant to a loss of freedom and happiness. Fathers caught up in these feelings may react with bouts of heavy drinking or other substance abuse, overwork, breaking time-related agreements, fits of depression, or even promiscuity. If the mother reports such behavior in her partner, ask her to bring him along to the next prenatal, or you may wish to make a special home visit. Deal tactfully with the male ego in this state of polarization by discussing

the matter dispassionately, taking a simple, objective look at relevant social patterning. If you try to delve emotionally (as is usually so easy and stimulating when counseling a woman), the average man will either withdraw or become defensive.

For their part, expectant mothers often struggle with conflicting role models of the self-sacrificing Madonna and the self-determined free spirit. The hormones of pregnancy further complicate matters, so that many women wonder how they will ever be able to care for a baby and have anything left for themselves. Sometimes a damaging cycle of fear, self-doubt, and repression sets in long before the birth. Do not let this slip by unattended, or the mother may suffer terribly from postpartum depression.

In lesbian relationships, the nonpregnant partner may feel alternately oppressed by impending responsibilities or compelled to reach new heights of sensitivity and perfection. Whatever their situation, expectant partners need to be told that it is possible to be a parent and be human at the same time, and that it is infinitely better to express emotions with spontaneous intensity than to vent them later as distorted or violent outbursts. Explain that parenting operates on the same principles of honesty and assertiveness effective in adult relationships. The more they relax and trust their instincts, the better they will deal with the expectations of other family members and society at large.

SEXUAL PROBLEMS

Sexual difficulties often stem from mistaken concepts of appropriate masculine or feminine behavior. Polarized gender roles have marked our culture since its inception, and even now, while subscribing to sexual equality, the feminine aspect is underexpressed in our society.

As regards sexual intimacy, most problems spring from an inability to integrate this polarity and effectively communicate needs and desires. Broach this subject with your clients by explaining physical and emotional changes trimester by trimester, including various sexual positions and other adaptations appropriate for different phases of pregnancy. This can help a mother more comfortably articulate what she desires from her partner, and vice versa. In this respect, discussion with other expectant couples is ideal because all are undergoing similar changes and adjustments.

Both partners should understand that a pregnant woman's desire for sex fluctuates dramatically. At no other time will the emotional aspect have so strong an influence on her response. In turn, her emotions will vary according to the stage of pregnancy through which she is passing. The first trimester can be a honeymoon of all-barriers-down intimacy and tenderness. Of course, ambivalence toward the pregnancy will temper these feelings. Nausea and fatigue may also interfere.

Once movement is felt, the mother may focus so intently on the baby that she becomes a bit withdrawn. But generally, high levels of estrogen, progesterone, and oxytocin (the "love hormone" associated with sexual arousal, nipple stimulation, and orgasm), plus increased pelvic circulation, serve to boost desire in the latter part of pregnancy. This is a time of balance, ease, and happiness for the mother, and her sexual response usually reflects this. If she complains that her partner is insensitive to her slower and more sensual pregnant pace, suggest she take more initiative or talk to him or her when they are not being sexual. As the baby grows, she may also need to try different positions for comfort.

As the birth approaches, the mother may once again withdraw to focus on impending labor. For sex to seem right at this time, she needs to know and feel that her partner is deeply connected to her and the baby,

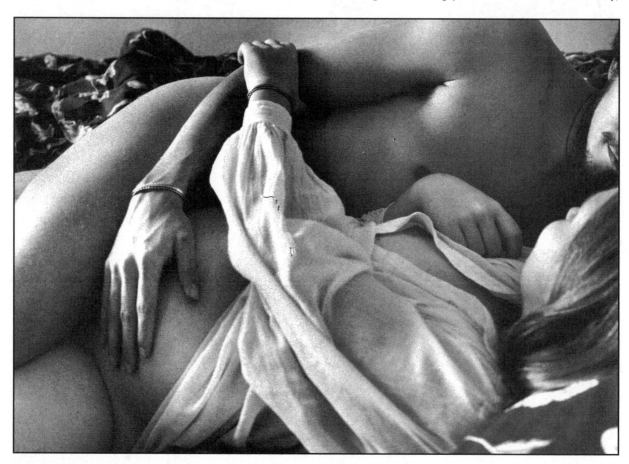

More than ever, it's about communication and closeness.

making love to them both. This is a very vulnerable time for the mother, and it is perfectly all right for her to be selective regarding the nature and frequency of her sexual encounters.

If the mother is not happily partnered or there are other issues that prevent her from having sex, explain that birth prompts the same kind of emotional and physical release as happens with orgasm, and that, barring signs of premature labor or other complications, masturbation is fine during pregnancy, right up to the moment the baby is born. Encourage her to keep her sexual circuits open, so she can fully respond to labor's intensity.

In fact, all couples should be apprised of the sexual nature of the birth experience. A graphic demonstration may serve to convey the idea—start with intense breathing, combine with an attitude of physical surrender, add a few moans or urgent demands, like, "Squeeze my shoulders . . . mmm," or, "There . . . push harder," and you will have made your point. This dramatization may move parents (and you) to embarrassed laughter, but you will have imparted more about the psychosexual nature of birth than they could get from any book!

Shy women afraid of their own passions may recoil at these suggestions. Make clear that labor is a body-centered experience that will call on her to take the lead. Help her redefine her sexuality as a sharing of her power, rather than her skill in submitting to or pleasing her partner. Encourage her to take sensual pleasure in hot baths, relaxed meals, massage, and so on. Physical practices of yoga or dance may help her get in touch with her rhythms, release tension, and find her own resources for feeling good. Again, masturbation is fine—many pregnant women report masturbating more than ever before, perhaps several times daily.

One of my favorite stories that illustrates the sexuality of birth involved a young couple and their three-year-old daughter on a rare warm and beautiful San Francisco afternoon. The mother set up her birth nest in the living room area, near the kitchen, and I still remember the breeze blowing through the white curtains as sunlight filtered through. Labor progressed quite rapidly but the mother stayed calm, with her daughter tucked comfortably beside her as crowning approached. Her husband sat between her legs, waiting to catch the baby, when suddenly she reached for him passionately, saying, "Kiss me, Jack," which he did as the head slipped out effortlessly. A truly gorgeous and unforgettable moment!

A mother's ease with her sexuality affects not only her labor, but her comfort with her baby, her rate of recuperation, and her commitment to breastfeeding. Help her to explore and celebrate her sexuality as much as possible.

ABUSE ISSUES

Sexual abuse may be defined as intimate contact in which a child or adolescent is used for the sexual gratification of someone older. The key to differentiating abuse from experimentation is what Anne Frye has termed the "power differential"; the abuser always has the upper hand.[33] The incidence is estimated to be 33 percent of women, although one study showed that 53 percent of pregnant teens had experienced sexual abuse.[34] Repressed memories of sexual abuse are likely to arise (1) during the perinatal cycle, (2) when a woman gets married or commits to monogamous relationship, (3) when her own daughter reaches the age when she herself was first molested, or (4) when her perpetrator dies. If the mother responds to relevant questions on the medical history form with some uncertainty but is willing to discuss her experience, ask the following:

1. Have you ever been tricked into an intimate situation you did not desire?

2. Has anyone ever touched you intimately against your will?

3. Have you ever been forced to have sex when you didn't want to?

4. Have you ever been forcibly held down or restrained for sex when clearly indicating you wanted to be free?

A woman with a history of sexual abuse may suffer from extreme PMS, chronic pelvic pain, constipation or vaginal infection, pain with intercourse, and eating disorders. There may be history of habitual abortion, hyperemesis gravidarium, or premature labor. She is likely to have an intense reaction to internal exam, speculum exam, breast exam, or even with blood draw. She may also suffer from **vaginismus,** an involuntary contraction of the vaginal muscles if any attempt is made at penetration.

Sometimes the abuse survivor develops a dissociative disorder and behaves in a fashion opposite of the above. During exams, she may splay her legs wide or open her labia far apart, but emotionally she is passive, detached, checked out, not there with you. In the extreme, a woman with a history of prolonged sexual abuse may develop multiple personality disorder. Here is a list of characteristics or behaviors common in women who have been sexually abused:

- Describes self as never having been a child

- Is extremely concerned with control

- Is overly willing to expose genitals to others

- Has unexplained pain with intercourse

- Has extreme ideas about sexuality

- Is hypersensitive to touch

- Is repeatedly exploited by others in relationships

- Is deeply estranged from family

- Has a general feeling of being "under it"

- Detaches from self and others

- Says nothing is ever wrong with life, always neutral

- Displays childlike behavior, dress, or appearance

- Has an unkempt personal appearance

- Has chaotic surroundings or habits

- Has overly controlled surroundings and habits

- Shows no personal boundaries

- Has no trust

- Displays anger inappropriate or out of proportion to the situation

- Is unable to appreciate others

- Blindly adores others

- Has fanatic religious or philosophical beliefs

- Jumps into situations or to conclusions

- Has difficulty with making decisions[35]

With regard to the birth process, certain impacts of sexual abuse are classic. Most abuse survivors have a tremendous fear of losing control, and cannot bear the thought of grunting, trembling, crying out, or feeling helpless in labor. Sensations in second stage may be particularly terrifying, as vaginal distension triggers memories of early violation. Cesarean is common. The abuse survivor may also have great difficulties with breastfeeding, particularly when her baby reaches an age where it begins to fondle the nipple or play at the breast.

Experts Penny Simkin and Phyllis Klaus observe that working with sexually abused women can be difficult because they are often needy, controlling, and/or angry.[36] Even if the midwife is doing everything in her power to be of assistance, an imagined slight may snowball into litigation. Particularly if the mother demonstrates any behaviors listed above, consider these guidelines for working with her:

1. **Don't withdraw.** Even if the mother is critical of your care or behavior, or behaves in a childlike way, stay present in a state of active listening.

2. **Validate the mother's perceptions.** Even though they may seem overblown or wildly inaccurate, you will do well to concur with her views.

This diffuses her anger, which might otherwise be directed at you, at her baby, or at herself.

3. **Once trust is established, negotiate.** If you are able to be patient with the mother and can win her trust, you can work to settle any disagreements or field any disappointments she may have regarding her care.

A woman who has been victimized by **rape** may have striking similarities to one who has suffered sexual abuse, depending on how well she has healed from her trauma. She too may be needy and angry, and so may suffer similar difficulties with labor unless she receives counseling during pregnancy. As you take her history, be ready to discuss residual fears, embarrassment, or feelings of powerlessness linked to her experience.

On the other hand, women who have done significant work to move through the traumas of sexual abuse or rape may be quite self-sufficient and responsibly interdependent. And they may have extraordinarily empowering birth experiences. This account from a survivor of childhood sexual abuse serves to illustrate:

> During the birth of my daughter I felt immense power. I could feel this hard, glorious ball filling my vagina, washing it clean of shame, proving its power and purity. I felt the heat from her head and the stretching of my tissues. I felt burning and stinging. Then I felt a feeling better than any orgasm I had ever had, as her sweet, slippery body left me. I immediately felt I'd do anything to feel that feeling again, that last moment of ecstasy. But by then I was caught in a wave of other ecstasies, the feeling of her warm body against mine, her soft purple skin turning pink in my arms.

Victims of **physical abuse/domestic violence** require special care. First and foremost, they must be apprised of their legal situation. In many states, health workers are obligated to report evidence of physical abuse to the local authorities, and the abuser will be arrested. Apart from the obvious physical danger, there are major emotional ramifications of physical abuse. If your pregnant client remains with her abuser, you must make some decisions on how to care for her. Even though her partner may wish to be present at the birth, you must separate her needs from her partner's desires. In many ways, you must treat her as you would an estranged or single mother. Be aware of the resources in your area and, as they say in abuse-recovery circles, "make yourself safe."

Particularly with a history of physical abuse, the mother may feel extremely protective of her unborn baby, keeping it inside her as long as possible. To some extent, this instinct is sound: the postpartum period is fraught with liabilities for her and the baby, as physically abused women tend toward self-abnegation, repression, frustration, and, unfortunately, child abuse. Get expert consultation or refer her to counseling as indicated.

PSYCHOLOGICAL SCREENING OUT

Despite your best efforts, a client may continue to have emotional problems that make you question the wisdom of home birth for her. Before jumping to conclusions, discuss your concerns with her counselor or other associate familiar with her case, who may see signs of improvement that you have overlooked. On the other hand, guard against excessive optimism. Give credence to the emotional aftertaste of working with a troubled client, and take pains to distinguish the exhilaration of extending yourself from her actual level of responsiveness.

If her case is borderline, discuss the situation with your backup physician before the birth is imminent. This will render any emotional problems in labor more comprehensible in the event of transport. Also discuss such cases with your peers, not only to benefit from their perspective but to forestall any rumors in case of an unhappy outcome.

Then again, if you have exhausted every resource at your disposal and still feel her progress to be inadequate, it is wise to excuse yourself from her care and appropriately refer her. Provide a list of recommended caregivers, including contacts for hospital birth. Not uncommonly, the mother is relieved at your decision, and it becomes evident that her lack of comfort with you (or perhaps with the prospect of birthing at home) was part of the problem all along. This amounts to psychological screening out.

It is important to note that the shock of being screened out may prompt the mother to rally her resources and make long overdue changes in her situation. Thus a client determined by one midwife to be psychologically at risk may be cared for by another and do just fine. Then again, if her emotions remain jumbled regardless of a changed situation, the mother's chances of developing complications are even greater than before and hospital birth is advisable.

The only way to learn psychological screening is by experience. I cannot remember a single workshop on this subject where a midwife has not presented a hair-raising case history capped with the final lament, "I knew from the start I shouldn't have worked with her." Those who have borne the consequences via malpractice proceedings will tell you that initial feelings of ambivalence are a warning every midwife should heed.

Once you have made a decision to risk-out, hold firm. If you have agreed to support the woman in hospital, remember that any last-minute improvements are probably due to increased security with more conventional plans. Do not be tempted to reverse yourself just because things are looking better. This takes the wisdom to let things be and to forgo your desire for a certain kind of personal involvement. The birth may not be any easier in the hospital than it would have been at home, but at least some of the weight is off your shoulders.

Notes

1. F. G. Cunningham, and others, *Williams Obstetrics,* 20th ed. (Stamford, Conn.: Appleton & Lange, 1997).

2. Claudia Panuthos and C. Romero, *Ended Beginnings* (Boston, Mass.: Bergin & Garvey, 1984).

3. Anne Frye, *Holistic Midwifery: A Comprehensive Textbook for Midwives in Homebirth Practice, Volume 1* (Portland, Oreg.: Labrys Press, 1998), 724.

4. Stephen G. Gabbe, Jennifer R. Neibyl, and Joe Leigh Simpson, *Obstetrics: Normal and Problem Pregnancies,* 4th ed. (New York: Churchill Livingstone, 2002), 230.

5. Jack Pritchard and Paul MacDonald, *Williams Obstetrics,* 15th ed. (New York: Appleton Century Crofts, 1976), 418.

6. Gabbe, Neibyl, and Simpson, *Obstetrics: Normal and Problem Pregnancies,* 1,272.

7. Henci Goer, *Obstetrical Myths Versus Research Realities: A Guide to the Medical Literature* (Westport, Conn.: Bergin & Garvey, 1995), 158.

8. Henci Goer, "Gestational Diabetes: The Emperor Has No Clothes," *The Birth Gazette* 12 (2): 1966.

9. J. S. Hunter and M. J. N. C. Keirse, "Gestational Diabetes," in *Effective Care in Pregnancy and Birth,* ed. Ian Chalmers and others (Oxford, England: Oxford University Press, 1989).

10. K. L. Boyd, E. K. Ross, and S. J. Sherman, "Jelly beans as an alternative to a cola beverage containing fifty grams of glucose," *American Journal of Obstetrics and Gynecology* 173 (6): 1,889–92, December 1995.

11. Anne Frye, *Understanding Diagnostic Tests in the Childbearing Year,* 6th ed. (Portland, Oreg.: Labrys Press, 1997), 319.

12. Kevin Dalton, "Home Telemetry: A Need for Reassessment of PET," report presented at the Royal College of Medicine, London, England, September 15, 1989.

13. Guyati, et. al., "Calcium during pregnancy could save lives," *Journal of the American Medical Association* 274 (14): April 1996.

14. G. Hofmeyer, A. N. Atallah, and L. Duly, "Calcium supplementation during pregnancy for preventing hypertensive disorders and related problems," *Cochrane Library* 4, 2003.

15. S. E. Maynard, J. Y. Min, J. Merchan, K. H. Lim, J. Li, S. Mondal, T. A. Libermann, J. P. Morgan, F. W. Sellke, I. E. Stillman, F. H. Epstein, V. P. Sukhatme, and S. A. Karumanchi, "Excess placental soluble fms-like tyrosine kinase 1 (sFlt1) may contribute to endothelial dysfunction, hypertension, and proteinuria in preeclampsia," *Journal of Clinical Investigation* 111 (5): 649–58, March 2003.

16. Frye, *Holistic Midwifery, Volume 1,* 958.

17. S. Kilpatrick and others, "Maternal hydration increases amniotic fluid volume in women with normal amniotic fluid," *Obstetrics and Gynecology* 81 (1): 49–52, January 1993.

18. Gabbe, Neibyl, and Simpson, *Obstetrics: Normal and Problem Pregnancies,* 827.

19. Doña Queta Contreras and Doña Irene Sotelo, Midwifery Today conference notes, Oaxaca, Mexico, October 2003.

20. Charles Lockwood, *New England Journal of Medicine* editorial 346 (January 2002): 282–84.

21. E. Morzurkewich and others, "Strenuous working conditions are related to preterm birth," *Journal of Obstetrics and Gynecology,* April 2002.

22. M. Jeffcoat and others, "Periodontal infection and preterm birth: results of a prospective study," *Journal of the American Dental Association* 132 (July 2001): 875–80.

23. H. Minkoff and others, "An association between the heat-humidity index and preterm labor and delivery," *American Journal of Public Health* 87 (1997): 1205–7.

24. S. J. Olsen and N. J. Secher, "Low consumption of seafood in early pregnancy as a risk factor for preterm delivery: prospective cohort study," *British Medical Journal* 324 (February 2002): 447.

25. S. M. Ludington-Hoe and S. K. Golant, *Kangaroo Care: The Best You Can Do for Your Premature Infant* (New York: Bantam Books, 1993).

26. Morzurkewich and others, "Strenuous working conditions."

27. Gabbe, Neibyl, and Simpson, *Obstetrics: Normal and Problem Pregnancies,* 931.

28. H. Oxorn, *Oxorn-Foote Human Labor & Birth,* 5th ed. (Norwalk, Conn.: Appleton & Lange, 1986), 712.

29. R. D. Eden, L. S. Seifert, A. Winegar, and W. N. Spellacy, "Perinatal characteristics of uncomplicated postdates pregnancies," *Obstetrics and Gynecology* 69 (1987): 296.

30. Verena Schmid, Midwifery Today conference notes, London, England, June 2003.

31. Suzanne Arms, MANA conference notes, San Francisco, Calif., October 1985.

32. Frye, *Holistic Midwifery, Volume 1,* 936.

33. Frye, *Holistic Midwifery, Volume 1,* 308.

34. T. Hoffman, N. Kellogg, and E. Taylor, "Early sexual experiences among pregnant and parenting adolescents," *Adolescence* 34 (1999).

35. Laura Davis and Ellen Bass, *The Courage to Heal* (New York: Harper & Row, 1998).

36. Penny Simkin and Phyllis Klaus, audiotape, Midwifery Today conference, Eugene, Oreg., 1996.

For Parents: Danger Signs in Pregnancy

Report to your midwife immediately if you notice:

1. **Vaginal bleeding.** In the first trimester, this may indicate threatened, spontaneous, or missed abortion (miscarriage); molar pregnancy; or ectopic pregnancy. In the second or third trimesters, this may indicate placenta previa, placental abruption, ruptured cervical polyp, or other causes.

2. **Initial outbreak of blisters in the perineal or anal area during the first trimester.** This may be herpesvirus; contact your midwife at once so a culture can be taken.

3. **Severe pelvic or abdominal pain.** In the first trimester, this may indicate a tubal pregnancy. In the last trimester, this may indicate placental abruption. Both are emergencies; contact your midwife at once.

4. **Persistent and severe midback pain.** This may indicate kidney infection/pyelonephritis; contact your midwife at once.

5. **Swelling of hands and face.** Particularly if your face looks puffy or your features coarse, notify your midwife immediately. This may indicate preeclampsia.

6. **Severe headaches, blurry vision, or epigastric pain (under ribcage).** This may indicate a preeclamptic condition becoming critical. Notify your midwife immediately.

7. **Gush of fluid from vagina.** If in the first or second trimester, this may indicate miscarriage. If in your late second or third trimester, this may indicate premature delivery. Contact your midwife at once.

8. **Regular uterine contractions before thirty-seven weeks.** This may indicate impending premature birth. Don't wait to see if they will abate; lie down and call your midwife immediately.

9. **Cessation of fetal movement.** This may indicate fetal demise. The baby should move several times per hour, more right after you have a meal. If fewer times than this, or fewer movements than usual, report to your midwife at once. ■

Chapter 4

ASSISTING AT BIRTHS

The first principle of attending births is to maintain an open mind and pay attention to what is happening in the present. Regardless of any prenatal turmoil or conflict, the birth is the main event and every effort must be made to come to it clear and clean of preconceptions. This quality of freshness will be well appreciated by the mother and her supporters— it is the spark for getting labor off to a good start.

EARLY LABOR

Every woman should know the signs of early labor well before her baby is due. Obvious signs that labor is impending include **the show** (pink-tinged mucus from the vagina), **spontaneous rupture of the membranes (SROM)** (the water bag breaks), or **regular contractions** (at most, twenty minutes apart).

Encourage all mothers to call at the first indication that labor might be starting. This gives you time to put your personal life in order and prepare to attend, even if the birth does not happen for several days.

Note that globs of mucus are often passed in the final weeks, but only if secretions are blood-tinged can you assume that cervical changes are occurring. Be sure the mother knows the difference between a normal show and excess bleeding, which might be related to placental problems. Sometimes the plug is lost and labor takes several days to commence. If so, advise the mother to go about her normal routine, eat high-quality, noncon-

stipating foods, and get plenty of rest. Explain that she doesn't have to do anything to get labor going: what matters most is that she take the best possible care of herself, relax, and let her feelings flow. Should she experience a prelabor burst of energy, be firm about her need

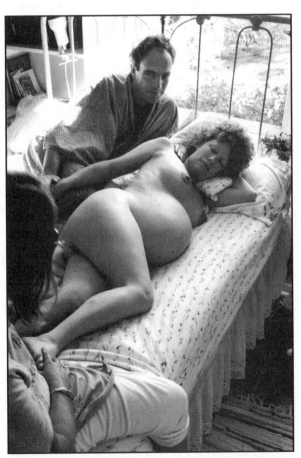

The midwife makes her presence felt by holding the woman's feet without intruding on the couple's privacy.

for rest (and sleep) to prepare for the work ahead. But share in her elation too, as this will help her release nervous tension and get into the process.

Less commonly, labor begins with the amniotic fluid leaking or gushing out completely. It may be difficult to be certain that what appears to be a slow leak is not just a bit of urine being passed involuntarily due to pressure from the baby's head on the bladder. Time will tell, and it is better not to place a speculum (or anything else) in the vagina if you suspect SROM, at the risk of precipitating uterine infection.

If the woman reports a gush of water with no more following, we call this a **hind leak.** It is caused by a tear high in the membranes, which releases just enough fluid to allow the baby to settle snugly down in the pelvis so that any further flow is prevented. But sometimes a bit of fluid does filter down and is trapped behind the intact membranes still encasing the baby's head; these are the **forewaters,** which feel like an intact but bulging water bag.

Apart from a hind leak, rupture of the membranes calls for certain precautions. Infection can occur if bacteria from the vagina enter the sterile uterine environment. But if the mother drinks sufficient amounts of liquid at regular intervals, her body will defend itself by increasing the production of amniotic fluid, which flushes the vagina and discourages bacteria from migrating upward. She must also be meticulous in her toileting and put nothing in her vagina. To ward off infection, 250 mg vitamin C can be taken every few hours. If you are not yet with her, have the mother check her temperature periodically and note the odor on her pad: it should smell clean and fresh. Tell her to report any changes immediately. The debate continues as to the maximum time membranes can be ruptured before infection is likely (see "Prolonged Rupture of the Membranes" in chapter 5).

Also have the mother contact you at once if she notes a green or yellow tinge to the amniotic fluid, which indicates that the baby has passed **meconium,** that is, its first bowel movement. This is due to relax-

ation of the anal sphincter, which may be caused by a lack of oxygen, or **hypoxia.** As meconium in the waters is suggestive of fetal distress, you must immediately attend the mother and check fetal heart tones.

In responding to ruptured membranes, place primary importance on helping the mother conserve her resources for active labor. There is no need to try and get labor going. If near bedtime or in the middle of the night, suggest she have a strong cup of relaxant herbal tea (such as hops or valerian) or a glass of wine (barring history of alcoholism) and get to sleep. Her partner might want to give her a massage, but again, no intercourse, finger-genital, or mouth-genital contact.

Labor beginning with contractions alone is a bit harder to confirm, as some women have rounds of uterine activity for weeks before actual labor. Typically called **false labor,** this negative term serves only to increase the frustration of stop-and-go contracting, which can hurt and lead to sleep deprivation. Put a positive spin on the situation and explain that although the fibers of the uterus are not yet synchronized (which must happen for dilation to occur), these contractions tone and strengthen uterine muscle and may also facilitate effacement and fetal descent. We may more accurately term this sort of uterine activity **warm-up labor.**

With warm-up labor, contractions may come every ten to twenty minutes, or even as often as every three minutes, but last less than forty seconds and never form a consistent pattern. In this case, suggest a glass of wine, which will slow or stop the process if the time is not yet ripe. Sensations similar to warm-up labor may also occur when the baby is large, unengaged, and then suddenly descends. This is called **lightening or dropping** and is often accompanied with considerable stretching of the lower uterine segment. The mother may think she is in labor, but upon further investigation you find that her "contractions" are more like twinges, with no particular pattern of dispersal or duration. Suggest she take a hot bath, do deep relaxation, and rest up.

True labor is characterized by contractions that gradually increase in intensity and occur closer and closer together. They may be erratic in spacing and duration at first, but if there is cervical (menstrual-like) cramping, chances are it is the real thing. Most women are eager to discuss their first contractions, giving you a chance to allude to labor's forthcoming intensity.

If labor starts in the morning, inquire of the mother as to whether she got enough sleep, then suggest a good breakfast and an outing with her partner in some natural setting (*not* the mall). Recommend that she pause when contractions come, leaning against something and releasing her pelvis and hips completely. Encourage her to keep eating and drinking, and take a nap in the afternoon if things have not changed (especially if her sleep the night before was limited).

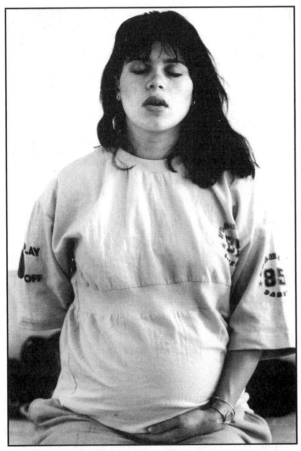

A picture of relaxation: note the loose mouth and easy jaw.

If labor starts in the afternoon, make sure she had a good lunch, and then suggest a hot shower or bath and a nap. In this case, the priority is rest rather than activity, as it is quite likely she will labor well into the night, particularly if this is her first baby. To help her rest, suggest hops tincture in tea or a massage. Remind her that she should plan to have dinner and should call you after she rests to check in.

If labor starts at night, have her follow the guidelines mentioned earlier for getting sleep. Also make sure she had a good dinner, and remind her to keep fluids by the bed—she should drink (and urinate) regularly.

This brings up the question of when to go to the birth. After your initial conversation, the mother will want to know when next to be in touch and when you will be coming. Tell her to call if anything changes or if she wants you there. Let her know that you are happy to help her through any rough periods, regardless of how early it may seem. Explain your willingness to come and go, and reassure her that there is no such thing as calling too soon.

First-time mothers often call at about 2 or 3 cm dilation to report some "really intense" contractions, aware they are early in the process and fearful of how much more painful it might become. This is a fairly universal response in reckoning with the forces of childbirth. Explain that as labor progresses, her body will release endorphins that will make the pain easier to bear, and as long as she continues to surrender, she will find resources for coping that she does not even know she has. You might suggest a hot bath or shower to help her get used to her sensations, or a massage from her partner. And remind her of the importance of relaxation; women often forget to use relaxation techniques in early labor.

However, there are certain indications to attend the birth immediately. Mothers with psychological issues in pregnancy may want an immediate visit for reassurance and may need some help getting settled. If the baby was high at the last prenatal visit and the mother calls to report that her waters have broken, immediately go and check fetal heart tones to rule out cord prolapse. Or if you have any question concerning the baby's ability to handle labor due to intrauterine growth restriction (IUGR) or postdatism, be there from the beginning to monitor fetal response. A report of meconium-tinged waters or decreased fetal movement necessitates your immediate presence to rule out fetal compromise. Maternal conditions of borderline hypertension or polyhydramnios should be monitored right from the start. In general, any marginal findings in the last weeks of pregnancy require earlier involvement and more diligent assessment during labor.

The birth environment also merits your attention. It is virtually impossible for a mother to relax and get into her labor if her home is chaotic; beware of loud partying noises in the background. You may need to help her clear the house of distractions, by explaining to well-meaning friends or relatives that it will be a while yet and she needs a chance to concentrate. Send members of the birth team on last-minute food runs, or have them do a bit of cooking for after the birth (or for now if the mother is still hungry). The birth room itself should be kept neat, well ventilated, and aesthetically pleasing, with ample fluids by the bed as well as massage oil, towels, a heating pad, and so on all laid out and ready for use. Many women use their natural nesting instincts to take care of this in early labor, but those who feel frightened may need help getting organized.

Otherwise, maintain good phone communication, and you may be able to guide the mother through early labor without having to make a visit. This can be crucially important if you have a very busy practice or are tired from a recent birth. Aspiring midwives often struggle with the concept of anything less than start-to-finish involvement in labor, confusing their role with that of the doula or birth assistant, whose job reaches a peak with the birth of the baby and then quickly eases off. In contrast, the midwife's responsibilities may not peak until well after the birth. Complications may require her to handle a shoulder dystocia, or resuscitate a baby, or manually remove a placenta, or attend to persistent bleeding, or repair a torn perineum. Because the midwife's participation is weighted to the latter part of the birth process, conserving her energy in early labor is essential. But this is only possible if she methodically attends to her clients' needs for support and information prior to the birth, in the context of prenatal caregiving.

When a mother calls to report increasing uterine activity, keep her on the phone for a few contractions. You can usually gauge the intensity of her labor by how long it takes her to recover after contractions end—a lengthy pause before she resumes conversation may be indicative of active labor. If she seems to be going deeper with each contraction, or the pause period before she speaks increases as you listen, go and attend her regardless of her (or her partner's) evaluation of labor's intensity.

Patterns of early labor vary dramatically from woman to woman. In general, those who commence with close-set contractions give birth sooner than those who begin with contractions every twenty minutes. But a mother can shift gears to active labor very suddenly, so be conscientious about staying in touch, and be sure to explain signs of active labor so she or her partner know when to contact you. If she is able to make a smooth transition from early to active labor on her own, she may very well call too late for you to make it to the birth on time. *In general, contractions a minute long, coming every five minutes, signal the onset of active labor.*

PHYSICAL ASSESSMENTS AND DUTIES IN EARLY LABOR

If you attend the mother in early labor, begin your labor record (see appendix E) with notes on how labor started and how it is progressing. Check the mother's urine for ketones (which indicate that she should eat something), take her blood pressure, pulse, and temperature, and palpate the baby for position and descent. Do these assessments between contractions so as not to disturb the mother. On the other hand, fetal heart tones must be taken during and immediately after a contraction in order to gauge fetal response (more on this in the next few pages). You may also wish to palpate the uterus during a contraction to assess the intensity of uterine activity. Chart assessments as soon as they are completed.

Vaginal exams are optional in early labor. They may be useful for establishing a baseline and letting everyone know what is going on, but in general, vaginal exams should be kept to a minimum. Many midwives feel that the physical and emotional impact of exams contradicts the mother's need to release down and out—and I agree. Still, do not let your commitment to nonintervention prevent you from doing an exam if the mother requests it, if she seems to need the information to get focused, or if her contractions begin to get weaker and further apart. Particularly as a beginner, you may check more frequently than is really necessary until you learn to read signs of progress in the mother's apperance or behavior. Nevertheless, check whenever in doubt.

Your goal in doing vaginal exams during labor is to be as gentle and undisruptive as possible, while quickly obtaining as much information as you can. Use sterile gloves with lubricating jelly (or a squirt of Betadine or other antiseptic if the membranes are ruptured and labor is well progressed). Start the exam the moment a contraction ends and you have the mother's consent. Begin by checking **dilation,** taking care not to stretch the cervix as you assess, and record in centimeters. (If the mother is dilated to 6 cm or more, see additional assessments under "Physical Assessments and Duties during Active Labor" later in this chapter.) Next, note the **quality of the cervical opening:** is it stretchy and yielding or tight-rimmed? If the latter and labor is very early, you can insert six to eight capsules of evening primrose oil high around the cervix, which should soften it in about twelve hours. If labor is already well under-

way and the tight-rimmed cervix seems to be hindering progress, apply pressure to the rim edge—it should break up under your fingers.[1]

Also note the **placement of the cervix:** is it central, anterior, or posterior? Typically posterior when the head is above −2 station, the cervix swings forward as the baby descends. Next, check for effacement by estimating the percentage of cervix that has been drawn up into the lower uterine segment. Finally, estimate the station of the head, and note how evenly it fills the pelvic cavity.

Interpreting your findings depends on how rapidly labor is progressing and how the mother is responding to it. At this stage, the most crucial assessments are of dilation, effacement, and station. If the mother is losing control at 2 cm, with her cervix just 25 percent effaced, she needs a change of scene to rest, relax, and integrate. If it is late at night, contractions are not very strong, and she is dilated just 2 or 3 cm with the baby high in the pelvis (−2 or above), sleep is the best idea for everyone involved.

If early labor is prolonged or there is a lull in progress, consider the baby's position. If posterior, the head may be deflexed and poorly applied to the cervix, and without adequate pressure on the cervix, contractions will be short and irregular, and progress very slow. This situation may self-correct with time; if not, you may be able to manually reposition the head when the cervix is more dilated. Meanwhile, encourage rest if possible; if not, suggest upright and forward-leaning positions to promote descent. (See more on this in chapter 5.)

ACTIVE LABOR

Sometimes you get the feeling that active labor is knocking at the door, but the mother is not ready to get up and answer. Up to 4 or 5 cm dilation (and sometimes beyond), women have the power to control the ebb and flow of contractions and, unless labor is precipitous,

Aseptic Technique and Universal Precautions

Utilization of aseptic technique and universal precautions is crucial to safe midwifery practice. Although these basic procedures are mentioned throughout the text, this sidebar is meant as a summary and ready reference.

Handwashing Techniques

To wash your hands properly, you will need soap, a sink with hot and cold water, a scrub brush with povidone-iodine, and paper towels or a clean hand towel. Proceed as follows:

1. Remove any rings with rough surfaces (you may wash under smooth rings). Move your watch several inches up your forearm or remove it.

2. Wet your hands and forearms to the elbows with warm water, taking care not to touch the sink.

3. Add soap to your hands and lather up.

4. Use one hand to wash the other, including the wrist, the forearm, the back side of the hand, as well as the fingers and the areas between them.

5. Cleanse under your nails with a nailbrush, fingernail of the other hand, or a nail stick.

6. Repeat for the other hand and arm.

7. Rinse your hands and arms and under the nails, then hold your hands up so water runs down to the elbows.

8. Pat hands and arms dry.

9. Use a dry portion of your towel to turn off the faucet, and dispose of the towel appropriately.

These handwashing techniques should be utilized before and after every examination of mother or baby. If performing a series of exams on different mothers and babies, wash hands between each exam.

Gloving and Ungloving Techniques

1. Wash and dry hands.

2. Peel down the outer wrapper of the glove package.

3. Set inside packet on a clean and dry surface, and open to expose gloves.

4. Pick up a glove at the folded cuff, touching only the inside of the cuff.

5. Pull the glove firmly over hand, being careful not to touch anything with gloved fingers.

6. Put on the second glove, repeating steps 4 and 5, above.

7. Adjust your fingers in the gloves; keep your gloved hands in sight and above your waist.

To remove gloves, grasp inside the cuff of one glove, turn inside out and remove, then carefully remove the other glove the same way, taking care not to touch the outside. Dispose of them immediately.

Universal Precautions

The **Centers for Disease Control and Prevention (CDC)** publish the document "Recommendations for Prevention of HIV Transmission in Health-Care Settings," which urges health-care workers to use blood and body fluid precautions with all clients, regardless of blood-borne infection status. The procedures outlined in this document are known as **universal precautions.** Copies of this document can be obtained from the CDC's National Prevention Information Network at (800) 458-5231. Below is a summary of universal precautions relevant to midwifery care:

1. Utilize barrier precautions, such as gloves, waterproof gowns or aprons, masks, protective eyewear, and mouthpieces for resuscitation, in order to prevent exposure of skin and mucous membranes (eyes, nose, and mouth) to blood, amniotic fluid, vaginal secretions, seminal fluid, and breast milk.

2. Make sure to use gloves for blood-collecting procedures, collecting cultures, vaginal exams, assisting delivery, handling of the newborn until he or she is washed and dried, and handling of underpads, clothing, or bed linens wetted with body fluids.

3. If hands or skin are contaminated, they should be washed at once, and a health-care provider consulted.

must deliberately let the forces of birth take over. To move into active labor, the mother must give up notions of how labor is "supposed to be."

If the uterus works up to a certain intensity and the mother fights against it, difficulties occur. This is often the case when a woman is rocking and moaning with very little dilation. Forced movement during contractions can exacerbate tension and hinder progress; help the mother by showing her how to be still and let her body "melt" while focusing on the rhythm of her breath. Once she lets go and makes this shift, frantic agitation gives way to peaceful resignation as endorphins are released.

As Michel Odent has reminded us, the act of giving birth is seated in the primitive brain, which releases of a "cocktail of hormones" to ease the way.[2] To benefit from this and tune into our instinctual birthing wisdom, we must first turn off the neocortex, our thinking and reasoning aspect. And how is this to be done? Consider factors that stimulate the neocortex: speech, bright light, and a sense of being observed (by others, by oneself, or by technology). Laboring women need a quiet, peaceful, private, and intimate environment—with their birth attendant knitting quietly in the corner or, better yet, in the other room. This is not sentimentalism; this is physiology.

Similarly, Ina May Gaskin has evolved the Sphincter Law, which simply states that cervical, vaginal, and rectal sphincters work best in an atmosphere of privacy—for example, in a room with a locking door where interruption is unlikely or impossible. None of our sphincters can be commanded at will to open or relax, and once in the process of opening, they can close down again with fear or self-consciousness.[3]

Thus, once the mother has moved to active labor, your role is to do all you can to not disturb her, and to make certain that no one else does. If all of the above conditions are met regarding privacy, quiet, and dimmed lights, and she is having difficulties, of course you should offer help. But rather than ask questions, use gentle touch and soft words of encouragement. If she is restless, offer to rub her shoulders or lower back. Transmit reassurance through your hands; it will ground her and give her focus.

If the mother complains of nausea, try stimulating the acupressure point known as PC-6, found on the inner wrist. Pressure on this point can also curtail vomiting—apply until she feels better, which may take several minutes. See that she has fresh air and an environment free from distractions.

The mother's position can also affect her comfort. Women who labor undisturbed instinctively know what is best, but again, offer help if indicated. If the baby is low in the pelvis, she may get relief lying on her side with pillow support and lower back massage. If the baby is not yet engaged, an upright and forward-leaning position will maximize the effects of gravity and evenly distribute pressure on the cervix to keep the contractions coordinate and effective. Walking serves the same purpose. If the baby is really high (–2 or –3 station) and posterior, hands-and-knees position with pelvic rocking or standing and leaning forward with one foot on a low stool can encourage rotation. Deep squatting should be avoided, as it closes the inlet.

Positive sensory stimulation via aromatherapy, music, candlelight, or immersion in water can be of great benefit. In fact, once the woman is in active labor,

she can get in the tub any time she likes. The water will help relax her voluntary muscles, which in turn will increase blood flow to the uterus and help it work more efficiently. The sense of weightlessness she finds in the water can increase her immersion in labor, allowing her to feel it through her entire body rather than just in her cervix or back.

If the woman's partner is eager to get involved but at a loss for what to do, give them privacy so they can find a way to work together. Being in the tub may be enjoyable for both of them, or if they feel the need to be up and active, they might put on some music and slow dance. Encourage them to be as intimate as they like, and reassure them that if you need to do an assessment—for example, listen to heart tones—you will knock first and wait for their okay.

Sometimes the atmosphere in the room becomes stale, and a walk outside is in order. A roomful of dozing friends and tired birth attendants can be depress-

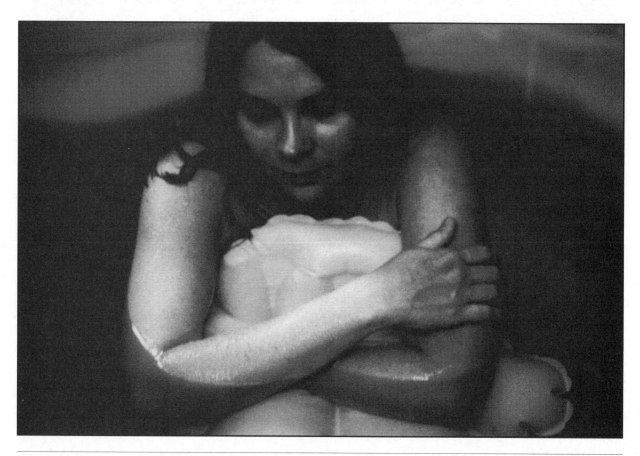

ing for the laboring woman. Clear people out to sleep elsewhere, open windows, fluff the bed, light candles, or serve up some food—all these are good catalysts for stimulating progress.

PHYSICAL ASSESSMENTS AND DUTIES DURING ACTIVE LABOR

What are the midwife's medical duties during active labor? She should **check maternal blood pressure hourly,** or every twenty minutes if it was borderline high in pregnancy or becomes elevated in labor. She must also **see that the mother is well hydrated and urinates hourly.** In fact, encourage the mother to eat as long as possible, drink fruit juice, or take an occasional tablespoon of honey to help prevent clinical exhaustion.

If labor has been prolonged for any length of time—three hours or so without apparent progress—**do a urinalysis to check for ketones.** Ketonuria indicates that the mother is dipping into her fat reserves for energy. A trace reading is acceptable, but higher levels indicate a disrupted electrolyte balance and the need for more fluid and calories. An intravenous solution of Ringer's lactate might be given in the hospital; at home, you can replicate this formula with something called **labor-aide.** Here is the recipe: 1 quart fluid (water), $1/3$ cup honey, $1/3$ cup lemon juice, $1/2$ teaspoon salt, $1/4$ teaspoon baking soda, and 2 crushed calcium tablets. Better yet, have the mother eat whatever she can; even a piece of toast will help immensely.

Take her pulse every few hours; it should stay within ten to fifteen points of her normal range. If it rises, **check her temperature.** Elevation of both combined with ketonuria indicates a level of exhaustion threatening to both mother and baby, for which transport is advisable. Clinical exhaustion is unusual in home birth, where the mother is free to eat and drink as she desires, but can become a problem if the mother has been vomiting and is unable to keep anything down.

Take fetal heart tones (FHT) every half hour. If anything unusual arises, listen continually until the problem resolves spontaneously or treatment is decided upon. To get a full picture of fetal response, always listen throughout a contraction and for fifteen to thirty seconds after it ends. A slight rise to the peak, with a return to baseline by the end, is normal. Labor places circulatory stress on the baby, and just as our heart rate accelerates with exertion, so should the baby's rate accelerate with contractions. Because you must make these assessments of increase and decrease quite rapidly, it helps to listen in six-second increments (easy to multiply by ten).

Heart rate consistently above 160 beats per minute (BPM) is termed **tachycardia.** This is cause for concern, as it may be a sign of fetal infection or maternal exhaustion. The baby's baseline must be considered, though—a rise above 160 BPM is serious for a baby with a baseline of 130 BPM, but if the baby's normal rate is 156 BPM, a rise to 170 BPM could be considered within normal range.

Sometimes FHT dip and bob dramatically during a contraction, with lows below 80 BPM and highs well above 160 BPM, in a pattern we call **variable decelerations (type III).** This is caused by cord entanglement or cord compression, the degree of which varies according to the strength of a contraction and the resulting tension or pressure exerted on the cord. Although not an immediate emergency, serious fetal distress may ensue if variable decelerations are ignored. The solution is quite simple—*have the mother try a new position*. This usually relieves pressure or traction on the cord and brings the FHT back to normal.

There are several more ominous heart rate patterns; one is **flat baseline with no variability** and the other is **late decelerations (type II).** Flat baseline indicates a baby on automatic pilot—the baby's autonomic nervous system cannot adjust its heart rate to the demands of uterine activity. Good variability is considered to be the most important indicator of fetal well-being in labor. You can usually tell if variability is absent without even timing the heartbeat—as one midwife explained, "When the FHT sounds like a metronome, you get an unnatural, creepy sensation." With late decelerations, the FHT is normal through the first part of a contraction but dips down at the peak, slowly returning to baseline as the contraction ends. Late decelerations may be linked to placental insufficiency or maternal ketoacidosis; in any case, there is not enough oxygen reaching the baby to see it through a contraction. If the baby is very compromised, the period of deceleration will extend past the end of the contraction—we call this **poor recovery.** If you pick up either flat baseline or late decelerations during first stage, give the mother oxygen and transport.

As contractions strengthen, it may be difficult to get heart tones throughout, particularly if using a fetascope. This is because the uterus contracts so firmly that it obstructs your ability to hear. But you will be able to listen for fifteen to twenty seconds at the beginning, and again at the peak when the uterus relaxes, and this is sufficient to identify the baby's response pattern. For example, if you hear the heart rate increase at the beginning of a contraction, and then find it at the peak to be noticeably slower, you have detected a late deceleration. Or, if you hear it accelerate at the beginning of a contraction, and find it at the peak to be slightly higher but gradually returning to baseline, this is a normal response.

At this stage of labor, the midwife's most important task is to **pay attention** to maternal and fetal well-being while remaining in the background. On the other hand, some midwives are too little involved, and in the name of nonintervention allow the mother to languish in an ineffectual position or struggle futilely with labor sensations, negatively affecting her strength and self-confidence. Try to find the balance between the mother's need to find her own pace in labor and your need to make responsible assessments and keep things on track.

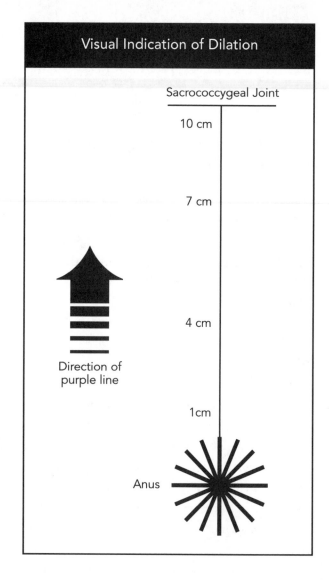

Visual Indication of Dilation

Also remember that the mother may need to slow labor periodically for integration. This is the plateau phenomenon, occurring at 4 cm, 7 cm, or again at 9 cm. Note that each of these is a turning point in terms of new sensation. Four cm marks the challenging transition from control to surrender. At 7 cm, transition contractions can be surprisingly long and overwhelming. Difficulties near full dilation reflect the confusion of bearing-down urges disrupting relaxation. Help the mother through a plateau by understanding its nature and giving her time to collect herself. An arrest of several hours is fine as long as the mother's condition is good, her morale is high, and the baby is doing well.

But if she consistently chooses nondynamic positions in an effort to keep her sensations manageable, remind her with humor that labor is not always comfortable, stronger contractions get the baby born, and she should go on while she still has the energy.

As labor intensifies, do your best to avoid internal exams. A wonderful technique for estimating dilation has recently come to light, based strictly on visual observation of the area immediately above the mother's anus. As she dilates, a dark red line will extend upward and between the cheeks of her buttocks[4] (see diagram "Visual Indication of Dilation" on the opposite page). Many midwives have found this assessment to be quite reliable, plus it supports forward-leaning positions. Or if the mother is upright, you may observe the development of a crease immediately above and parallel to the pubic bone, which will extend fully across the lower abdomen when she is complete.[5] You can also assess descent by observing or palpating the area immediately above the pubic bone—if there is no bulge of head left or you feel shoulders rotating, you can assume the baby is passing through the spines.

Then why do internal exams at all? If the energy of labor feels static—that is, it seems that the mother is dealing with more than a plateau, or if your gut tells

you it is necessary, or if the mother insists—do so for additional information. You may be able to **identify fetal position** and **assess degree of flexion** in addition to the usual evaluations, which can aid your understanding of the mother's labor pattern.

To assess position, the cervix must be dilated to at least 6 cm, or the lower uterine segment thin enough to feel the landmarks of the baby's head, that is, the **sutures** and **fontanelles,** behind it (see "Fetal Skull" diagram, below). Of these, the sagittal suture is generally most prominent as it is most subject to molding; as you sweep your fingers across the surface of the head, it feels like a bony ridge. Follow the suture line and feel for a fontanelle at one end or the other (if the baby is term, only one fontanelle will be in range). If the head is flexed, you will feel the posterior fontanelle; it is the smaller of the two, triangular and about the size of a fingernail. The anterior fontanelle is diamond shaped and more like a thumbnail; if you feel this, the head is deflexed (not uncommon in early labor if the baby is posterior). Based on the way the sagittal suture is running and the location of the fontanelles, you can determine the baby's position.

Certain situations may prevent you from determining the baby's position, such as tight forewaters,

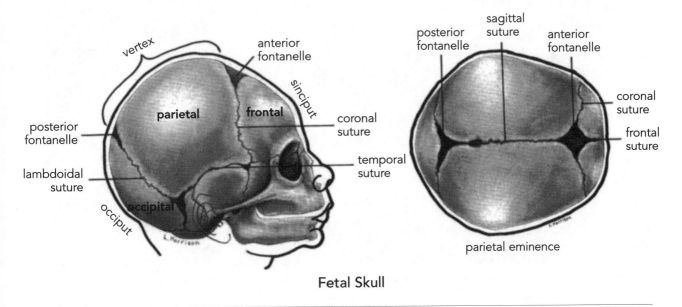

Fetal Skull

or swelling atop the baby's head known as **caput.** Caput indicates head compression and is often associated with extensive moulding; take it as a sign that increased pelvic relaxation is in order. Also note how well the cervix is applied to the head; it should feel smooth against it. If it is loose like an empty sleeve, the head is either mal-presenting or not fitting well into the pelvis (see chapter 5, "Cephalopelvic Disproportion").

You may not be able to get all this information in one exam. If necessary, check again after the next contraction, using a fresh glove. And here is a trick of the trade for beginners—once the cervix has dilated to 6 cm, assess dilation *not by the size of the opening, but by how much cervix is left*. The reason for this is simple: the cervix need not dilate to 10 cm to be fully open for a six-pound baby, whereas one weighing eleven pounds will need more than 10 cm to pass though. Thus, if you feel 2 cm of cervix before reaching vaginal wall, the mother is 8 cm dilated; if you feel just 1 cm, she is dilated to 9.

TRANSITION

Labor intensifies dramatically as the mother reaches a deep level of surrender. Her behavior is characterized by great concentration and quietude, creating the illusion that time has stopped. At this point, attendants may find it difficult to stay alert, particularly if labor has been going on for many hours. This is a good time for the mother's partner to take a break, and for the midwives to spell one another. The mother is usually so immersed in her work that she hardly notices these comings and goings.

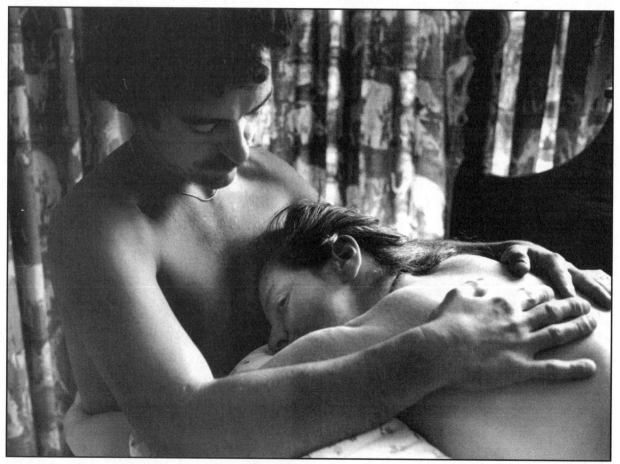

Skin-to-skin contact is tremendously reassuring to the laboring woman.

To observe women at this time is a privilege; most have a certain softness about them as social masks fall away and deep beauty is revealed. The sleepy, faraway place between contractions is reported by many to bring bliss and renewal. Birth attendants must respect this phase of labor for what it is: a peak, out-of-body experience that prepares and rejuvenates the mother for the back-in-the-body, reentry phase of pushing and birthing.

This shifts with transition, the "I can't do this anymore" point near full dilation. It may be heralded by symptoms of restlessness, complaining, shift in focus, or loss of control. The mother should be upright, as maximum pressure on the cervix will speed the last bit

---

Cardinal Spiraling Movements of the Baby during Labor

It is crucial to understand that the baby actively participates in birth; its movements are essential to labor's progress. But because we cannot visualize these, the precise movements the baby makes have been based more or less on speculation. In *Holistic Midwifery (Volume II)*, Anne Frye presents a compilation of fascinating research on this subject, most notably, observations made by X-ray.[6] In light of this, I have revised the standard cardinal movements to her "Cardinal Spiraling Movements of the Baby during Labor," as follows:

1. **Flexion.** Flexion generally occurs as the head enters the pelvic brim. The spine flexes (curves) too, which helps the head flex as much as possible.

2. **Descent.** Descent continues throughout labor due to decreased intrauterine space and pressure exerted at the fundus.

3. **Engagement.** As the widest part of the head clears the pelvic inlet and engages at the ischial spines, increased pressure on the cervix stimulates labor.

4. **Internal rotation of the head.** In response to the oval-shaped musculature of the pelvic floor (not the ischial spines, as was formerly thought), the head rotates to OA or OP, which facilitates passage through the midpelvis.

5. **First internal rotation of the body and shoulders.** The shoulders follow the head and enter the pelvis in the transverse diameter.

6. **Engagement of the shoulders.** As the head descends through the ischial tuberosities, the shoulders engage in the pelvis.

7. **Spinal extension.** As the head moves down, the baby has room to stretch its body so the back becomes less curved.

8. **Second internal rotation of the body and shoulders begins.** As the head begins to distend the perineum, the body rotates to the oblique (usually back to whichever side it was on originally) to negotiate the spines and midpelvis.

9. **Birth of the head by extension of the lower neck and spine.** Pelvic floor muscles hold sinciput and the face back as the head crowns, and extension of the spine further supports flexion. As the head slips past the pubic bone, the perineum retracts around it, and the face is born.

10. **Restitution of the head.** The neck untwists as the head realigns with the shoulders.

11. **Second internal rotation of the shoulders and chest completed.** The shoulders rotate to the antero-posterior diameter.

12. **External rotation of the head.** The head rotates in concert with the shoulders and chest.

13. **Birth of the shoulders and delivery.** The anterior shoulder slips under the pubic bone, and then the posterior shoulder is born first, by lateral flexion of the body.

14. **Birth of the arms, torso, and legs.** The baby slides out in a spiraling motion. This is especially noticeable in water birth, where warm water may trigger primitive reflexes that cause the baby to actively make a spiraling exit.[7] ■

of dilation and prevent edema. Suggest standing, with partner support during contractions. Or she can sit on her heels, leaning forward with knees apart. Squatting with a forward lean (thighs parallel to the floor) is perfect for opening the midpelvis, although it may cause a dramatic increase in sensation. If the mother has an urge to push, suggest a less compelling position, like hands-and-knees (with the hips lower than the shoulders). Avoid advising her not to push, as she may interpret this to mean holding back. Instead, encourage her to listen to her body and do what it tells her to do.

Understand that transition sensations are basically impossible to integrate. Transition means turning point, change—this is not a time of having it all together! Conflicting messages from her body—one of "squeeze and bear down"; the other, "no, it hurts, let go and open"—can completely disrupt the mother's concentration. Convey your understanding of this, and she may feel easier about expressing awkward or explosive emotions. It is especially important now to watch her body language—make sure her shoulders and neck are loose and relaxed and that her focus is low in her body.

PHYSICAL ASSESSMENTS AND DUTIES IN TRANSITION

Whenever there is a marked shift in the strength of contractions, check fetal heart tones more frequently to see how the baby is adjusting. The FHT should be assessed every twenty minutes. Your surveillance of the mother remains about the same, with attention to her fluid intake and elimination. Help her get a sip of tea or water as each contraction ends and before she slips away (bendable straws make this easier). Your most challenging task at this point is to avoid disrupting her comfort and concentration. For example, she may have to lean back slightly in order for you to obtain clear fetal heart tones with your fetascope, which can be rather disorienting. If you have a Doppler, you may wish to use it now.

The membranes often rupture spontaneously as contractions intensify. What should you do if you find the fluid stained with meconium? This depends on the color and consistency of the fluid: **old meconium** creates a yellow tinge, and is evidence of a brief episode of hypoxia much earlier in labor or in the days preceding it; **fresh meconium** is particulate and green or brown like pea soup, indicative of recent or current fetal distress. With fresh meconium, immediately listen to fetal heart tones for several contractions, tracking even the slightest deviation from normal. Unless the baby sounds absolutely perfect, with a healthy acceleration response to each and every contraction, consider transport. Particularly if this is a first baby, the mother's second stage could be somewhat prolonged, exacerbating any underlying causes of fetal distress and meconium in the water.

With the unrelenting rhythm of contractions, don't forget to keep track of the mother's progress. But if you can tell by her breathing and expression (or the dark red line) that she is moving ahead, forgo an internal exam. Particularly when a first-time mother says, "I have to push," try to assess by external signs only. Why avoid an internal exam at this point? According to midwife Gloria Lemay, "First, because it is excruciating for the mother. Second, because it disturbs a delicate point where the body is making many fine adjustments and the woman is accessing a very primitive part of her ancient brain. Third, because it [creates] performance anxiety . . . that can muddy primip [first labor] birth waters."[8] If the mother pushes only at the peak of contractions, or with every other one, she still has some dilating to do.

On the other hand, if this is a second or subsequent birth, the mother will probably make a smooth transition from dilating to pushing, and the baby could come quickly. Prepare by **straightening up the room and clearing the floor area** (crucial in the event of an emergency). Make sure there are no open flames or lit candles, in case you need to run your oxygen. Remove blankets from the bed and set them aside so they do not get bloodied or wet (a good idea even if the birth is to be in the tub, as circumstances may change at the last minute). If you are assisting alone, here is a tip from an experienced midwife: place several strips of masking tape on your pant legs to make notes in case of emergency. This saves you from having to fumble with the chart or worry about getting it dirty.

Scrub up well with Betadine or other soapy antiseptic, using a nailbrush and working well up your forearms. Then **set up for delivery,** laying out a disposable underpad or sterile towel on which you place your tray of instruments, bulb syringe, and DeLee suction device, extra pairs of long cuffed gloves, four-by-four sterile pads, and, if she is not birthing in the tub, a bowl of hot water (with a squirt of Betadine added) for perineal compresses. Tear off the tops of the gauze pads so you can reach them without handling the outside wrapper. Have syringes and medications for controlling hemorrhage (pitocin and methergine) readily accessible, and herbal or homeopathic remedies close at hand. Set up your oxygen and resuscitation unit (if you have not done so already). Have the mother's supplies (washcloths, baby blankets, and towels) laid out, as well as a bowl for the placenta.

Setting up during transition is also wise if the mother has a small baby and generous pelvis, or if either the current or previous labors have been precipitous. And one last but critical point—*make certain that the mother urinates before entering second stage.* A full bladder can hinder descent and lead to postpartum hemorrhage.

SECOND STAGE

Second stage begins when the cervix is, at last, fully dilated. Typically, contractions ease from the back-to-back intensity of transition and become further apart. If labor has been long or difficult to this point, the mother may even have a time-out and get some sleep as her uterus rests and regroups for the work ahead. This should be encouraged, as stimulating the uterus at this point can lead to problems later, not the least of which is postpartum hemorrhage.

In order to assist a woman in second stage, we must understand what is occurring physiologically. According to midwife Jean Sutton, a key role is played by the **rhombus of Michaelis,** a kite-shaped area of the lower spine with points at the waist, coccyx, and sacroiliac joints. This area has the potential to open dramatically in second stage, increasing the front-to-back dimensions of the pelvis by several centimeters. But this can only happen if the mother is leaning forward with her knees lower than her hips—kneeling and resting her upper body against something, or sitting on the toilet or a birth stool with legs extended. In this position, the back of the baby's head contacts the G-spot, which triggers the sacrum to open. As this occurs, the mother will instinctively (1) grab forward for support, (2) spread her knees apart and let her belly sag, and (3) arch her back and wriggle her lower body.[9] This series of movements, which Michel Odent has termed the **fetus ejection reflex,** brings the baby down.[10] Corroborating this, Sheila Kitzinger has reported that Jamaican midwives believe a baby will not be born until the mother "opens her back."[11]

When a woman lets go this way and gets a strong, spontaneous urge to push, she will probably feel relief and excitement at moving from passive surrender to active participation. This is the most striking energetic shift in labor, the time when the mother's identity and body consciousness return anew, accompanied by bursts of energy and enthusiasm. On the other hand, if the mother struggles with her first pushing urges, remind her to relax her shoulders, or massage them to release tension in her chest and throat. Encourage her to make sounds, too ("Let it out, and keep breathing"). Some women make loud, moose-like bellowing noises with each exhale, but whatever sounds the mother makes, suggest she keep her throat open. She may well scream out with her first involuntary pushing urge, as a natural rush of adrenaline is released at this point. Just make sure her jaw is relaxed. And keep in mind that the feeling of a baby's head pushing through the vagina is some incredible stimulation! Give her your gutsy appreciation, and do your best to help her settle into her sensation.

Debate on the best method of pushing should be over and done with by now. The hospital convention of forced, sustained bearing down has been linked to fetal bradycardia, increased episiotomy rates, and need for neonatal resuscitation.[12] Jean Sutton notes that in New Zealand, before forced pushing became the norm, women in hospital almost always gave birth in left-lateral position, which at least allowed the back to open.[13] In contrast, semirecumbent or supine positions favored in hospital today do just the opposite.

If the mother is free to assume a physiologic position when second stage begins, her pushing efforts will be sensitive and variable according to what each contraction demands. This helps her conserve energy while assuring maximum oxygen flow to the baby. As long as the baby is fine, the mother should

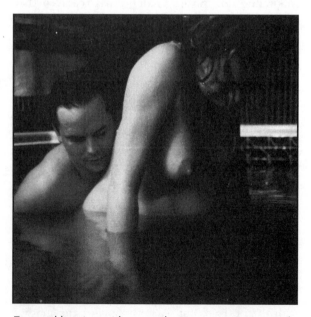

Forward leaning with second stage contractions and partner support.

set the pace. Contractions usually vary in intensity until the head is at +2 station; after this, pressure on the pelvic floor and the urge to push remain fairly constant contraction to contraction.

It is important to appreciate what is happening with the baby too. During labor, fetal catecholamines (noradrenaline and adrenaline) rise to prepare the baby for the challenging transitions at birth. Head compression intensifies catecholamine release, particularly of noradrenaline, which helps protect the baby from asphyxia by bringing more blood to the heart, brain, adrenals, and placenta. Endorphin levels rise too, which help offset the potential negative effects of soaring adrenalines. In other words, just as the mother is primed for birth by vaginal stimulation and increased oxytocin, the baby is also stimulated and prepared.

When the head first begins to show, ask the mother to blow through (pant with) a contraction. This will enable you to see how rapidly descent is taking place, while giving her a chance to try this technique before the actual moments of delivery when it is much harder to integrate. If she pants through a contraction and there is no descent, it may be a while before the birth. She may wish to get up, move around, or assume a new position. But if the baby moves dramatically in spite of minimal efforts on the mother's part, get ready!

If there is an arrest of progress at this point, or if the mother is tightening up involuntarily with pushing, it is probably because she is overwhelmed. Under these circumstances, Valerie El Halta has suggested this surprisingly effective remedy: have the mother get in knees-chest position. Although this may seem counterproductive, it eases pressure on the head, which can then complete its accommodations to the pelvis without undue stress from the vaginal muscles. With this, it is not uncommon for the head to suddenly descend to the perineum, and the mother can resume an upright position.[14]

PHYSICAL ASSESSMENTS AND DUTIES DURING SECOND STAGE

Depending on the position and size of the baby, the mother's pelvic dimensions and internal muscle tone, and whether this is a first or subsequent birth, second stage can be a breeze or rather trying for the baby. The greater the degree of head compression, the more likely the baby is to be compromised. To assess this, check the FHT every few contractions, during and immediately after each ends. Once the head is on the pelvic floor, listen with every contraction. Babies do have their limits if subjected to hours of extreme head compression, so listen well and often, and stay focused on facilitating progress. Strong pushing is seldom the answer, but change in position, deeper breathing, or greater relaxation can help.

Typically, head compression causes **early decelerations (type I).** With this pattern, fetal heart tones decelerate as the contraction begins, reach a low point as it peaks, and return to baseline as it ends (in other words, mirror the contraction). In the early part of second stage, dips of ten points are considered normal. Dips of twenty points are not uncommon with perineal dilation, nor are occasional dips to 80 BPM as birth approaches. But consistent dips to 60 BPM will render the baby hypoxic before long, and thus necessitate immediate delivery or transport if the birth is not imminent.

As important as the severity of the dip is recovery as the contraction ends. If recovery is poor, **bradycardia** may result. Moderate bradycardia (FHT above 100 BPM) is considered normal in second stage, but severe bradycardia (FHT below 100) necessitates quick delivery or immediate transport. For either bradycardia or severe early decelerations, give the mother oxygen by mask, six liters per minute.

A pattern of early decelerations is unusual before the head reaches the pelvic floor, and may be due to extreme muscle tension linked to a history of sexual abuse (known or unknown). The mother manifesting this pattern usually becomes agitated; if so, let her know she is safe. Suggest an upright position, perhaps standing so she can move freely and feel more in control. Help her with pelvic relaxation techniques, position change, and breathing through contractions. Do not be frightened if she panics; help her move through this.

On the other hand, a prominent sacral vertebra or sharp ischial spine can also cause head compression by reducing the midpelvis. Once the head gets past this point, heart tones should return to normal. If you suspect disproportion between the baby's head and the mother's pelvis, see chapter 5, "Cephalopelvic Disproportion," for suggestions.

Variable decelerations can also occur in second stage, indicating cord nipping, pinching, or entanglement. Occasionally, cord sounds (swishing at the same rate as the FHT) are heard in the vicinity of the baby's torso. If the head is still high, have the mother change position. But if the head is well down, listen constantly and be prepared for cord around the neck with clamps and scissors open and readily accessible.

Sometimes the first strong pushes cause the membranes to rupture. If you find the water stained with meconium but heart tones are normal, do not panic. Be ready to do a gentle but thorough suctioning of the baby's mouth and throat with a DeLee trap (plastic tubing with a catch compartment) as soon as the head is born and before the body delivers. This is important, as meconium aspiration may cause neonatal pneumonia (see "Meconium Aspiration" in chapter 6).

In case of **prolonged second stage**—more than two hours of urge-to-push contractions—have the mother take ample fluids and tablespoons of honey to boost her energy. If there is no physical impediment to progress and her emotional state is good, be patient. She may become quite tired, though, and so should be encouraged to rest completely between efforts.

At the other end of the spectrum is **precipitous delivery.** Particularly if the mother has given birth several times within the past few years, one push may bring the head to the perineum, and the next, the entire baby from head to toe! Far from being the boon it appears, a short, vigorous second stage can cause postpartum hemorrhage. The mother misses the integration of pushing and may struggle to greet her baby while in a state of emotional shock. If you anticipate a precipitous delivery, suggest a hands-and-knees or side-lying position during transition so second stage will commence more slowly. This may give the mother a few more moments to integrate her sensations, and you, a bit more time to prepare for the birth.

ASSISTING DELIVERY

Delivery positions should be discussed prenatally, as many women have definite ideas and preferences. The most popular positions are hands-and-knees, kneeling, squatting, or standing. The supine position is contrary to the laws of gravity and bad for the baby, due to compression of the maternal vena cava and reduced blood flow to the placenta. Side-lying with one leg raised can reduce strain on the perineum, which is important with a history of deep perineal scarring or precipitous delivery. Hands-and-knees is particularly good for mothers with big babies, or for those who have pushed for a long time with the head low. Squatting or standing allow the mother to see what is going on, and touch or lift the baby up as it is being born.

The mother may instinctively choose a position just as the birth is about to occur, so it is best to be ready for anything. One mother recalled pushing happily in hands-and-knees throughout second stage, until her midwife insisted she switch to semi-sit for delivery. Perhaps the midwife had never assisted a woman in hands-and-knees, but the mother felt quite disoriented by the change and believed that her subsequent loss of control and extensive tearing with the birth were due to this last-minute shuffle. Every midwife should visualize and prepare to assist birth in a variety of positions, so she can comfortably follow the mother's lead.

Once the birth is imminent, the time of utmost concentration has arrived. No matter how many births a midwife has attended, there can be nothing matter-of-fact about assisting at this sacred moment, especially if she lets her participation be guided by love. Every birthing is unique! There are skills for making it run smoothly, but the midwife's main responsibility is to open fully and respond with devotion. Not only is she an assistant to the mother and her supporters, but handmaiden to the forces of creation.

One of the hallmarks of midwifery care is trauma-free, tear-free delivery. Although approaches to preventing tears are many, nothing takes the place of a mother's internal awareness in easing her baby out. That said, perhaps the most helpful and appreciated technique for preventing tears is the **application of hot compresses to the perineum** (unless, of course, the

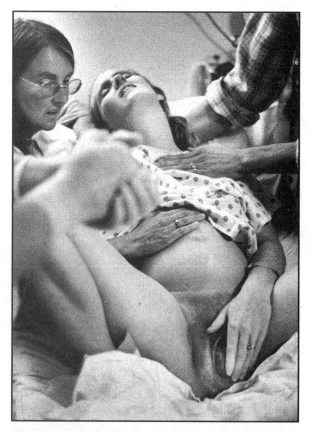
The magical wonder of touching your baby for the first time.

woman is birthing in water). Hot compresses stimulate·circulation, promote relaxation, and provide relief from burning at maximum stretch. Use sterile gauze pads or clean washcloths soaked in hot water with a squeeze of Betadine or other antiseptic agent. Hot compresses can help a mother involuntarily contracting her outlet muscles to relax and focus and are crucial if the perineum blanches with descent. Rarely, pressure of the head on the rectum may cause the mother to pass fecal matter. Wipe with tissue, and if your gauze pad or washcloth becomes contaminated, immediately replace it with another.

As you attend to the mother's perineum, remember to check the FHT. Early decels to 60 BPM or severe bradycardia indicate that the baby should be born at once. Inform the mother that she must get the baby out quickly, and that you need her full attention and cooperation. Tell her to let go completely and follow your lead on when to push. Sometimes this advice is enough to dissolve the last bit of resistance, and the baby births spontaneously with the next contraction.

Otherwise, you may need to do an **episiotomy.** This is an extreme measure, not to be undertaken lightly. But if the mother has tried her hardest to get the baby out and it is crashing, it is your only option. In terms of timing, an episiotomy should be performed only if the perineum is stretched to at least half of its capacity, but the head is not yet crowning. Inform the mother of the situation and obtain her consent. As a contraction ends, position two fingers inside the perineum to protect the head, insert scissors between them and, as the next contraction brings the head forward, cut straight down about an inch. At this late stage, the episiotomy should cause little bleeding, but apply pressure with a gauze pad if necessary. The tissues will be vulnerable to tearing beyond the apex, so give counterpressure and support to the base of the wound. (Note that lidocaine infiltration is optional as the perineum is quite numb by now, but you may wish to infiltrate the area if there is time— see "Suturing Technique" in chapter 5.)

To return to the normal sequence: note that as the baby nears crowning, it may be difficult to get heart tones with a fetascope. As it moves lower still, heart tones may become inaudible. This coincides with perineal stretching, which usually lasts for just a few contractions but sometimes takes longer. You can use your Doppler at this point, but there is another indicator of fetal well-being you can use as well—**the color of the baby's scalp.** Once, while attending a hospital delivery, I heard the obstetrician say, "I'll hang my hat on pink scalps." Pinkish-blue is good, blue is less favorable, and white-blue is ominous. The rate of venous return when the scalp is gently depressed is also significant. Both these assessments indicate how much oxygen the baby is getting.

As long as the baby is doing well, the heart tones are fine, and the scalp color is reassuring, you can relax and wait for the birth. As the head distends the perineum, have the mother breathe lightly and remind her to keep releasing down and out. If she complains of the burning or tingling characteristic of extreme stretching, tell her to pant.

Another critical factor in avoiding tears is **maintaining flexion** of the baby's head. If the mother is taking her time and is birthing in an upright position, pelvic floor muscles promote this automatically. But if the head is at all deflexed or the baby is coming quickly, **apply counterpressure** to the perineum when crowning begins, holding back the forehead so the smallest possible diameter passes through. (If the baby is OP, reverse these maneuvers.) Take care not to push toward the urethra, or tears in this sensitive area may result. Particularly if the head is large or is crowning rapidly, **guard the urethral area** by positioning the wrist of your free hand by the pubic bone, extending your fingers down across the head to **control the rate of expulsion.**

If in spite of all this, if the perineum blanches and a tear appears inevitable, have the mother **push the head out between contractions**—she will feel more

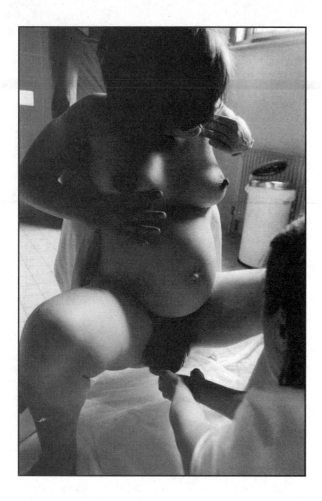

needs to be birthed quickly, and one that may need some help getting started. Wipe excessive amounts of blood and mucus or meconium away from the eyes, nose, and mouth (this is usually not necessary if the baby is born underwater). If the baby is gurgling or choking with respiratory efforts, suction with a large rubber ear syringe. Squeeze all the air out first, and insert no more than a few inches or you will stimulate the gag reflex at the back of the baby's throat, which can suppress its attempts to breathe.

Suction on the perineum is considered mandatory if the baby has passed meconium in labor (which would also preclude water birth). However, a recent study of two thousand infants with meconium staining, randomized to be suctioned or not, showed no significant differences in outcome between the two groups, suggesting that meconium aspiration (MAS) is probably caused by an earlier incident of severe depression in utero.[15]

Nonetheless, suction on the perineum is standard of care. It is definitely a good idea if it appears that the baby may need resuscitation. Use a DeLee trap for this. Check to see that the lid is screwed on tightly so the device will work properly, then insert the tubing about four and a half inches into the baby's mouth. Withdraw slowly while sucking sharply and repeatedly (see illustration on "Using the DeLee Mucus Trap," opposite page). Tell the mother not to push, and have your assistant hold the shoulders back until you are finished. If you are still bringing up meconium as you remove the tubing, repeat the procedure.

Next, **check around the neck for the umbilical cord.** Slip your finger (pad side out) along the back of the baby's neck, and if you find cord simply pull it over the head. If there is not enough slack to slip it over the head, try making a loop large enough for the shoulders and body to birth through. If there is not enough slack for this, tuck the baby's face against the mother's thigh and support the body as it somersaults out. If none of these is possible because the cord is double-looped or

relaxed and in control, and your efforts will be more successful without the added force of contractions.

Very rarely, an arrest occurs in the perineal phase. The head appears ready to birth with the next contraction, yet no progress occurs for ten, fifteen, even twenty minutes. This may be due to muscle tension associated with sexual abuse, a very big baby, or unconscious resistance caused (ironically enough) by the fear of tearing. Whatever the cause, **help the mother feel the baby's head.** This often brings a moan of surrender, and birth soon follows. If she doesn't want to touch the baby, **arrange a mirror so she can see the head.** Or have her push between contractions, for more control.

As soon as the baby's head is out, do a quick appraisal of color and presence. Note the vitality level of the baby. Look for signs of stress: a white-blue head with a clenched mouth usually indicates a baby that has no slack whatsoever, you must cut it. This should only be done in dire necessity, as cord blood is vital to newborn stabilization. Tell the mother not to push, and have your assistant hold the shoulders back. Clamp the cord with two curved hemostats placed several inches apart, cut between them using blunt scissors, and unwind the cord from the neck. You have now cut off the baby's oxygen supply, so it must be born immediately.

Otherwise, there is no need to hurry delivery of the shoulders as long as the baby's color is good. But if the head becomes suffused with blood (turns purplish), encourage the mother to push the baby out at once (see " Shoulder Dystocia" in chapter 5).

To **assist the birth of the shoulders and body:**

1. If the mother is semi-reclining or deep-squatting, make your hand into a bowl shape and gently hold the perineum until the anterior shoulder appears, then lift to a forty-five-degree angle so the posterior shoulder can birth without causing a tear. Once the shoulders are out, encourage the mother to reach down and bring the baby out.

2. If the mother is on hands-and-knees or kneeling forward, reverse the above directions and pass the baby through her legs or help her turn over to receive it.

3. If the mother is standing, kneel beneath her and make your hand into a C-shape (fingers toward her pubic bone, thumb at perineum) and place around the back of the baby's head. In this position, your palm holds the perineum until the anterior shoulder appears, then your entire hand lifts the shoulders toward the mother as the other reaches up to support the body.

Once the baby's body is exposed to air, cover immediately with three flannel blankets (preferably oven-warmed) to maintain its temperature. The two essentials for stabilizing the newborn are **warmth** and a **clear airway.** Make certain the baby is breathing well—if so, its color will be good; if not, suction and stimulate by rubbing its back. Promptly change the first set of blankets, which are usually dampened with fluid. Help the mother get comfortably positioned so

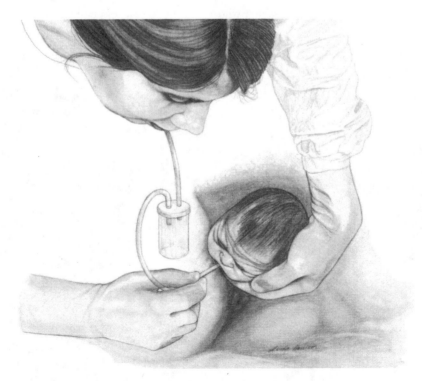

Using the DeLee Mucus Trap

that she and the baby can fully relax. See that she is warm and has something sweet to drink, then ease back and give the new family a chance to bond. Keep an eye on the baby's color and responsiveness, and don't forget to do Apgar scores at one and five minutes (see appendix H).

These are the mechanics of spontaneous delivery. But every birth is unique, depending on how passionately the mother has labored, how alert or tired she feels, and how happy she is to be having this baby. For the woman who has really found her way with labor, the moments of giving birth are a time of complete concentration and focus. The pressure of the head on vaginal nerve endings causes overwhelming sensation. And what a release as the head is born! Then, as the body surges out, the mother feels the exquisite details of her baby's form, followed by waves of relief. Some call this the orgasm of birthing.

And yet, as the baby emerges, sudden emptiness can come as a bit of a shock. It is of greatest importance that the mother has access to her baby at once, so this shock does not deepen into numbness that will hinder her ability to bond. The practice of removing the baby for suctioning and cleaning also disrupts its need for immediate contact with its mother. No exceptions to this—even the baby born "floppy" should be lifted onto the mother for stimulation or resuscitation.

On the other hand, I used to rush the baby into the mother's arms, but I have now stopped doing so for several reasons. First, I noticed that women who birthed in a deep squat, with the baby coming directly onto blankets beneath them, took a few moments before picking up their babies. Similarly, mothers giving birth in the water generally touch and examine their babies a bit before holding them close. Then I watched Dr. Lennart Righard's video, *Delivery Self Attachment,* in which a just born baby placed on its mother's abdomen instinctively crawled to her nipple and latched on without help![16] Therapist Raymond Castellino postulates that our rush to put the baby in its mother's arms and get it nursing as soon as possible may come from our own unresolved birth traumas.[17] Why not place the baby on the mother's belly and allow it to come to her, or let her lift and embrace it when she is ready?

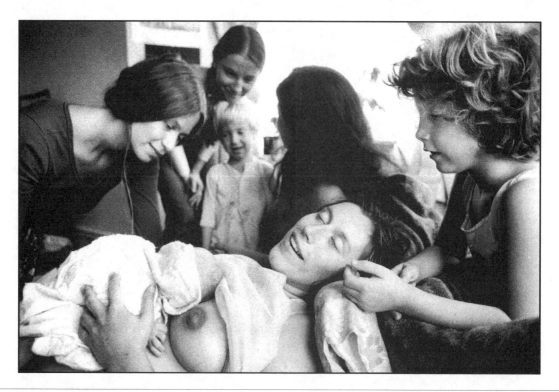

Herbs and Homeopathy during Labor

by Shannon Anton, CPM

Most labors do not require the assistance or intervention of herbal or homeopathic allies. However, some labor circumstances can be aided by a skilled attendant utilizing these remedies appropriately. This support is offered primarily to preserve the precious energy of the laboring woman.

Early Labor

If early labor is intense like transition, with contractions three minutes apart (and especially if the woman is shivering), try homeopathic **Cimicifuga** 200C. Labor may seem to diminish but is finding a more effective pattern. This support greatly preserves the woman's vital forces. If not yet regular, but unrelenting and not given to rest, promote regular contractions with homeopathic **Caulophyllum** 200C.

If on again, off again in nature, and especially if the woman is more whiny and clingy than usual, or needs a lot of validation that what she feels is emotionally normal, try homeopathic **Pulsitilla** 200C.

Active Labor

If one in which the woman appears to be scrambling away from herself and her contractions, try homeopathic **Sepia 200C.** If the cervix is 100 percent effaced, about 3 cm dilated, the os feels like a loop of thread, and labor appears very active or transitional, prepare for the birth as if it was imminent and give homeopathic **Gelsimium** 200C. Frequently, the cervix eases open to complete dilation. If the woman is not yet fully dilated but feels an urge to push, give **Arnica** 200C to prevent cervical swelling.

If there is a strong urge to push at only 6 to 7 cm dilation, or there is a cervical lip, try homeopathic **Sepia** 200C and **Arnica** 200C, followed by Sepia 200C every ten to fifteen minutes. I rely on these remedies absolutely and find them to be among the best kept secrets of homeopathy for labor.

If dehydration or exhaustion occur, consider homeopathic **China** or **Carbo Veg,** or **Ustilago** 200C. In addition, an enema of warm water and **honey,** or a dose of **royal jelly** taken orally can

greatly revive for the short term. Another good remedy is **Essence of Chicken,** found in Asian groceries and apothecaries.

Second Stage

If during second stage, contractions come less and less often, give homeopathic **Caulophyllum** 200C to keep labor going and to prevent postpartum hemorrhage. Each dose should have a noticeable effect. Repeat as necessary to establish a regular pattern of contractions. Homeopathic **Aconite** is invaluable for helping women release fear or anxiety in labor. However, not all women benefit from crying or talking out their feelings; some are truly more internal in their process of release. Aconite 200C supports quietude and letting go.

Homeopathic **Arnica** is excellent when pain in labor seems out of proportion to the strength of contractions. Arnica can also render contractions more regular and effective. If the cervix is unyielding or swollen, Arnica 200C can alleviate irritation and reduce swelling. I give Arnica 200C to most mothers in my practice as soon as they feel bearing down urges in second stage, dosing again as soon as possible after the baby is born. I rarely see swelling of the perineum postpartum. I suggest that my clients continue to take Arnica 30C for the first few days postpartum for soreness and body fatigue.

The Immediate Postpartum

I rely on two herbs during third stage: **Angelica** and **Shepherd's Purse.** I carry both in tincture form and keep them next to my pitocin. I find these herbs sufficient to handle most blood loss following birth. In case of sudden, torrential hemorrhage, I give an IM injection of pitocin as well as the appropriate herb. In some instances, I am sure it was the herb that stopped the bleeding, as the pitocin would not yet have had time to enter the mother's circulation. Nonetheless, with any dramatic blood loss, I give both.

continued →

Angelica tincture helps bring the placenta when the wait is prolonged. I give a dropperful under the tongue with a swig of water following. Remind yourself (and the mother) that Angelica brings the placenta "like an angel." Use also for partial separation of the placenta.

Shepherd's Purse tincture is best used after the placenta is out and you are certain it is complete. Because it promotes clotting so expertly, Shepherd's Purse can cause clots to form immediately as the placenta separates, which may lead to uterine distension and additional blood loss. If you are not sure the placenta is complete, use Angelica to bring on more contractions.

If you are confronted with a vaginal tear that has ruptured a small vessel, apply direct pressure to the tear and give a dropperful of **Trillium,** or Birthroot tincture. Trillium constricts small blood vessels and works perfectly in this application. You may find it unnecessary to tie off the vessel with suture.

NEWBORN RESUSCITATION: HOMEOPATHIC REMEDIES

While CPR and oxygen are essential, homeopathy is always appropriate and sometimes critical in newborn resuscitation. Ifeoma Ikenze, pediatrician and homeopath, taught me most of these applications. In my experience, their potency has been lifesaving. I keep these remedies near my drug box, with red labels to make them easily identifiable. To give a remedy to a newborn, tuck one pellet in the cheek of the baby's mouth. A dose is assimilated by contact with the mucous membranes. In critical situations, repeat the dose in a minute or two. I have never heard of a baby aspirating a homeopathic remedy, even with use of an ambu-bag.

Respiratory arrest. If there are minimal or no respiratory attempts, and the baby looks bluish or feels slightly cold, give **Carbo Veg** 1M.

Circulatory collapse. If the baby is pale as a ghost, floppy, cold, or weak, give **Camphora** 1M.

Weak heart rate. If the baby appears lifeless and pale, with no respirations, give **Arsenicum** 1M.

Mucus or wet lungs. If the baby is gray-blue, choking or gurgling, if suction does not clear mucus, or if the lungs sound moist and sticky, give **Anti-monium** 200C. Dose and repeat, along with percussion. Consider blow-by oxygen or steam from the shower. **Aconitum** 1M is for the baby that is struggling and warm, perhaps crying inconsolably as if from a great fright, with rapid heart rate and respirations, and color red, not blue. This baby appears to be shocked by the abruptness of birth and may have difficulty integrating all the stimuli. Another solution is **Rescue Remedy,** given orally or on the soles of the baby's feet. **Arnica** 200C is a wonderful remedy for extreme molding or caput. If the mother chooses not to give vitamin K, homeopathic Arnica is appropriate.

MATERNAL DIFFICULTY WITH URINATION

A new mother may have difficulty urinating immediately after birth. It's important to make sure she is able to empty her bladder, as a distended bladder can interfere with her uterus staying contracted. Her bladder may also be injured if it becomes too distended. Homeopathic **Arnica** 200C can help reduce swelling of the urethra. Also try turning off the lights, dribbling water in the sink, having her put her hands or feet in warm water, or putting a few drops of **Peppermint oil** in the toilet before she tries to urinate. Give her privacy but make sure she has support should she become faint. Keep in mind that Peppermint oil will antidote any homeopathic remedies she has taken. This is usually fine, but if using homeopathic Arnica, dose again after she's settled back into bed.

FAINTING IN THE IMMEDIATE POSTPARTUM

Giving birth creates incredible changes in a woman's body. Getting to her feet, or even sitting upright, can cause dizziness and fainting. If so, place her in shock position and try this old, reliable but strange remedy: **burnt hair.** Take a lock of hair from her partner or closest relative present. Burn the hair to cinders and place the crunchy bits under her tongue. Believe it or not, this will stabilize her dramatically. Some women benefit from a pinch of the **placenta** under the tongue. You may want to try a dose of **Rescue Remedy.** Or, using a soft bristled brush, stroke from her feet to her knees, then from her knees to her hips. Strong **black tea** will also help normalize her circulation. ■

THIRD STAGE

As soon as the baby is stable, the mother will want to rest. A drop in adrenaline levels moments after the birth makes it difficult for her to stay upright. This is fine but continue to attend her until third stage is completed, that is, the placenta is delivered. (Note: If the mother is not kept warm, adrenaline will remain high, which can disrupt placental separation by opposing oxytocin.)

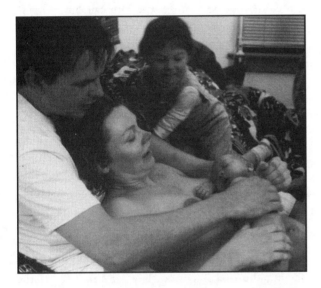

The key to a safe and uncomplicated third stage is **watchful observation.** Many a bonding period has been disrupted by an overzealous midwife intent on getting the placenta out as soon as possible. Then again, many a hemorrhage has been precipitated by a nonattentive attendant missing signs of concealed placental separation. Watchful observation means exactly that: the midwife's participation is indicated by key signs and signals rather than by rote.

The umbilical cord should not be cut until it has stopped pulsing. If there happens to be a true knot, loosen it for maximum blood flow. Cord blood stimulates lung function and provides critical perfusion in the brain and other vital organs during the baby's transition to breathing. Some midwives feel that keeping the cord intact until the placenta has birthed prompts the mother to remember that her work is not yet completed.

Or perhaps this is to be a **lotus birth,** in which the cord will not be cut at all (placenta and baby are kept together until, several days later, the cord dries and detaches).

If the cord is to be cut before the placenta is birthed, make certain it has stopped pulsing completely (check the base where it joins the baby), then place one clamp near the mother's vagina and the other about eight inches away. Have her, her partner, other family member, or your assistant cut between the clamps, several inches from the one nearest the baby.

Now, watch for **signs of placental separation.** If the cord has been cut, keep an eye on the clamp nearest the mother; it will move downward as the placenta detaches, and the cord will appear to lengthen. Also watch for excessive bleeding. In general, there is very little blood loss until the characteristic gush-flow of placental separation. Rarely, the placenta separates only in the center, with no blood evident at the outlet because margins remain attached. The uterus will then increase in size and become boggy, and if the mother continues to bleed, she may go into shock. To rule out a concealed separation, rest a hand on the fundus as soon as the baby is out, and keep it there until the placenta delivers. This is known as **guarding the uterus.** Do not massage or prod, as this can result in partial separation and hemorrhage. In other words, no "fundus fiddling"; keep your hand still.

I recently taught a workshop on third stage to midwives in London, where physiologic birth has become all the rage. Several participants complained that in spite of doing "everything right," i.e., hands off the woman while waiting for the placenta, several of their clients had gone into shock from concealed bleeding. This happened because the midwives had been taught that guarding the uterus was too invasive. I say, let common sense be our guide—guarding the uterus can be done with great subtlety, and the information provided by this procedure can be lifesaving.

ASSISTING PLACENTAL DELIVERY

The placenta usually delivers twenty to thirty minutes after the birth, although it may take an hour or more. Nine times out of ten, it separates all at once. As you notice the cord lengthening, the mother may look at you a bit anxiously, reporting that she feels "something." This is an opportune time for her to squat, as delivery of the placenta is best accomplished with the mother in an upright position. If she is too exhausted and does not feel like moving, you can assist her. Encourage her to focus on getting the placenta out, and ask her to push.

Standard of care in hospital is to use **controlled cord traction** to get the placenta out. But beware: If the placenta is not separated and you pull on the cord, you run the risk of **inverting the uterus** (that is, turning it inside out), which could kill the mother. If you wish to use cord traction to assist the placenta out, you must first make sure it is fully separated by donning a clean glove and gently **following the cord to the cervical os.** *Only if the placenta is immediately behind the cervical opening (or in the vagina), may you use controlled cord traction to remove it.*

To perform controlled cord traction, hold the uterus in place by pressing the edge of your hand in above the pubic bone and up toward the mother's head. As you apply traction to the cord, guide the placenta along the L-shaped curve of the birth canal—first down and then out. Do this when the uterus is contracted and with the mother's pushing efforts.

Sometimes separation occurs just moments after the birth, but the membranes remain adherent until the placenta drops to the cervix and its weight detaches them completely. If the placenta is born but the membranes are lagging (rare if the mother squats), coax them out by holding the placenta with both hands and moving it in a give-and-take motion. Or twist the placenta around repeatedly so that the membranes form a rope, then coax outward. Should the mother happen to be standing when the placenta comes, it is important to support it as it delivers, for membranes may shred or tear if they are not yet separated and the placenta is allowed to fall any distance.

The placenta may deliver either fetal or maternal side first. If the fetal side presents, we call this **separation by the Shultz mechanism.** This correlates to fundal implantation of the placenta with separation beginning at the center. If the maternal side presents, we call this **separation by the Duncan mechanism.** This correlates to low implantation of the placenta with separation starting at the edges. Students often remember these distinctions with slang terms: *shiny Shultz* (glossy membranes) and *dirty Duncan* (meaty maternal side).

As soon as the placenta is out, check immediately to be certain the uterus is well contracted, and give it a few quick squeezes to expel any clots that may have formed behind the placenta (this is unnecessary if the mother is in a squat, as internal organs naturally compress the fundus). Continue to maintain watchful observation, keeping an eye out for any bleeding and feeling the uterus periodically for firmness. If the uterus feels soft or asymmetrical in shape, or excess bleeding is noted, rub up a good contraction and encourage the mother to nurse the baby. You might also give her several droppers of shepherd's purse and blue cohosh tinctures.

Slow trickle bleeding must be watched very carefully. Make sure the mother's bladder is not distended, as this can interfere with the uterus clamping down. Another potential cause of bleeding is **retained placental fragments**—examine the placenta thoroughly to be sure it is complete. You can do this right at the bedside, while you keep watch on the mother.

First examine the maternal side of the placenta, which is comprised of lobes called **cotyledons.** Start by pulling away any clots, then hold the placenta in your hands so that it opens convexly, exposing the rents between cotyledons clearly. Then cup it together

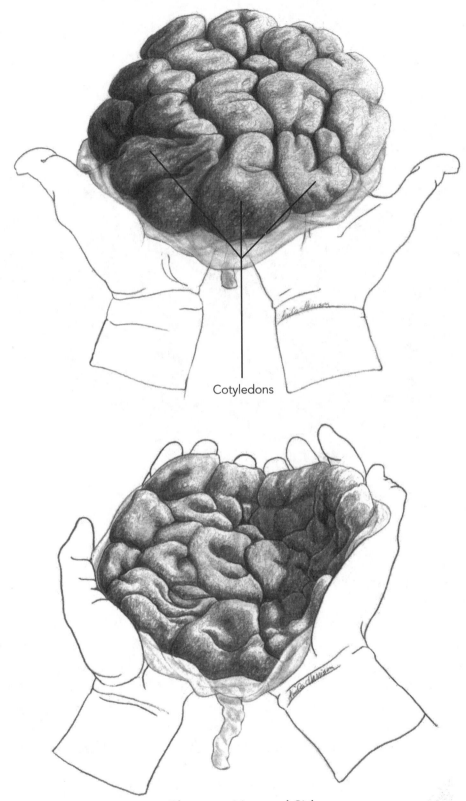

Cotyledons

Placenta: Maternal Side

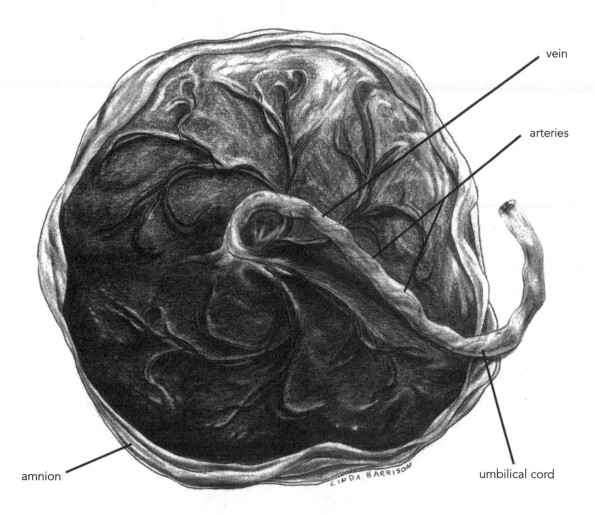

vein

arteries

amnion

umbilical cord

Placenta: Fetal Side

and see if the edges of the rents join evenly and match up. Check the edges of the placenta to make sure they blend cleanly into membrane and nothing appears to have been torn away.

Turn the placenta over to check the fetal side. If the cord has been cut, note how many vessels are present—there should be three holes (two arteries and a vein) visible at the end. If there are only two, the baby may have anomalies not immediately apparent and the pediatrician should be notified. The bluish-white substance in which the vessels are suspended is called **Wharton's jelly.** The amount of this varies, but it should be present at the juncture of the cord and the placenta. If the vessels are suspended in membrane

alone, you have discovered a relatively rare **velamentous cord insertion.** Next, determine where the cord joins the placenta: **central insertion** (at the center) or **marginal insertion** (at the edge).

Also check for vessels running from the edge of the placenta into the membranes, leading to a separate bit of placenta called a **succenturiate lobe.** If vessels are found to terminate with a hole in the membranes, it is probable that the lobe is retained and will likely cause postpartum hemorrhage. It must be removed manually, either by you or at the hospital (see page 164 for more on third-stage hemorrhage).

It is essential to understand that clots or fragments retained in the uterus will prevent it from clamping down completely and therefore must be removed before blood loss can be controlled. Neither massage nor pitocin will make a lasting difference with these obstacles in the way. This brings us to the cardinal rule for handling postpartum hemorrhage: **determine the cause of bleeding** before taking action. Should blood begin to flow steadily or in spurts, it is time to resort to emergency measures (see page 167 for more on fourth-stage hemorrhage).

If this is a lotus birth, you must do something to preserve the placenta until the cord separates from the baby. Some midwives suggest sprinkling the placenta with salt, but Frye cautions that this tends to make it sticky and difficult to handle. Instead, she advises rubbing powdered rosemary thoroughly into the maternal surface.[18] The placenta can then be wrapped in an underpad and its own receiving blanket or bundled in with the baby.

If the cord has already been cut, use a disposable clamp and recut several inches from the navel. Get the baby and the mother warm, cozy, and cleaned up. Before facilitating breastfeeding, see that the mother is comfortable—this is very important. If she has slouched down in her pillows, help her into a sitting position with support under each elbow to allow her to cradle the baby easily. Bring her something to drink, like juice at room temperature or tea with honey to boost her energy. Once she is relaxed and alert, she will nurse and bond more readily, which will help keep her uterus well contracted.

CHECKING FOR TEARS

Once the placenta is out and the mother is stable, she will want to know if she has torn, and you will be anxious to resolve this for yourself. Discard the bloodied underpads beneath her and replace with several fresh ones. If necessary, gently wash her perineum with warm water. Arrange good lighting—a high-intensity lamp works well—then open some sterile gauze, put on sterile gloves, use the gauze to part the labia, and see what you can see. Check for any abrasions, obvious tears around the urethra and perineum, or internal muscle splits at the floor of the vagina (see "Assessment and Repair of Lacerations and Episiotomy" in chapter 5 for further instructions).

Even if the mother needs repair, this need not be done immediately. As long as her uterus is firm, the placenta is complete, and the baby has good color and responsiveness, sit back for a moment and rest. As you do so, offer heartfelt words of praise for the birth and the baby. This can help alleviate any self-consciousness the mother or her partner may have about their behavior during labor. As the new family relaxes and draws closer together, give them privacy, go out to the kitchen for a break, and have something to eat or drink as well.

Tell the mother to call out if she feels herself bleeding or feels at all weak or dizzy. Check her uterus and blood flow every ten to fifteen minutes, and bring her more juice and something to eat. As her band of supporters begins to disperse and she is ready to get up—perhaps to go to the bathroom—make sure someone stays with her. Then attend to cleaning up, changing the bed linens, straightening the room, and so on.

NEWBORN EXAM

Because of HIV and hepatitis risks, wear gloves for the newborn exam unless the baby has been bathed and is free of maternal secretions. Before you begin, make sure the mother has had a chance to fondle and bond with the baby and has nursed at least once. Do the exam right on the bed, where she and her partner can watch. The baby will be more relaxed if the room is warm. If the room is at all cool, place a heating pad on low setting under a towel or several receiving blankets to create a cozy exam surface. Unwrap the baby gradually, exposing just the area to be examined. Explain each step as you move along. You will be checking the baby from head to toe—first the front side, then the back. (See "Newborn Examination" in appendix H.)

Begin by **checking the baby's heartbeat.** Listen closely for anything unusual (such as arrhythmia) and then time it carefully. The heart rate often drops a bit after delivery; normal newborn rate is about 110–150 BPM. Next, **note the baby's general condition and activity level** with a brief description—for example, "pink, vigorous, strong cry" or "good color and muscle tone, quiet." Any general concerns regarding the birth or the baby may be noted here—for example, trauma with delivery, need for resuscitation, and so on.

Then **check the skin.** Note the color; a bright-red tone is associated with prematurity and a condition known as **polycythemia** (excess red cells). This finding necessitates a hematocrit or referral to the pediatrician. Premature babies typically have **lanugo,** or a fine covering of hair, on various areas of the body; make note of the amount and location. **Desquamation** (peeling skin) is common with postmaturity and no cause for alarm in and of itself, but it may alert you to more serious problems associated with this condition (such as dehydration or hypoglycemia). A yellow tinge to the skin indicates **jaundice,** which is abnormal at this stage and should be referred to a pediatrician immediately, as should **circumoral cyanosis,** a blue ring around the mouth linked to heart, circulatory, or intercranial pathology. Babies of Russian, Mediterranean, African-American, or Hispanic parentage may have **Mongolian Spots,** dark-blue splotches at the base of the spine, which are normal and usually vanish in time (you can wait until turning the baby over to check for these). Also note any birthmarks or hairy moles. If vernix is present, massage it into the baby's skin or it may cause inflammation, particularly in the skin folds.

It is important to **check the head carefully for excessive molding, bruising, or swelling.** All of these indicate some trauma during labor or delivery. Normal molding causes the head to assume an elongated, abnormal shape, but tends to diminish within a matter of hours. **Caput,** or generalized swelling on top of the head, may result from extreme molding. **Cephalhe-**matoma appears as an abnormal, lumplike swelling confined to a particular area of the head (it does not cross suture lines) and is associated with internal bleeding between the scalp and the skull. Cephalhematoma, bruising, or excessive molding are signs of significant trauma, necessitating administration of vitamin K. The baby should be seen by a pediatrician as soon as possible.

Check the eyes for red spots or hemorrhages of the sclera caused by pressure in the birth canal. Also look for evidence of jaundice—the whites of the eyes should be white, not yellow. Check to see if the pupils are equal in size and reactivity when exposed to light. Check for tracking by moving your finger back and forth close to the baby's face. Check the shape and spacing of the eyes, noting any irregularities. With the mother's consent, **instill medication;** erythromycin ointment is standard and is effective against both gonorrhea and chlamydia. (Note that this procedure is mandated by law. The prevalence of chlamydia and its typically asymptomatic presentation argue for the routine use of eye prophylaxis, but it is nonetheless a matter of choice. If the mother declines, she must sign a waiver.)

Next check the **ENT** (ear, nose, and throat). **Check the ears** for normal shape and reactivity to sound. Also note ear placement—the top of the ear should be level with the corner of the baby's eye. Low-lying ears are associated with kidney problems or other anomalies; if you discover this, have the baby seen immediately. If the baby has not been bathed, you must reglove before **checking the lips and palate** to prevent maternal secretions from entering the baby's mouth. Use your little finger and feel carefully around the roof of the mouth and back to the throat, making certain the palate is intact. In so doing, you will stimulate the sucking reflex—note its strength in the reflexes category. Also check the frenulum (under the tongue) for normal length.

Checking the thorax for retractions is usually done right at the time of birth. A positive finding indicates respiratory distress, which should have long since been dealt with. But if the baby had meconium or thick mucus at birth, make sure that there is no lung damage or obstruction. Observe how the chest and stomach move when the baby breathes—ribs and belly should inflate and deflate smoothly together. If the skin pulls tight between the ribs, or the chest and the abdomen move in a seesaw fashion, the baby has retractions and should be seen by a pediatrician at once.

Next **check the abdomen.** Occasionally you will discover an **umbilical hernia,** appearing as a bulge at the base of the cord stump. Contrary to popular belief, this is not caused by a particular method of handling or tying the cord, but is a congenital defect that can be remedied by surgery when the child is about two years old. Also feel the belly for masses or swelling; all should feel smooth and even (it is easier to do this if you flex the baby's knees toward the abdomen with one hand while checking with the other). Lastly, listen with a stethoscope for the presence of bowel sounds.

Check femoral pulses by lightly placing fingertips (both index fingers) in the left and right groin areas. You should feel pulsing on either side, and the pulses should be the same (symmetrical). If not, the baby may have a congenital heart problem; contact the pediatrician immediately. (If you have trouble performing this evaluation, you may be compressing the vessels so much that you can't feel the pulse. Try using a lighter touch.)

Check genitals carefully to be sure that all essential parts and openings are present. Girls frequently have vaginal mucus, which may be blood tinged due to high hormone level effects. Boys should be checked to see that both testes are descended. Do this by placing your finger at the top of one side of the scrotum to close off the inguinal canal, feel carefully for the testicle, and repeat on the other side. If the scrotum is edematous and difficult to palpate, shine a flashlight against it to visualize the testicles. This is particularly important if the baby was breech, as torsion of the scrotum may cause testicles to be lost unless the problem is detected within several hours of the birth.

Several **reflexes** have usually been demonstrated by now: **sucking** with palate check and **swallowing** with breastfeeding. To verify the **palmar** (or grasp) reflex, let the baby grab your little fingers—you should be able to lift its back slightly off the bed. Next, hold the baby to face you, support both back and head, and tip it slowly backward to activate **Moro's** (or the startle) **reflex**—arms and hands should extend evenly. Also check **Babinski's reflex** by stroking a foot from bottom to top with your thumb—the toes should fan out. Place your thumb at the base of the toes, and they should curl as you activate the **plantar reflex.** You can also check the **stepping reflex** by holding the baby in a standing position—it should take a few steps forward. The presence of normal reflexes indicates neurological health and maturity.

Now turn the baby over and **closely examine the spine.** Note Mongolian spots and record with other findings regarding the skin. Check for straightness and complete fusion, looking for any sinuses (openings), especially in the sacral area. Even the tiniest opening indicates a condition called **spina bifida,** which can lead to major infections like meningitis; report immediately to the pediatrician. If the opening is large and there is a protrusion through it, the condition is more severe. Cover with sterile gauze soaked in warm saline, notify the pediatrician, and transport.

Then **check the lungs,** listening through the baby's back. Position your stethoscope up near each shoulder, and then again at midback on either side of the spine. Count respirations and chart. The lungs should sound clear, air resonating as if in a hollow chamber with no rattling or scratchy noises. This is particularly important if there has been any meconium at delivery; if such is the case and the baby's lungs sound obstructed, try percussion and steam (see "Meconium Aspiration" in chapter 6) or contact the pediatrician immediately.

Check the anus by observation; it is not necessary to insert a thermometer to check for patency. Even if the baby has not passed meconium, it will often have a plug visible at the opening; this is also proof of patency.

Of great interest to parents and friends are the baby's **weight and measurements.** Measure the head circumference at the widest point, from occiput to frontal bone, and record in centimeters (average measurements are 34–37 cm). Then measure the chest; the difference between head and chest should be no more than a few centimeters. If the head is much larger, there may be an abnormal amount of fluid in the cranium, which should be checked immediately by a pediatrician. If the chest measurement is the same or larger than that of the head, and the baby is over nine pounds, the mother may have had some degree of glucose intolerance and the baby should be checked for hypoglycemia. Measure the baby's length by setting the tape alongside its body with top edge level with the tip of the head, then stretch the leg out and measure at the heel. Chart in both centimeters and inches. To weigh, use either a standard baby scale or the more convenient hanging type, which has a hook from which the baby is temporarily suspended in a stork-style bundle. Don't forget to subtract the weight of the blankets. Chart in both pounds and grams.

Finish by **checking the extremities.** Begin by counting fingers and toes, noting uniform length and checking for webbing. Note symmetry of muscle tone in the arms (largely accomplished already by checking Moro's reflex). This is crucial if there has been a tight squeeze with the shoulders, which could cause nerve damage known as **Erb's palsy** or injury to the clavicles. Check each clavicle by palpating from the sternum to the shoulder—if there is a fracture, you will note an unmistakable crinkling sensation called **crepitus.** Administer vitamin K and contact the pediatrician.

Finally, **check the hips** by doing the "click test." Rotate the legs firmly in their sockets, while your fingers rest on the hip joints and feel for clicks that might indicate dislocation. Then flex the knees to the abdomen, and as you press them gently, feel once more for any clicking or unnatural movement of bone slipping out of the socket. If you find anything unusual, turn the baby over again and check hip creases from the backside. These should be symmetrical; if not, contact the pediatrician.

Wrap the baby in dry blankets. If it is content, this may be a good time for the mother's partner to hold it while she takes a shower or stretches her legs a bit.

POSTPARTUM WATCH

Your postpartum watch should last at least two hours, or until the mother's blood pressure, pulse, temperature, and lochia flow are within normal range for at least an hour. She should urinate before you go, and have

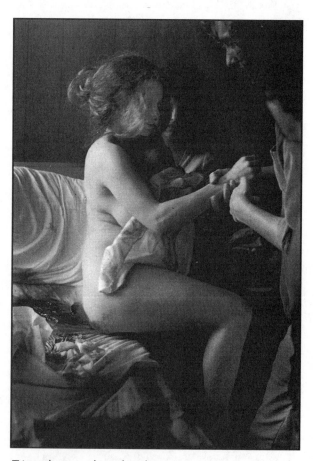

Triumphant and tender, the new mother gets up with her baby for the first time.

something to eat and drink. Make sure she has nursed successfully and understands that although her milk will not come in for a few days, **colostrum** is sufficient for the baby's needs until that time. Go over your post-partum instructions carefully (see appendix K), making sure that everything is clear and that both the mother and her partner understand normal and abnormal new-born behavior. Leave copies of the Birth Record (appendix G) and Newborn Examination (appendix H) for the pediatrician. Encourage them to call anytime, about anything, at any hour. If they seem at all uncom-fortable with you leaving, wait a little longer.

You should also be sure that you are in stable con-dition before going. Particularly after a grueling labor or complicated delivery, you may be absolutely exhausted and should rest and relax with your assistant or mid-wifery partner before attempting to drive. A midwife from my area had the great misfortune of falling asleep at the wheel on her way back from a birth; her car hit a tree and she sustained major injuries. Those first few hours after the birth fly by; *make a habit of getting some-thing to drink or eat immediately* so you are ready to go when it is time.

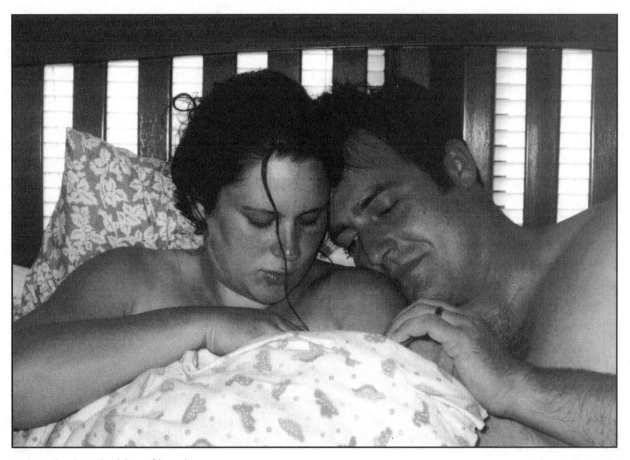

Parents bask in the bliss of bonding.

For Parents: Golden Tips for Assisting in Labor

Here are some special ways to help your partner during labor:

1. If labor begins at night and is light, help her back to sleep with a massage.

2. If labor begins during the day, take her to a place you both love where you can get used to labor together.

3. Help her to eat as long as possible; prepare (or buy) her favorite foods.

4. Wear something she likes, and keep in close, relaxed physical contact with her.

5. As labor progresses, help her relax by encouraging her to let her body "go limp," and stroke her gently to reassure her.

6. Breathe with her if she starts to panic.

7. Don't be embarrassed to use common endearments, even with your midwives around.

8. Don't be offended if she wants privacy. Many women need some time alone to make adjustments during labor—some more than others. Let her be.

9. In transition, speak tenderly to her between contractions, and maintain physical contact if it seems to help.

10. Once she is pushing, get your body close to her somehow so she feels your reinforcement (or, if she does not want this, that's okay too).

11. Let her know when you can see the baby's head, and help her reach down and touch it.

12. Tell her you love her, especially after the baby comes out. ■

Notes

1. Anne Frye, *Holistic Midwifery (Volume II)* (Portland, Oreg.: Labrys Press), manuscript pages.

2. Michel Odent, "The Dehumanization of Birth," lecture, California Association of Midwives conference, 2003.

3. Ina May Gaskin, *Ina May's Guide to Childbirth* (New York: Bantam Dell, 2003), 170.

4. D. L. Byrne and D. K. Edmunds, "Clinical methods for evaluating progress in the first stage of labour," *Lancet* 335 (8681): 122, 1997.

5. Frye, *Holistic Midwifery (Volume II)*.

6. Kyle Steele and Carl Javert, "The Mechanism of Labor for Transverse Positions of the Vertex," *Surgery, Gynecology, and Obstetrics* 74 (4): 477, 1942.

7. Frye, *Holistic Midwifery (Volume II)*.

8. Gloria Lemay, "Pushing for First-Time Moms," *Midwifery Today* 55 (Fall 2000).

9. Jean Sutton, "Birth without active pushing: a physiological second stage of labor," in *Midwifery: Best Practice,* ed. Sara Wickham (London, England: Elsevier Science Limited, 2003), 91.

10. Michel Odent, "The fetus ejection reflex," *Birth* 14 (2): 104–5, 1987.

11. Sheila Kitzinger, *Ourselves as Mothers* (New York: Bantam Books, 1993).

12. Roberto Caldeyro-Barcia, "The Influence of Maternal Bearing-down Efforts During Second Stage on Fetal Well-being," *Birth and the Family Journal* 6 (1): Spring 1979.

13. Sutton, "Birth without active pushing," 90.

14. Lemay, "Pushing for First-Time Moms."

15. Wisnell, et al., "Delivery room management of the apparently meconium-stained neonate: results of the multicenter, international collaborative trial," *Pediatrics* 105 (2000): 1–7, 2000.

16. L. Righard and Kittie Frantz, "Delivery Self Attachment" (video), Sunland, California: Geddes Productions, (1995), based on the study by M. Alade and L. Righard, "Effect of delivery room routines on success of first breast-feed," *The Lancet* 336 (1990): 1,105–7.

17. Raymond Castellino, private conversation, with author 1996.

18. Frye, *Holistic Midwifery (Volume II)*.

COMPLICATIONS IN LABOR

Complications arising in labor are challenging to any midwife, no matter how experienced. Prenatal problems are not so pressing, as there is usually time to consider, consult, and reevaluate from visit to visit. But in labor, decisions must be made both carefully and quickly.

Close and vigilant attention is the key to detecting complications at their inception. When complications develop, one of the attributes of a good midwife is the ability to consider the total picture, while pinpointing the area on which to focus a remedy. Beyond that, sensitivity and objectivity must be combined to determine whether a particular course of treatment is proving effective. Interventions may also bear side effects, which must also be tracked throughout labor and the postpartum period.

Above all, commitment to the principle of nonintervention cannot be used to excuse hesitation in complicated circumstances. There is a delicate balance between the mother's right to give birth undisturbed, to proceed at her own pace and find her way, and the midwife's responsibility to use her knowledge and skill so stamina and safety are maintained to the end.

The impact of maternal emotions on labor cannot be overestimated. There are certain instances when emotional problems portend physical danger, yet there is still safe leeway for turning the tide and getting labor back on course again. By the same token, emotional breakthrough can render progress that is nothing short of miraculous.

The art of handling complications may be approached as follows:

1. Determine the possible cause or causes of the complication.

2. Test your diagnosis through further observation plus discussion with your midwifery partner and the mother.

3. Modify your diagnosis if need be, suggest a remedy, and, with the mother's agreement, implement it.

4. Follow up with close and careful checks on vital signs and progress to determine effectiveness and results.

5. Watch carefully for any side effects and reevaluate as indicated.

It helps tremendously if the entire birthing team is intent on working together. If you sense a noncommittal attitude from the mother despite your best counsel and encouragement, it may be that the birth is not meant to happen at home. Waiting in limbo is dissipating, particularly when labor forces are struggling to move ahead. If the mother concurs that transport is a good idea, the move to the hospital should be made as quickly as possible.

Sometimes a mother requests transport not out of fear or desperation, but because she senses that something is about to go wrong. Never try to dissuade her from her instincts in this regard.

Transport is a complication in itself, especially if labor has been long and everyone is tired. The mother often needs help getting dressed, packing a bag, making childcare arrangements (if necessary), and notifying key friends or relatives. Her partner may be moved to tears out of sympathy, out of sadness for the loss of their home birth dream, or out of sheer frustration and exhaustion. Some get angry, others go numb. Meanwhile, you must contact the obstetrician and call the hospital to arrange for admission. Trying to be lucid and articulate while stressed out or suffering from sleep deprivation can be quite a challenge. It helps to have your chart in order, so questions from hospital personnel can be kept to a minimum when you do arrive (you should update it in the car if necessary). A one-page transport summary sheet is also helpful (see "Transport Record from Home Delivery," Appendix F).

When life-threatening emergencies arise, the focus is on survival, with little time for integration. But in the majority of transport situations, you have opportunity to give reassurance, support, and hope to the mother and her partner on the way to the hospital—definitely one of the greatest services a midwife can render.

PROLONGED LABOR AND MATERNAL EXHAUSTION

To address this subject, we must first pose the question: What makes labor prolonged? What is the difference between a labor that is simply long, and one that is prolonged? And how did we get into this mess of defining labor in terms of its length in the first place?

The trouble began with birth in hospital, where the prompt turnover of beds became of practical and financial concern. Next came practitioner impatience—physicians with over-busy schedules, or with better things to do than wait around for women to give birth, wanted to define how long was too long. One such was Emanuel Friedman, notorious for the development of the Friedman Curve, which, based on averages, defines optimal length and rate of progress for first and subsequent labors. According to his research, first labors average 6.4 hours in the early phase, 4.6 hours in the active phase, and 1.1 hours in second stage; with subsequent pregnancies, these figures are cut by 50 percent. More significantly, normal dilation was defined as one centimeter per hour for first labors, and two per hour for subsequent births.[1, 2]

Needless to say, Friedman's work has been misinterpreted and misused. If birthing in the hospital, mothers working through a perfectly normal plateau phase, or experiencing a lull in progress due to lack of sleep or nourishment, or whose large or posterior babies need some extra time to descend, are all too often diagnosed with "failure to progress." Many unnecessary cesareans are performed on this basis, even though recent studies show average labor lengths double those of Friedman's.[3]

From the midwife's point of view, labor is prolonged only when clinical exhaustion threatens. More about this condition in a moment, but note that it occurs after the fact—and this is the tricky part. With a commitment to a minimum of vaginal exams, it is critical that we keep our senses open, watching for contractions that are monotonous in rhythm, labor energy that feels static instead of dynamic, or a mother who is stressed or out of it rather than passionately engaged. Our concern is less a matter of labor's length than of energy-sapping arrests in the process.

Arrests in labor can have a number of causes, both physical and emotional. Often the two are interwoven, and you must sort through numerous factors to arrive at the central issue. For example, if you are assisting a mother with a large, unengaged posterior baby, it is not uncommon to see an arrest of progress at 6 cm due to lack of descent and insufficient cervical stimulation. The mother may also be fearful of labor, or may become frustrated and impatient as time goes by, but in this case, no amount of counseling or encouragement can override fetal malpresentation as the principal cause of arrest.

To take this subject in chronological order, a long early phase of labor is no cause for concern if the mother is handling contractions well and continues to eat, rest, and sleep. This may sound simple, but all too often mothers become so excited by and reactive to early contractions that this critical balance is lost. If the mother is not sleeping, recommend hops tincture or a glass of wine to assist. Women birthing in hospital get little or no advice in this respect, and typically arrive at the labor ward utterly exhausted and only a few centimeters dilated.

In general, early labor should not interfere with normal life. If the mother is well rested, encourage her to go for a walk, to a movie, or to visit friends. If she is only a few centimeters dilated and is panting, groaning, and plugging away, she needs help winding down so she can conserve energy and keep her sense of humor for the hard work ahead.

Occasionally, you may have the confusing case of a mother who appears to be in active labor, with contractions coming every five minutes, lasting up to a minute. But after a few hours, contractions taper off, and internal exam reveals her to be only 2 or 3 cm dilated. Typically, women with a strong athletic component or highly intellectual nature tend toward this pattern, which is based on the inability (at least at this juncture) to let go and cross into the active phase. Uterine inertia often results; if so, a complete break for everyone is the best solution. Labor will start up again after a period of rest— and dilation may take place quite quickly.

This may leave the midwife thinking, "What was I doing here, anyway? Maybe I just should have waited at home!" Strong contractions rightfully prompt assessment of the baby, but if the mother is not yet ready to move ahead, a meal and some sleep are in order. The chance to be completely alone, with a taste of true labor behind them, will often set a couple to discussing unresolved conflicts or their more immediate needs for intimacy. This sets the stage for rapid progress in the next round.

Early in my practice, I attended a birth classic in this pattern. For twelve hours (mostly at night) the mother walked, squatted, was in and out of the shower, drank labor-promoting teas, and so on. It felt odd but liberating to be sitting around the following afternoon in limbo, sharing a glass of champagne (we went ahead and opened it) and simply relaxing together. My partner and I decided to go home and after six hours were called back to find the mother dilated to 7 cm, handling her labor well and birthing shortly thereafter. When we asked her what had happened, she replied, "Well, after you left we got in bed and talked a lot, fell asleep, and then it just started up again really strong."

Up to about 5 cm, labor may come and go, and the plateau that leads from early to active labor may last for quite some time. Just remember that a plateau is not an arrest. Arrests become a concern only when a woman reaches 6 cm, because now the uterus is hard at work and tends to persist regardless of maternal tensions. At this point, if the mother resists the forces of labor, she may reach a state of **clinical exhaustion** long before her uterus takes a break. Clinical exhaustion is diagnosed with a combination of **ketonuria, elevated temperature,** and **elevated pulse.** This condition is also known as ketoacidosis, in that the mother's blood becomes abnormally acidic and less able to carry oxygen. Unless this condition is reversed, fetal distress will result.

If signs of clinical exhaustion manifest, remedial measures of nutrition and hydration should be implemented immediately (see labor-aide, page 113). The baby must also be monitored more closely for signs of distress, unless labor has tapered off and the mother is resting. This brings us to the cardinal rule for handling prolonged labor: *If labor begins to slow down, do not try to stimulate it!* Diminishing contractions indicate that the uterus is fatigued, thus the mother must be encouraged to eat and rest in order for it to rebound. If you make the mistake of forcing the uterus when it is crying out for rest, prolonged second stage, fetal distress, and postpartum hemorrhage are likely to result. Have the mother eat some toast, yogurt, anything that appeals to her. Then give her a glass of wine, shot of brandy, or dropperful of hops tincture in juice or tea to help her get some rest. Typically, women are not able to sleep at this stage of labor, but can rest deeply even if light contractions persist.

It must be understood, however, that merely treating the symptoms of arrest will not rectify the situation—you must try to determine the cause. Begin by doing a thorough internal exam to ascertain any impediments to fetal descent. It is important to remember that the cervix can open to 6 cm without pressure from the presenting part, but after that, the head (or butt) literally dilates the cervix the rest of the way by passing through it. Pressure on the cervix also strengthens contractions and must also be uniform for labor to intensify. Check the position of the head and how it is presenting very carefully. Posterior babies are often somewhat deflexed, which increases the circumference of the head and may hinder descent. If this is the case, or if the baby is large for the mother's dimensions, **asynclitism** may also be noted.

Asynclitism usually occurs when the baby has trouble negotiating the pelvic inlet and then compensates by leading with one side of its head only. Upon internal exam, the suture line is found either to be running high or low in the pelvis, rather than directly across the cervical opening (see illustration "Fetal Asynclitism," page 147). Asynclitism is also linked to polyhydramnios and a small baby, as the baby is apt to descend rapidly and can easily land in a cocked position when the water breaks. Asynclitism and deflexion

of the head lead to asymmetrical pressure on the cervix and arrest at 6 cm. To treat these conditions, please see the following section in this chapter on cephalopelvic disproportion (CPD).

Another cause for delay may be **cervical edema.** If noted at 6 cm, with the cervix not well applied to the head, rule out the malpresentations just cited. Prone positions can also lead to edema by causing compression of vaginal tissues adjacent to the baby's head, impairing venous return from the cervix. If edema occurs around 8 cm and the mother has been favoring prone positions, the cervix should thin out rapidly once she is upright. On the other hand, if she has been upright and labor has been particularly painful or intense, edema may be better alleviated by having her lie on one side for a while, and then switch to the other. Even if the cervix is relieved of pressure one side at a time, edema will gradually resolve.

Sometimes a **cervical lip** is the last obstacle to complete dilation. This is swelling of the anterior portion of the cervix (the rest being fully retracted), due to the head pinching it against the pubic bone. It is most common with persistent posterior babies. Try repositioning the mother, as just described. For a stubborn lip, place ice in the finger of a sterile glove and hold against the cervix. Once the swelling is reduced, or if the lip is soft enough, you may try to push it back. To do so, position your fingers at the edge of the lip and with the next contraction, push the lip over the baby's head as it descends. Hold it behind the pubic bone, and then have the mother bear down. If the lip is gone, you've succeeded; if not, try again. This may be somewhat painful for the mother—it helps if she is in a semi-squat. It is okay to exert a bit of pressure with this maneuver, but never force the cervix or it may tear.

Sometimes **tense membranes or a tight forebag** can retard descent and cause an arrest in progress, typically at 7 or 8 cm dilation. You may wish to perform **artificial rupture of the membranes (AROM),** but first, make sure the head is low enough in the pelvis to prevent cord prolapse (as a rule, it must be at 0 station, but a larger head may fill the pelvis snugly at −1 station). If the head is too high for AROM, the mother must walk, relax, and wait until it descends. Be forewarned, this may take hours, so be sure she drinks plenty of water, takes tablespoons of honey, eats if possible, and keeps her bladder empty.

To perform AROM, don a sterile glove, squirt a bit of sterile gel over your fingers, and splint an **amnihook** between them, keeping the tip protected. As a contraction ends, insert your fingers and push the hook to the bag, then pull down on the handle to lift the tip, and pull back toward you to snag the membranes. Carefully draw the hook back between your fingertips and remove all slowly. It is best to do this with the mother propped upright. Be sure to take heart tones immediately afterward and chart.

You may occasionally be tempted to perform AROM earlier in labor. I once made the mistake of doing so with a mother only 4 cm dilated, hoping that descent would result and additional pressure on the cervix would stimulate progress. This decision was made after thirty-eight hours of erratic contractions, with another twelve hours of regular, moderately strong ones. A tense bag of waters was forming, and the baby's head (which was small and engaged) was not well applied to the cervix. The mother had a generous pelvis with no abnormalities, so I reasoned the forebag was holding the baby up. Surprisingly enough, rupturing the membranes did not bring descent. The real problem was that the mother was still early enough in labor to have active control; she used her excellent abdominal and vaginal vault muscles to hold the baby up so she would feel less pressure on her back. The result of this intervention was to create yet another problem—prolonged rupture of the membranes (PROM), which, according to the standard of the day, necessitated transport and pitocin augmentation.

Arrests in second stage are far less common than in first stage and have already been addressed at some length in chapter 4. Here too, Friedman's Curve has had its effect on the standard of care, in that descent is expected within a certain time frame and in consistent increments. But progress in second stage does not take place in a steady stream any more than it does in first stage. Generally, the baby remains at +1 or +2 station until the head has been sculpted by the vaginal muscles to fit through, at which point it often descends quite rapidly. Then again, if you know the mother to have a narrow pubic arch, close-set tuberosities, or a prominent coccyx, see the discussion on cephalopelvic disproportion in the next section.

Once you have determined that there are no physical obstacles impeding progress, consider both psychological and environmental dynamics. There are many factors that might cause a mother to resist opening up or letting the baby down. By now, emotional problems revealed at prenatal visits should have given specific clues as to what has gone awry, but here is a general list of possibilities:

1. Mother not feeling enough love, communication, or faith from her partner.

2. Partner unable or unwilling to let go and give, due to inhibitions with self or history with the mother.

3. Worries for both about becoming parents; for the mother, loss of personal attention she enjoyed during pregnancy; for her partner, moving from limbo to new levels of responsibility.

4. Awareness of sexual dysfunction awakening with the physical-emotional intensity of labor, including unknown history of sexual abuse.

5. Disharmony in the environment—too many people, too many comings and goings, no sense of privacy, or a family friend or relative who is undermining or threatening the mother in some way.

6. Baby feeling hesitant, uncertain of parents' feelings or its own about being born.

These problems may be largely resolved by facilitating intimacy between the mother and her partner. Demonstrate helpful ways to touch and massage the mother during contractions, and model a loving and tender tone of voice. Encourage both parents talk to the baby. Once they are working comfortably together, take any necessary vital assessments and leave them be for a while.

As for the environment, the labor room can get rather stale after a while, so freshen things up if need be. And too, if the couple feels a veritable party impinging on their privacy, friends within earshot of their bedroom door, how free will they feel to be intimate? Clear out well-wishers kindly, explaining that it may be many hours before the birth takes place and now is the best time for a break.

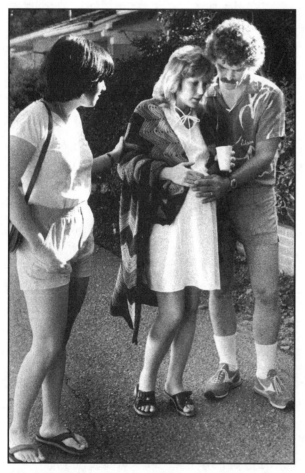

Pep up a lagging labor by getting out in the fresh air.

The mother may also want complete privacy but be unable to say so. Women are so accustomed to accommodating the needs and wishes of others that they may equate the desire to be alone with selfishness. Or they could be afraid of hurting their partner's (or midwife's) feelings. Make the suggestions and see how the mother responds.

Sometimes a complete change of scene is in order. Especially if active labor is just beginning, the mother may benefit from a walk to a nearby park, beach, or wooded area, if not in her own backyard. Being in touch with nature can do wonders for her morale. Someone on the birth team should accompany her, and whoever is left behind should straighten up the room, remake the bed, bring in fresh tea, water, flowers, and so on while she is out. But do keep in mind that emotional release is a major catalyst to progress. In the absence of physical impediments, the mother who fully surrenders all psychological resistance can dilate very rapidly. I have seen a number of women go from 5 cm to complete dilation in less than an hour—spilling out fear and anxiety one minute, easing into sensation the next, and suddenly feeling like pushing. *Don't take the mother out for a walk if you sense this kind of release is about to happen!*

Unacknowledged sexual abuse is most likely to manifest in an intense reaction to pressure on pelvic floor muscles, especially if descent is rapid. The reaction is unmistakable—the mother literally draws her energy and body upward as if trying to get away, and she may look absolutely panic-stricken. Do what you can to soothe her, perhaps getting her in water if she is not already, having her place her hand over her vagina (making clear that nothing is entering from outside and that she is in charge), or having her look in a mirror as the head begins to show. Don't be thrown by the intensity of her reaction. Stay strong, stay open, and let her know she is *safe!*

One of my students told of a birth with a very long second stage; the mother had pushed for more than three hours and was becoming exhausted when the midwives began talking to the baby, telling it to come out. At this, the father broke down and said that it was his fault, his ambivalence, and the baby was born shortly thereafter.

With any emotionally based arrest, continue to check for signs of maternal exhaustion while encouraging the mother to eat and drink. If she becomes depleted, emotional arrest can quickly deteriorate into pathology. Make sure she urinates frequently, as a full bladder can hinder relaxation and descent. Take blood pressure and fetal heart tones regularly, as emotional tension can impact both. Be frank with both the mother and her partner about any counterproductive behaviors. If physical symptoms of emotional distress begin to manifest, discuss the possibility of transport. This may elicit determination or despair, but a decision must be made promptly. Give the mother and her partner a bit of time to consider their options, be encouraging but firm, and the appropriate course of action will soon become evident.

CEPHALOPELVIC DISPROPORTION

Cephalopelvic disproportion is a condition in which the baby's head cannot readily pass through the mother's pelvis. As *Myles Textbook for Midwives* states, "Disproportion can be pelvic or cephalic in origin, due to small pelvis, a large fetus or a combination of the two."[4] It may also be a result of malpresentation—for example, if a posterior baby for whom the mother has plenty of room presents an excessively large diameter of its head due to deflexion, disproportion may result. Other relevant factors include the degree to which the fetal skull is moldable, the amount of flexibility in maternal tissues and joints, the strength of uterine contractions, and the mother's resolve. If she is upright and relaxed, her uterus is working efficiently, and she is well supported, even a moderate degree of CPD can be

overcome. It has been said repeatedly that the best pelvimeter is the baby's head, which is obviously true.

Thus CPD cannot be diagnosed before labor, but if the head bulges over the pubic bone in a rare condition known as **fetal overlap,** it may be suspected. Should the head be easier than usual to palpate in the final weeks of pregnancy, check for overlap by pressing the head toward the sacral promontory and down into the pelvis. If you find "give" front to back with room for descent, rest assured. But if space seems limited, plan to monitor labor closely. Yet another option is to induce labor (see later in this chapter for suggestions).

Failure to engage before labor cannot be considered diagnostic either, as large babies frequently stay at −2 or −3 station until strong contractions bring them down. Sometimes extremely strong or weak abdominal tone prevents the fetus from aligning with the inlet so that it can descend. Only 1 to 2 percent of all cases of CPD are due to a genuine discrepancy between the size of the baby and that of the mother's pelvis—usually, it is a problem with fetal malpresentation or misalignment.

During labor, CPD can occur also at the midpelvis or the outlet. Pelvimetry performed during pregnancy should have alerted you to any reduced dimension, helping both you and the mother prepare for labor. A pelvis with a roomy inlet but flat, heavy sacrum may render descent and engagement difficult. See that the head is well flexed in the last few weeks of pregnancy, and encourage the mother to squat (with thighs parallel to the floor) for ten to twenty minutes a day to open and stretch midpelvic dimensions as much as possible. Have her sit in forward-leaning positions with her knees dropped down, for example, straddling a chair facing its back, or at the edge of a chair, leaning forward. Or, if the pubic arch is reduced, the head may be forced downward so that lacerations occur, or delay at the height of head compression may lead to fetal distress and episiotomy. In this case, squatting (as above) forward-leaning positions, vaginal awareness, and visualization are crucial preparations for labor.

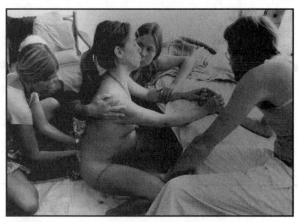

Squatting position for midpelvic CPD.

It is also important to remember that the birth canal is comprised not only of bones, but of musculature as well. The more we learn about the physiology of labor (see "Cardinal Spiraling Movements of the Baby during Labor" in chapter 4), the more we can appreciate the importance of healthy and flexible vaginal tissues. To quote Anne Frye:

> Observations regarding the influence of the pelvic soft tissues on the birth process are highly relevant to the midwifery model of care. The soft tissues are more easily influenced by maternal distress or relaxation, leading to correspondingly more difficult or easier labors. The flexibility of the pelvic joints is also influenced by the mother's emotional state. That the pelvic soft tissues (rather than the bones) are the primary influence over the movements of the presenting part in the average pelvis underscores the relationship between the maternal emotional state and the physical aspects of labor, and explains the ability of maternal activities and position changes to dramatically alter the course of labor for the better.[5]

Thus it is not uncommon to find a minor degree of CPD suddenly overcome not only by fetal rotation or repositioning, but with changes in maternal position or attitude.

How do we diagnose CPD during labor? First, it must seem a reasonable suspicion based on foreknowledge of the baby's size and the mother's dimensions.

Inlet disproportion is signaled by arrest at 6 cm dilation, lack of descent past –3 or –2 station, asynclitism, and cervix not well applied to the head. Particularly ominous is the cervix hanging like an empty sleeve. Another oddity of inlet CPD is the tendency of the cervix to reclose; I can recall several cases in which the cervix, hanging loosely during a contraction, spastically tightened up a centimeter or more as the contraction ended. This happens because the cervix has nothing to hold it open, neither the head nor adequate strength in the lower uterine segment. The result is weakening, incoordinate contractions, with maternal symptoms of asymmetrical, spastic pain.

Midpelvic disproportion presents quite differently. The head generally engages without trouble, dilation proceeds normally, but second stage is prolonged. Typically, the baby is stuck in **deep transverse arrest,** meaning that the head gets wedged behind the ischial spines and cannot rotate to the antero-posterior position.

Outlet disproportion also leads to prolonged second stage, but more commonly affects the perineal phase, causing severe early decels or bradycardia, delayed delivery, and tears of the bulbocavernosus muscle or perineum.

What about remedies for CPD? These depend on the dimension of the pelvis where the disproportion occurs. If at the inlet and caused by malpresentation (deflexion or asynclitism) you can attempt to manually reposition the head. This is more likely to work with intact membranes, as the baby can more readily move in response to your manipulations. Have the mother assume knees-chest position to make the best use of the effects of gravity. To **correct asynclitism,** press firmly on the protruding parietal bone to dislodge the head, and then center the sagittal suture line. To **secure flexion,** see directions and diagrams under "Posterior Arrest" (in the next section in this chapter).

If the head is too high to reach, have the mother try **duck-walking.** Much as it sounds, she must walk

Fetal Asynclitism

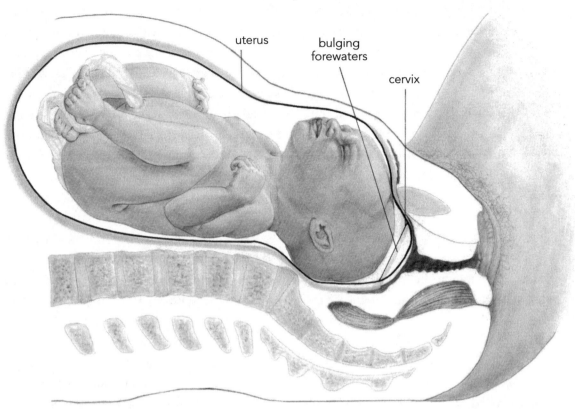

Relative CPD caused by a posterior position and a deflexed, asynclitic head.

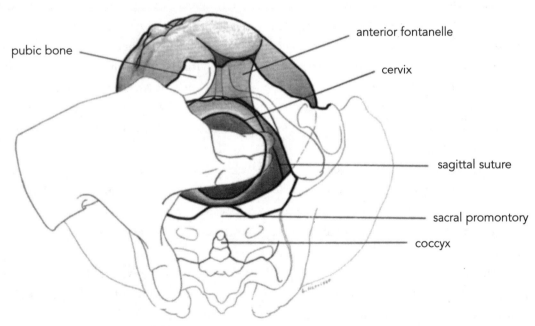

Correct asynclitism by centering the sagittal suture.

in a standing squat position by shifting her weight from one foot to the other. This helps open the pelvis, at the same time encouraging the baby to reposition itself. For similar effect, have the mother climb stairs two at a time. Pauline Scott and Jean Sutton recommend a **hip twist-and-lift** movement—the mother stands, throws one hip and leg forward, bends and straightens leg to pointed toes, and repeats on the other side (this is also useful for compound presentations).[6] Ruth Ancheta and Penny Simkin suggest **the lunge:** for this, place a chair on a carpeted floor (so it cannot slide) next to the mother on whichever side her baby is lying. Have her face forward and place the foot nearest the chair onto its seat, with toes pointed to the opposite side. She then leans into a lunge with each contraction, moving slowly back to standing as it ends.[7]

There are other maneuvers in which the mother is passive that may help. One is the **rebozo technique,** which requires a full-length, sturdy shawl (*rebozo* in Spanish). Stretch the rebozo out on the floor and have the mother lie with hips and lower back across it. Stand over her, straddling her body at thigh level, and pick up both ends. Encourage her to relax completely and then pull the ends alternately, rocking her briskly from side to side. In a Native American variation, the mother lies in a blanket with strong men at the corners, who then lift and toss her around.[8] The Chinese accomplish the same with **chunging,** an ancient technique that involves two or three people placing their hands on the mother and vigorously shaking her all over (she should be in a standing, forward-leaning, and braced position, perhaps against a wall).[9] Yet another possibility is to take the mom for a bumpy car ride—which all too often does not happen until transporting to the hospital, when it might have been effective in keeping the birth at home if tried earlier.

For midpelvic disproportion and cases of deep transverse arrest, you can attempt to flex and rotate the head to OA position (see "Posterior Arrest" section, next). You can also try the **pelvic press.** This should be performed with the mother in a standing squat or a kneeling, forward-leaning position. It will require some physical strength on your part, so get ready. If she is kneeling, find some padding for your knees and kneel behind her; otherwise, stand behind her and place your hands on her iliac crests (hip bones) and press them together as firmly as possible or until you feel some movement. Pressure on the iliac crests flexes the symphysis pubis and sacral iliac joints, opening the midpelvis so the head can rotate and descend. As you do this, have the mother bear down, even if she is not quite complete. Hold the press for the next few contractions. Have your partner check heart tones immediately after each contraction. Results are often quite remarkable.

The pelvic press is also useful for outlet disproportion, as it opens the pubic arch and increases the bituberous diameter. Once the head is beginning to show, a deep squat position (knees up against the abdomen) serves to accomplish much the same; it can increase the outlet dimension by 20 percent. Use hot compresses to deepen pelvic relaxation and work carefully during delivery to maintain flexion of the head.

Inlet CPD is usually the most difficult to address, particularly if you cannot reach the head to reposition it. If duck-walking, stair-climbing, the lunge, or hip-twist do not effect descent, you must wait it out. In the meantime, make sure that contractions are as strong as possible by seeing that oxytocin levels are high. Ways to do this include nipple stimulation, kissing, sex-play, and herbal tinctures of blue cohosh. The mother's powers are critical in these circumstances! Make sure she is well hydrated, changes position often, has privacy if she desires, and feels free to make sounds (open throat, open vagina). Should contractions begin to diminish, stop all efforts to stimulate labor and support the body in getting refueled and rested, with a snack, a glass of wine, and plenty of pillows. When labor starts up again, go into stimulation mode, and after an hour or so, recheck to see if the head has come down.

In terms of time, there are limits. With a very long wait for descent in active labor—days, not hours—the lower uterine segment can get so thin that uterine rupture is a real possibility. But maternal exhaustion or fetal distress generally necessitate transport long before this could occur. The bottom line—mother and baby can only endure so many rounds of hard labor. If CPD is confirmed and all reasonable efforts to correct it have failed, take the mother to the hospital while she still has energy left. Pitocin augmentation may strengthen contractions enough to effect vaginal birth but can also be traumatic for mother and baby, so transport while both are still in good condition.

After so many hours of difficult labor, pain relief may also be of benefit. Particularly if paired with pitocin, complete pelvic relaxation via epidural may cause the bones to give just enough to let the head pass through, thus averting a cesarean. Still, this decision may cause deep disappointment for the mother, both in labor and postpartum. The midwife can help by assuring her that the pain of obstructed labor, with bone wedged against bone, is different from that of ordinary labor and much more intense—she is not "copping out."

If pitocin and pain relief do not work, at least the mother may be content with knowing that she has tried everything. Seeing a woman through a rough labor that ends in a cesarean is difficult at best, but stay focused on providing emotional support as you guard her physical well-being. Do all you can to see that her incision is double-stitched and that the cord is left pulsing as long as possible to ease the baby's abrupt transition. The pediatrician must be contacted, and the mother will need your immediate care postpartum. Get her up and walking as soon as possible (with staff clearance and support) to speed the healing process and help eliminate painful gas. Encourage her to nurse on demand, and see that she has healthy food and drink brought to her at the hospital (you or your assistant should also visit daily). And help pave the way for her homecoming by coordinating the assistance of family and friends.

Years ago, I served as doula for a woman with an undiagnosed, nine-pound breech. Her physician recommended a cesarean, and she agreed. Both the father and I were present in the operating room. The mother received an epidural but was unable to tolerate the sensation of numbness in her chest; she felt like she couldn't breathe. So she asked for general anesthesia and was put out. Her husband held the baby immediately, she was taken to recovery, and the baby was taken to the nursery where the father and I took turns rocking and holding it. During the next few days, the mother went through periods of intense depression and paranoia. Even though she had the baby with her, she felt incapacitated, vulnerable to hospital staff, worried about her two-year-old son at home, and extremely disappointed in her experience. One night, she was so upset that she asked me to come stay with her at the hospital. We did a lot of talking in the weeks and months that followed. She repeatedly asked questions about the birth, wanting not just reassurance but exact observations of the baby's behavior, the finest nuances, every little detail I could provide. A year later I received a picture of myself holding her baby girl in the nursery, along with this letter:

Dear Elizabeth,

It is a year on the 11th. Thank you so much for all that you gave me. What words can I use to tell you that without you my birth experience would have been really cold, my hospital stay a nightmare, but most of all, I would not have had a true witness to the birth, and how beautifully and perfectly you filled these needs. How I counted on you!

I hope that I am able to give something so wonderful into the great supply of love in the Universe.

POSTERIOR ARREST

Posterior arrest occurs if a baby in LOP or ROP position gets stuck at the pelvic inlet during active, first-stage labor. A posterior baby may pass through the pelvis without trouble, but all too often, the occiput snags on the sacral promontory and the head deflexes, impeding descent. The resulting lack of pressure on the cervix causes contractions to become irregular, inco-ordinate, and weak. Posterior arrest typically occurs at about 6 cm dilation, with station of –3 or –2. Occasionally, cervical edema develops and further compounds the problem.

Findings by internal exam are similar to those with large baby and small inlet, i.e., true CPD. But with continuity of care, you should know enough about the mother's dimensions and baby's size to set this possibility aside. Assuming there is adequate room and that malpresentation has caused relative CPD, it is necessary to do something to reposition the head and effect rotation. What are your options?

In the past, the only solution I knew was transport for pitocin augmentation, with the hope that stronger contractions might force descent and rotation. Of course we would first try everything we could at home: positioning the mother on hands-and-knees, having her walk, trying nipple stimulation, having her take cohosh tincture or pulsitilla (homeopathic remedy) to stimulate stronger contractions, and so on. It was frustrating to repeatedly encounter this problem, and to know in advance that our efforts would probably be futile and we would end up in the hospital.

No matter the cause, whenever there is malpresentation at the inlet, the problem is getting the head low enough to do something about it. But now, with a better understanding of optimal maternal positioning, the prognosis is not so grim. A forward-leaning position, with one foot (on the side where the baby is lying) placed on a small stool or stair, flexes and opens the sacroiliac joint, giving the baby more room to turn. The forward lean is very important, in that the baby's posterior shoulder is typically on the other side of the sacral promontory and *cannot rotate unless the mother gets her weight forward,* well over and in front of her ischial tuberosities.[10] Counterpressure and cold packs can be applied easily in this position, and she can also try rocking her hips to encourage the baby to rotate.

Or you might use the rebozo technique, adding a sharp jerk every few shakes on whichever side the occiput is resting. Try first with the mother on her back, and if unsuccessful, use the method described for turning a breech during pregnancy, but with mother in knees-chest position (see page 81). According to Dona Queta Contreras, a traditional healer and midwife from Oaxaca, Mexico, this motion sets up a current in the amniotic fluid that helps bring the baby around, along with opening the first chakra (for grounding and connection to the earth).[11]

Meanwhile, the mother will be experiencing significant pain in her back. I've heard it said that back labor is "anterior labor times ten"; be that as it may, pain relief is critical. Hot compresses with firm counterpressure can help, particularly if pressure is exerted with a downward thrust. To accomplish this, place the heel of the hand at the sacral promontory with fingers pointing toward the coccyx and press firmly in and down. In extreme cases, consider the use of sterile water blocks, or papules. This procedure involves four subcutaneous injections of 0.15 cc sterile water (using a tuberculin syringe) in the sacral area (at both dimples near the promontory, and an inch below on either side). Although this causes a very painful burning sensation for about twenty seconds, subsequent pain relief generally lasts from forty-five minutes to three hours. This alone may facilitate descent and spontaneous rotation.

Even if these suggestions do not turn the baby, they may open the pelvis enough to bring it within reach. At this point, you may wish to try **manual rotation.** The following technique is based on the work of an Australian obstetrician, R. H. J. Hamlin, who claimed success with more than a thousand attempts.[12] (Please refer to diagrams on page this page.)

Begin with an internal exam to make certain the baby's position. You will not be able to find the posterior fontanelle if the head is deflexed, but you should feel the anterior fontanelle near the pubic bone. Once you have found it, you can undertake maneuvers to flex and rotate the head. But first, you must slightly disengage it, that is, dislodge it from the plane in the pelvis where it is wedged. Do this by spreading your fingers on either side of the sagittal suture and pushing upward on the parietal bones. With this alone, flexion and rotation may occur spontaneously.

If not, have the mother fully recline. Your assistant should sit facing you, alongside the mother and next to the baby's back. Dislodge the head again, then exert steady, even pressure on the bony edge of the anterior fontanelle and rotate it to a transverse position. Now flex the head by pushing the fontanelle toward the side wall of the vagina (as if to tuck it back inside the mother), until it is almost out of range of feeling.

Quickly reach for the posterior fontanelle, secure an edge, and prepare to complete rotation to anterior. As you turn and flex the head, your assistant can help by grasping the baby's shoulder and backside, lifting and pushing its body to the anterior position. At the same time, the mother should be instructed to roll over slowly in the direction you are turning the baby. This makes it easier for the assistant to access the baby's back and further facilitates rotation. Once the mother has turned to her side, immediately check fetal heart tones. If all is well, have her sit fully upright, then stand and assume a forward-leaning position to secure the baby in place.

How much force do you need to use? Hamlin uses the image of "dialing a telephone," but this is a bit misleading, as there is considerable effort involved in maintaining flexion during rotation maneuvers. If you feel strong resistance at any point, attempt no further.

If you are working without an assistant, I strongly suggest that you perform these maneuvers with mother

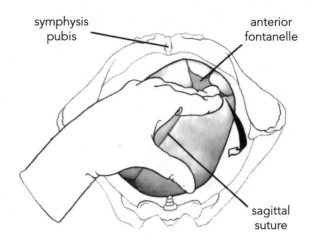

ROP to ROT

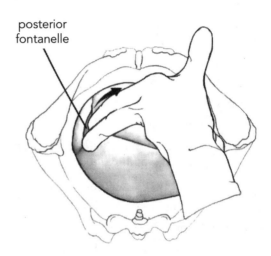

ROT to ROA

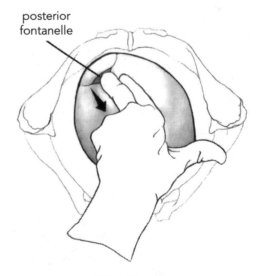

ROA Flexing

in knees-chest position. Knees-chest has advantages of increasing pelvic space and encouraging the baby to disengage (via the effects of gravity). For this reason, knees-chest may be your best option if the membranes have ruptured. Ordinarily, amniotic fluid provides room for the baby to move in response to manipulations, but when most of it has escaped, the uterus gets snug around the baby and makes it much more difficult to rotate.

If you do succeed in rotating the baby, have the mother maintain a forward-leaning, upright position, and check heart tones with every contraction for the next twenty minutes. Then do an internal exam to be sure the baby is still in place. Sometimes the baby reverts to its original position, and it appears that your efforts have been for naught. Do not be discouraged; you may need to make a few more attempts. With each, the baby should flex and descend a bit more, eventually staying in place.

Yet another rotation technique you can try involves (1) dislodging the head slightly, (2) placing two fingers, slightly spread out, on the sagittal suture line, and (3) turning them to rotate the baby. If the baby cannot be rotated to the anterior despite numerous attempts, consider turning the baby to OP—at least it can descend this way.

Here is an interesting case history. This mother was two weeks postdue; her baby was large and in ROP position. She had a long latent phase of twelve hours, with three more to dilate from 4 to 6 cm. The head was at −2 station and sharply asynclitic, with the right parietal bone presenting. The cervix hung loosely, and I couldn't even feel the sagittal suture as it was tucked behind the pubic bone. After a few more hours, cervical edema began to develop, but the head had come down a bit and the suture line was now within reach. With the mother's agreement, we attempted internal rotation and managed to turn the baby to ROA. It promptly rotated back to ROP but gained a centimeter of descent. An hour later and with good contractions,

we tried once more, and this time the baby settled at ROT, −1 station. With yet another try, the baby rotated to ROA, spontaneously flexed its head, and descended to 0 station, at which point we performed AROM to secure engagement. Fetal heart tones were fine throughout, and the baby was soon born in excellent condition. The mother found the procedure to be quite uncomfortable, but said that given the choice between it and transport, there was no question in her mind.

To minimize trauma, attempt rotation in a timely fashion when mother and baby still have the fortitude to handle it.

FETAL DISTRESS

Abnormal fetal heart patterns during labor have already been covered in chapter 4. In the event of transport for nonacute fetal distress, electronic fetal monitoring is likely. This may be external, internal, or a combination of the two.

There are two components of **external monitoring,** both belted to the mother's belly: an ultrasound unit to assess fetal heart patterns and a pressure transducer placed at the fundus to record uterine activity. With **internal monitoring,** which renders more accurate readings, an electrode is attached to the baby's head, and an internal pressure catheter is placed through the cervix and into the uterus to determine the actual strength of contractions. Internal monitoring is more likely when pitocin is used, particularly if there is fetal distress. Invasive as it is, internal monitoring alone shows whether the uterus is relaxing completely when contractions end. If it is not, reduced circulation can exacerbate fetal distress—and the pitocin should definitely be turned down or off.

In noncrisis circumstances, fetal heart auscultation and fundal palpation with contractions can be substituted for the assessments made by external monitoring. This is significant in that external monitoring generally confines the mother to bed, although some

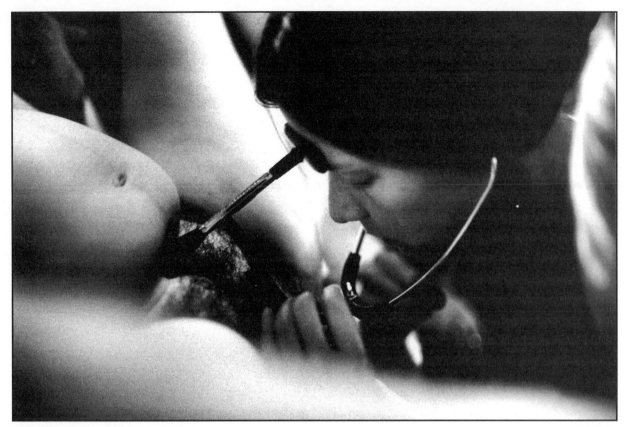

Using the fetascope.

hospitals now use **telemetry,** a remote monitoring unit that allows the mother to be up and moving (there are also watertight units that let the mother be submerged). Telemetry can be used with either external or internal monitoring systems.

Some hospitals utilize **scalp sampling** to further assess the baby's well-being. A small sample of blood is taken from the baby's head, and the pH is tested to determine whether or not the baby is acidotic, that is, truly hypoxic. Readings at or above 7.26 are considered normal. Fetal scalp sampling more truly identifies fetal distress than does fetal monitoring—not that the monitor readings are inaccurate, but some babies tolerate stress better than others. Thus, even in the presence of an ominous fetal heart pattern, labor may safely proceed if the scalp sample is within normal range. In short, fetal scalp sampling can make the difference between a cesarean or vaginal birth.

Some obstetricians use **fetal scalp massage** in lieu of fetal scalp sampling. Massage should be performed for about ten seconds. A fifteen-point acceleration lasting fifteen seconds is said to indicate a pH of at least 7.26.

CORD PROBLEMS

There are several types of cord problems that can reduce blood flow to the baby and cause fetal distress. **Cord nipping** occurs when the cord is periodically pinched between the head and pelvic bones, causing variable decelerations in the fetal heart rate (FHR). During first stage, repositioning the mother can shift pressure off the cord and brings the FHR back to normal. A remedy for variable decels in second stage is to press on the mother's abdomen where the baby's back is located—this frequently shifts the baby off the cord. It all depends on how low the cord is lying—if the head is able to move past it entirely, the FHR will return to normal. Otherwise, nipping may progress to **cord compression,** particularly in second stage.

Cord compression is usually due to **occult prolapse,** in which the cord is low enough in the pelvis to be increasingly compressed by the head as it descends, but not low enough to be at the os or in the vagina. If compression is severe, bradycardia will develop. Listen assiduously, as persistent bradycardia constitutes a crisis with very little leeway. Reposition the mother in knees-chest, and give oxygen at six liters per minute. Check the FHR with each contraction. If there is no improvement after four or five contractions and birth is not imminent, transport.

If it is a case of severe **cord entanglement**—that is, the cord is wrapped repeatedly around the neck or limbs and body—descent will probably be inhibited and you may hear cord sounds (a swishing like placenta or maternal artery, but at the baby's rhythm) over the FHR. A very tight cord around the neck can even deflex the head. The bottom line is persistent bradycardia, necessitating either birth or transport.

The obstetric disaster of **complete cord prolapse** is associated with polyhydramnios, multiple pregnancy, breech or compound presentation, and transverse lie—conditions where the presenting part is either high in the pelvis or fitting poorly at the inlet. Thus cord prolapse tends to happen in early labor (except with twins, when the second baby is most likely to be affected). Cord prolapse is occasionally diagnosed in the last few weeks of pregnancy with the discovery of pulsations at the cervix or through the lower uterine segment that are synchronous with the FHR. This finding necessitates immediate hospitalization and a cesarean to save the baby.

If the cord prolapses when membranes rupture during labor, call the paramedics and place the mother in a knees-chest position with your fingers inside her cervix, holding the head up and away from the cord. Do not remove your fingers until surgery is underway. Place the cord gently back inside the vagina if it is exposed. If there is not room, have someone bring you a washcloth soaked in warm water with a pinch of salt, then wrap the cord and cover with a plastic bag (rough handling of the cord or exposure to air can cause spasm and constriction). Give the mother oxygen at eight liters per minute. If you must transport her yourself, lay a chair back down on the floor and ease her on to it, then lift and tip her head lower than her hips (keep her in this position in the car).

Complete cord prolapse occurs very rarely, as many of the conditions listed above contraindicate home birth. But if the head is high in the pelvis near term and the mother reports labor's onset with rupture of the membranes, immediately go and check fetal heart tones.

MATERNAL HYPERTENSION

If the mother's blood pressure was elevated in late pregnancy, check every twenty minutes in early labor. You may be pleasantly surprised to find it decrease, as labor can be therapeutic for gestational hypertension. But if readings continue to rise, transport.

Bear in mind that hypertension in labor may progress to preeclampsia. Urinalysis for protein is somewhat unreliable in labor, as even with a clean catch, cells in the amniotic fluid may wash down and give a false positive reading. Instead, check for clonus/hyperreflexia and transport at the first sign. Hypertension in labor also increases risks of placental abruption and fetal distress, so check heart tones more frequently—every twenty minutes. Also push fluids, as dehydration can exacerbate the problem.

Herbal remedies may help to stabilize or lower blood pressure on the spot. The best is tincture of hops, one of the most effective sedative herbs known. The tincture form ensures potency (much stronger than tea) and quick assimilation (placed under the tongue, it absorbs directly into the bloodstream, whereas tea or anything else taken by mouth digests very slowly in labor). Tinctures of hawthorne, skullcap, and passion-flower are also useful, as is bathing with Epsom salts (magnesium sulfate).

If blood pressure is stable in early labor but rises at transition, place the mother on her left side to maximize oxygen delivery to the baby and give her oxygen at six liters per minute. Based on how rapidly labor has progressed and whether or not delivery seems imminent, make a decision on the advisability of transport. But do not be alarmed if blood pressure rises to 140/90 with second-stage exertion.

In the event of transport, standard procedures for hypertension include intravenous mag-sulfate for the mother and continuous fetal monitoring of the baby. Magnesium sulfate may reduce blood pressure somewhat but primarily serves to prevent changes in brain activity that could lead to convulsions. It can also slow labor, necessitating pitocin augmentation, and is associated with risks of pulmonary embolism and postpartum hemorrhage. Nevertheless, apart from the nuisance of IV and monitor hookups, the mother can still have a spontaneous, beautiful birthing if the hospital staff is amenable. The probable course of events should be discussed with the mother and her partner as soon as the problem develops, so they will be adequately prepared.

Any woman with borderline hypertension either prenatally or in labor is at risk for an even greater rise in blood pressure after delivery. Preeclampsia can develop suddenly in the immediate postpartum—be on the lookout for this.

PROLONGED RUPTURE OF THE MEMBRANES

Prolonged rupture of the membranes (PROM) is challenging to address, in that there is wide disagreement on just how long is prolonged. Although it is normal for membranes to rupture at the onset of labor, the concern is that the baby is now at risk for infection because the uterus is no longer closed to organisms present in the vagina. In this respect, PROM is merely a potential complication. The standard of care is to wait no more than twenty-four hours before inducing labor, and some physicians start even earlier to make sure the baby is born before twenty-four hours have elapsed.

The problem with this approach is that it does not incorporate factors of the mother's health, her personal cleanliness, or her environment as relevant to her risk status. Women planning home birth are usually in top condition, and it is a proven fact that risks of infection are much less at home than in the hospital, where patients are routinely exposed to virulent strains of microorganisms for which they may have little or no resistance.[13]

In 1996, a major study on PROM was conducted at the University of Toronto, involving 5,041 women from Australia, Britain, Canada, Denmark, Israel, and Sweden. At random, half had their labors induced, and the others were free to wait for up to four days for labor to start spontaneously. In terms of outcome, there was very little difference between groups—in both, about 3 percent of babies developed infection, and about 10 percent were delivered by cesarean.[14] Because this study was conducted in hospital, it is safe to assume that the risk of infection is even lower for women birthing at home (no accommodations were made for the health status of the women, either).

Yet another study published in the *American Journal of Obstetrics and Gynecology* more than two decades ago indicates that the risk for infection with ruptured membranes increases dramatically *twenty-four hours after the first vaginal exam*.[15] This makes sense, for how can we expect to move fingers (or speculum, for that matter) through the vagina without bringing potentially infectious organisms to the cervical opening? Thus it is crucial to avoid vaginal exams and cultures for as long as possible when the membranes are ruptured. The only exception would be to visually inspect the cervix and vagina for herpes lesions, if the mother has any history.

In my experience, it is not unusual for mothers to go twenty-four hours after the water breaks without even starting labor. But in order to minimize risks of infection, here are some commonsense guidelines for the mother (also given in chapter 4):

1. No tub baths until advanced, active labor.

2. No hand-mouth-genital contact.

3. Use utmost care when using the toilet, wiping backwards and washing hands both before and after.

4. No underwear, just clean loose clothing, and preferably no sanitary pad unless flow is considerable, in which case the pad should be changed often.

5. Have plenty to drink, in order to replenish amniotic fluid and keep system flushed.

6. Increase dosages of vitamin C, up to 2 g per twenty-four hours, or 250 mg every three or four hours.

7. Eat good-quality, nonconstipating foods, to keep energy levels high.

8. Take temperature readings every three or four hours, reporting any elevation at once.

Your backup physician may want daily blood-work for white blood cell counts and elevated banded cells (generated in response to acute infection). It is also possible for the mother to be only minimally infected, with the baby decidedly septic. If this is the case, fetal tachycardia will result. Once membranes have been ruptured for twenty-four hours, check fetal heart tones regularly.

Your response to ruptured membranes should include close phone contact with the mother during the immediate postrupture period to check on her morale and to make sure she is following guidelines for avoiding infection. Avoid exams and internal manipulations until they are absolutely necessary—definitely not before the mother is in advanced active labor. If

you must check, use Betadine or other antiseptic solution with a sterile glove and avoid inserting your fingers into the os.

If the mother is known to be group B streptococcus (GBS) positive, the guidelines change considerably. The Centers for Disease Control recommend that women with this status receive antibiotics if membranes are ruptured for more than eighteen hours. As mentioned in chapter 2, this is a matter of informed choice. If the mother wants antibiotics, you can administer them by IV. If she declines antibiotics, a pediatrician should see her baby as soon as possible.

Whenever risks for neonatal infection are increased, make certain the mother understands normal newborn behavior. An experienced pediatrician colleague says the first sign of newborn infection is usually failure to nurse. Any baby who acts listless or irritable should be checked at once by a pediatrician.

UNUSUAL PRESENTATIONS

Vasa previa. This is an exceedingly rare complication in which placental or cord vessels present over the cervical os. This can happen with a velamentous cord insertion, or if vessels extend beyond the edge of the placenta, running through the membranes immediately above the cervix to an accessory, **succenturiate lobe** of placental tissue. If the membranes rupture at this location, the mother will hemorrhage and the baby could die. This complication may be detected in late pregnancy with the discovery of a pulse near the cervix, particularly if unusual changes in the FHR are noted after the exam. If not discovered in pregnancy, vasa previa is usually identified in early labor. Otherwise, if membranes rupture and bleeding is noted, give the mother oxygen and rush to the hospital.

Face presentation. This is quite rare, occurring 1 in every 250 deliveries. In fact, careful prenatal palpation should have alerted you to this long before labor. With face presentation, the deflexed head is quite noticeable unless the baby is posterior (in which case the occiput is out of range). If you discover this before the head is down in the pelvis, make an attempt to secure flexion (see page 55). Bear in mind, however, that face presentation is sometimes caused by cord around the neck tightening and deflexing the head as the baby descends, so proceed slowly, with continual assessment of the FHT.

Another cause of face presentation is inlet CPD. Do your best to make certain this is not the case, lest you waste precious time and energy at home on a seriously obstructed labor.

The mechanics of face presentation require that the baby be born OP, that is, chin up. Although labor may begin with the baby anterior, descent cannot occur in this position because the brow will impinge on the symphysis. When the face first begins to show, hold back the baby's brow by applying counterpressure to the perineum until the chin escapes—it must not get caught behind the pubic bone. Obviously, the occiput will put extra strain on the perineum. Tearing is common with face presentations; you may not be able to prevent it. Suction is usually necessary because the baby is facing up and may thus get a nose full of fluids as the head births. Have resuscitation equipment ready.

The newborn will probably have considerable bruising and swelling, a clear indication for arnica and vitamin K. Also watch for breathing difficulties due to tracheal edema.

Brow and military presentation. These deflexed positions of the head can be remedied prenatally during the last few weeks of care. If they are discovered in labor by internal exam, you may be able to flex the head with internal maneuvers. See the earlier section, "Posterior Arrest," for instructions.

Compound presentation. Most frequently, this means that a hand is presenting alongside the head, a condition known as **nuchal arm.** Compound presentation is usually not discovered until the head is birthing;

it all depends on how far down the hand extends. If you find it before the head and arm are engaged, try Scott and Sutton's hip twist-and-lift movement—the mother stands, throws one hip forward, bends and then straightens leg to pointed toes, and repeats on the other side.[16] The biggest problem if compound presentation persists is the likelihood of perineal lacerations, as the head and arm together create an unusually large circumference. You may be able to avoid this by gently pinching the baby's finger well before the head crowns, which may cause it to retract its hand. If this doesn't work, prepare to extract the arm so the shoulders can be born. The easiest way to do this is to grasp the hand and manually restitute the head while bringing the arm across the chest and outward (see page 158).

Membranes presenting at delivery. This is not strictly a presentation problem but an unusual quirk of delivery. If the membranes present—that is, they bulge from the vagina as the head descends—they usually rupture when the head begins to distend the perineum. But sometimes, the break occurs higher up and away from the head, leading to a condition known as **delivery in the caul,** in which membranes envelop the face as it is born and will obstruct breathing unless removed. Some midwives routinely break presenting membranes to prevent this from happening, but the mother may resent this intervention, particularly as there are cross-cultural beliefs that birth in the caul brings good luck. Once thing is certain: the sensation of pushing a full water bag plus a baby is quite intense! If the mother complains or asks you to break the water, just be sure to warn her immediately before doing so, as the release of pressure can come as quite a shock.

If the bag is left intact and the baby is born in the caul, you must immediately hook a finger into the membrane below the chin and peel it back over the face so the baby can breathe. My daughter was born in the caul, and my midwife used a sterile receiving blanket to catch and lift the membrane edge, to which it adhered. Whatever you do, be sure and quick.

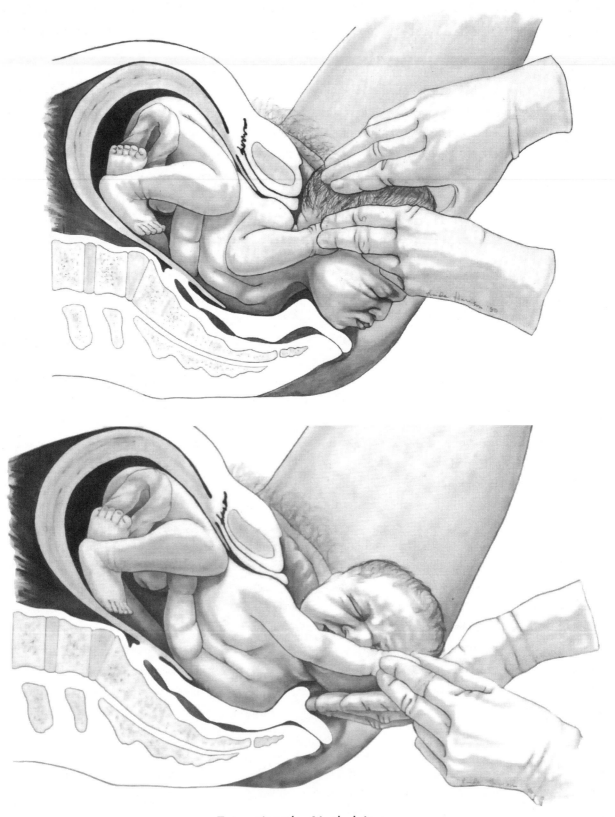

Extracting the Nuchal Arm

SHOULDER DYSTOCIA

Shoulder dystocia is a serious complication that can jeopardize the baby's life. It occurs when the anterior shoulder is impacted behind the pubic bone, usually because the shoulder girdle is too broad to negotiate the anteroposterior dimension of the pelvis. Because the baby is stuck in the birth canal, chest compression impairs venous return from the head and can lead to intercranial bleeding, brain damage, and death unless the problem is remedied swiftly and competently.

It is easy to panic with this complication, but less likely if it has been anticipated beforehand. The mother with a baby large for her pelvic dimensions is a prime candidate for shoulder dystocia. Nevertheless, it is important to remember that if the head can pass through so can the shoulders, although you may need to do a bit of maneuvering to make this happen.

Here is the usual course of events. An unusually large head passes over the perineum, then pulls back or retracts against it—this is the **turtle sign.** Due to tension on the neck, **restitution does not occur.** Both these occurrences are due to shoulders too high in the pelvis to allow the head normal freedom of movement. At this point, **the baby's color rapidly deepens to dark purple.** Despite the mother's pushing efforts, nothing changes and a diagnosis is made.

Immediately have the mother roll over to the hands-and-knees posture. Movement alone will often shift the baby and bring the shoulders spontaneously. If not, this posture will promote pelvic relaxation and enhance your ability to maneuver. Go directly to the **screw maneuver.** Reach inside the perineum for the posterior shoulder, place two fingers in front of it (at the juncture of the chest and armpit), and push backward to the oblique diameter of the pelvis (about thirty

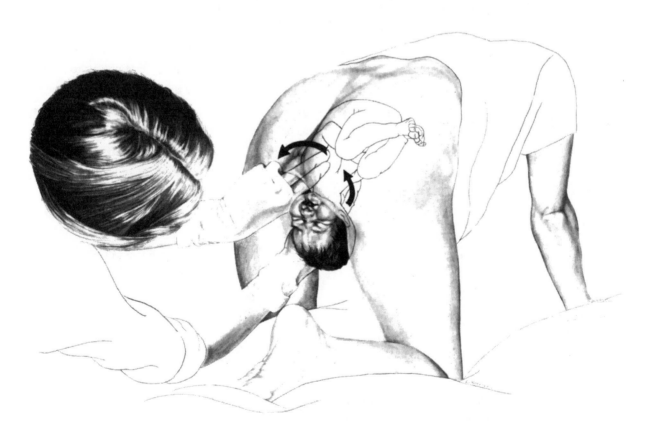

Managing Shoulder Dystocia

degrees). This dislodges the anterior shoulder and frees the baby to birth spontaneously.

An alternative to hands-and-knees is the McRoberts position, in which the mother is fully supine with her knees hyperflexed. This posture lifts the pelvis off the bed or floor, increasing flexibility of the joints and available room to maneuver. Have an assistant gently lift the baby's head up toward the mother's pubic bone, or do this yourself as you place two fingers behind the posterior shoulder and move it to the oblique position. Usually this will bring the baby, but if not, extracting the arm will further reduce the girth of the shoulders. To do this safely, splint the arm with two fingers, sweep it across the chest, grasp the hand, and complete the maneuver.

In either position, **suprapubic pressure** can help dislodge the anterior shoulder if applied in conjunction with your efforts. Suprapubic pressure should be applied at an angle, in the direction you are turning the shoulder rather than straight down. Do not confuse this with fundal pressure, which will only impact the shoulder further unless given in conjunction with firm suprapubic pressure (more on this in a moment). Some midwives slip an infant mask on the baby and give oxygen at six liters per minute as soon as shoulder dystocia is evident, which may improve the baby's condition at birth.

The worst case of shoulder dystocia I ever encountered was forewarned by another midwife. She visited me a few days prior to the experience and told me of a shoulder dystocia she had recently handled where nothing, not even the screw maneuver, had worked. "Well, what did you do?" I asked, and she said, "We pushed, pulled, and prayed until finally, the baby came out." This sounded like a panic scene I would just as soon avoid, but sure enough, a few days later . . . .

This mother was of small stature. She had been artificially inseminated, and knew nothing about the father. At her last prenatal, fundal height was 40 centimeters. After a long labor, the head birthed smoothly and without a tear, but I had to push the perineum back over the chin and there was no restitution. As the face rapidly turned purple, we had her move to hands-and-knees.

My senior apprentice was assisting; this was to be her first catch. She tried the screw maneuver but could not reach the posterior shoulder. She called for suprapubic pressure and tried again, but no change. So I stepped in and tried the screw maneuver and at the same time called for both fundal and suprapubic pressure. I figured that as long as we had strong suprapubic pressure to keep the anterior shoulder from being further impacted, fundal pressure would bring the baby down enough so that I could reach the posterior shoulder. This worked; I rotated the baby to the oblique and it was born. Although it was quite depressed and needed resuscitation, it was fine shortly thereafter (Apgars 2 and 8). But the mother tore all the way through her rectum; I had done an episiotomy out of panic and it extended badly.

My junior apprentice said later that she had seen the "Angel of Death," and it certainly felt to me for a time like we might lose the baby. But as I surrendered to my fear, adrenaline shot through me and I used it to help me complete the maneuvers. And yes, I guess I prayed, or at least offered up my total concentration.

Along these lines, students often ask how much time they have to get the baby out with this complication, and I always answer, "None." There is no time to waste on ineffectual procedures or on trying to figure out what to do—one must act immediately with the most potent response possible.

On another occasion, I was comanaging a planned hospital birth with one of my favorite backup obstetricians. This mother had experienced a difficult posterior arrest and transport with her first birth and chose hospital birth this time in case she wanted pain relief. She started out in the alternative birth room and progressed to about 6 cm, then opted for an epidural and was transferred to labor and delivery. She dilated rapidly to complete but slowed dramatically in second stage.

The physician was concerned but decided to leave the room because he noticed she did better when he was away. Although she was hooked to a fetal monitor, I suggested she squat on the floor by the bed, and the baby crowned immediately.

I called for assistance as the head was born, and it soon became apparent that the shoulders were stuck. Both the physician and I were quite disoriented. He was used to handling this with the mother reclining, and I was used to having her roll over to hands-and-knees, which the tangle of monitor tubes and wires prevented. As I was hands-on, he advised me to "pull down, down, down" on the head, until fearing I would damage the neck, I said, "No, you do it, you know what you're doing." Apparently he did not, because he began twisting the head this way and that, and I realized he was panicking. Suddenly, my mind cleared—I pushed his hands aside, applied suprapubic pressure, and directed him to go for the posterior shoulder, with which the baby promptly delivered.

Later, as he was completing the chart he pointedly asked me, "What would you call that delivery position?" The mother had actually been sitting on the lap of my partner who was kneeling behind her, so I suggested the term "supported squat."

"Hmm," he responded, "Sounds good . . . and that was suprapubic pressure with rotation to the oblique, was it not?" A nice gesture of acknowledgement, to top off a most challenging comanagement experience.

Purportedly, it may happen that you can reach the posterior shoulder but cannot rotate the baby. Based on my understanding of the mechanics of shoulder dystocia, this seems incomprehensible—after all, if the head has just passed through the vagina, the tissues should be pliable enough to turn the body easily. Perhaps this occurs more often in hospital when forceps or suction has been used, and the tissues have had little time to stretch and relax. Or perhaps the shoulders and chest are extraordinarily large and the fit is truly tight. In any case, **breaking the baby's clavicle** will collapse the shoulder girdle and effect delivery. Although this is a horrifying prospect, it is obviously preferable to brain damage or death. To break the clavicle, position two fingers against the anterior surface of the collarbone, place your thumb behind the bone and then push forward between your fingers (one doctor who used this procedure relayed that the clavicle "snapped like a matchstick"). As long as you break the bone outward, you avoid the risk of puncturing the baby's lungs. The baby should be seen by a pediatrician immediately, but do not worry—clavicles heal very readily.

Check any baby who has had shoulder dystocia carefully for bruising, injuries to the clavicles, or Erb's palsy due to nerve trauma. The latter is usually caused by pulling on or twisting the head—not maneuvers I recommend, for if the shoulder is stuck behind the pubic bone, what possible good can these do? Erb's palsy may be detected with an asymmetrical Moro's reflex (see "Newborn Exam," in chapter 4). Severe dystocia is an automatic indication for vitamin K. Consult a pediatrician at once if anything is abnormal.

This is often a "crash and burn" complication for the midwife; it can take a while to recover from such a close brush with death. In the first few hours postpartum, you will probably be completely exhausted from running so much adrenaline. Be very careful—it is almost impossible to drive immediately after handling a complication of this magnitude, so eat and rest (or sleep) before getting on the road.

SURPRISE BREECH

Even if you have decided you cannot assist breech births, it is wise to practice and memorize an emergency routine. How does surprise breech occur if the midwife has palpated assiduously? If the baby is extremely posterior, the sides of the head may feel remarkably like the iliac crests of the hips. Firm maternal abdominal muscle, excess fat, or extra amniotic fluid may also confuse your evaluation of fetal position. When in doubt, do an internal exam—the feeling of hard round head is quite distinct from that of the soft, irregular butt. If you are still unclear, order an ultrasound.

On rare occasions the vertex baby turns breech at the last minute, especially if high in the pelvis at term. Suddenly you have a surprise breech on your hands, and may not have time to transport. Be ready for this.

Assisting Breech Birth

1. **Warm up the room!** This is critically important in breech birth, as the baby's body will be exposed to air for an extended period.

2. **Have the mother in an upright position.** Standing, standing squat, or sitting on a birth stool or at the edge of the bed all work well.

3. **The mother must not push until the body is born.** If the mother pushes before this, she may bring the baby down before the cervix is dilated enough for the head to pass through. Once the body and cord are exposed to air, the baby will attempt to breathe, thus it is crucial that the head be free to deliver at this point. Although it may be stressful for the mother to hold back during pushing urges, she must pant-blow through most of her labor.

4. **Once the baby has birthed to the umbilicus and the legs are out, check for tension on the cord.** If it is tight against the baby's belly, insert a finger between the belly and cord and apply gentle traction to create a bit of slack. If it is under the pubic bone, move it gently to the side. But avoid handling if possible, as this can cause spasm and constriction of vessels.

5. **Unless the room is very warm, wrap the baby's body in two warmed receiving blankets to prevent stimulation of respiratory efforts.**

6. **If the breech is frank or complete and delivery of the body is arrested, nudge the legs to the antero-posterior position.** Do this by placing a finger at the illiac crest, then rotating gently. This should prompt further descent of the body. If not, and the baby arches sharply toward the mother's pubic bone, extract one leg by splinting it and bringing it across the body.

7. **After delivery of the shoulders, make sure the baby is OA.** If you must rotate the baby, grasp at the hipbones only, as undue pressure on internal organs could cause serious damage.

8. **Allow the baby to hang until the nape of the neck appears (or jaw line, depending on whether you are in front or in back of the mother), then support the body and slowly ease the head out.** This protects the head from being born too quickly, which can cause an abrupt and potentially traumatic change in intercranial pressure.

9. **Remember that babies born breech more often need extra suction, stimulation, or blow-by oxygen to help them get started.**

Note that many of these maneuvers can be modified if the baby is born in water. Certainly, waterbirth alleviates the concern about keeping the cord and body warm to delay breathing until the head is born. Water also provides support that makes it easier for the baby to negotiate its way out with less assistance from you.

An excellent reference on breech birth is midwife Maggie Banks's *Breech Birth: Woman-Wise,* available directly from the publisher Birthspirit on line at www.birthspirit.co.nz.

AMNIOTIC FLUID EMBOLISM

Embolism is the entry of foreign matter into the bloodstream. When this material enters the lungs, it causes obstruction or constriction. If amniotic fluid/fetal cells enter the mother's bloodstream, embolism can occur.

The exact cause of amniotic fluid embolism (AFE) is unknown. Possible factors include procedures of abortion, amniocentesis, and amnioinfusion. Hyperstimulation of the uterus has been implicated for the past thirty years (since pitocin has been used). More recently, Cytotec has been implicated, as it greatly hyperstimulates the uterus and thus may open microscopic hemorrhage sites to allow AEF to occur, particularly in VBACs with single-layer repair. Marsden Wagner has speculated that this may be a factor in the relatively high rate of maternal mortality associated with the use of Cytotec in labor, notwithstanding the difficulty of obtaining hard data due to gag orders on precourt settlements.[17]

There is also conflicting evidence to suggest that AFE *causes* hyperstimulation by setting off a catecholamine reaction. Whatever the mechanism, maternal mortality is 60–80 percent. Thankfully, this complication is rare, with incidence ranging from 1 in 8,000 to 1 in 30,000 births.

Symptoms generally occur when the mother is in hard labor, and include gasping for air, a drop in blood pressure, depressed cardiac function, hypoxia, seizures, and DIC. This calls for immediate transport. If born within fifteen minutes, 67 percent of babies survive intact.[18]

Treat the mother for shock, providing warmth, with feet elevated. Administer CPR with oxygen, and have your assistant run an IV. Or, if the mother has given birth, apply bimanual compression as she is likely to bleed out, and transport.

HEMORRHAGE

Hemorrhage is a complication we would all rather avoid. That is why it is crucial to take an exhaustive medical history and do thorough prenatal screening, including appropriate lab tests, so women likely to hemorrhage may be identified and treated, or risked-out in advance. All women should have a complete blood count at the initial visit, with a repeat at the onset of the last trimester. An adequate HCT/HGB reading ensures maximum resilience if bleeding does occur with delivery.

History of postpartum hemorrhage does not automatically contraindicate home birth; it depends on what caused the bleeding. If the mother recalls, "I was fine right after the birth, but then the doctor pulled on the cord . . . it really hurt, and I started to bleed a lot," you can assume third-stage mismanagement was primarily at fault. Additional information about subsequent measures required to stabilize the mother—such as medications or transfusion—will give you a more complete picture of the extent of the hemorrhage and the woman's recuperative abilities. Nevertheless, any history of postpartum hemorrhage or excessive bleeding following injury, surgery, or dental work should be investigated via lab tests for clotting factors. These tests are numerous and complex to interpret, so get medical consultation on this.

Yet another possible cause of, or precursor to, postpartum hemorrhage is close-set child spacing, that is, the mother has given birth to several children in quick succession without adequate time to fully recover. Childbearing and breastfeeding can take their toll on a woman's body; if abdominal muscle tone is not adequately restored postpartum, the uterus may not be able to contract effectively during labor or after delivery. Take a good look at the woman; observe her general appearance, energy level, and vitality. On this basis, recommend exercises to strengthen the abdominal muscles, or brisk walking or swimming to stimulate circulation. You may also wish to suggest appropriate herbal or homeopathic remedies. Cayenne pepper (three to six capsules daily) boosts circulation and revitalizes the system. She might also take alfalfa tablets regularly during her last weeks, as alfalfa is rich in vitamin K (which facilitates the clotting process).

Intrapartum bleeding. There are two principle causes of bleeding during labor, placenta previa and placental abruption. Rarely, bleeding may be caused by uterine rupture, or by rupture of a vessel with vasa previa (addressed in "Unusual Presentations," earlier in this chapter).

Placenta previa. This has already been defined in chapter 3. For review, this term refers to placental implantation low in the uterus, either over the cervix or at its edge, so that separation and bleeding occur automatically with effacement and dilatation. It is commonly diagnosed in the last trimester of pregnancy by painless spotting or bleeding, and appropriate management is determined at that time.

Placental abruption. Also discussed in chapter 3, this is premature separation of the placenta—that is, separation before birth occurs. This poses grave danger to both mother and baby: the more the mother bleeds, the more the baby's oxygen supply is reduced. The only way to control blood loss is by immediate cesarean, unless the abruption is marginal or the mother is in second stage and about to give birth. Here are the symptoms:

1. Severe, persistent abdominal pain (different from the ebb-and-flow sensation of contractions).

2. Abdominal tenderness (abdomen rock hard to the touch).

3. Fetal distress (with FHT pattern indicating hypoxia).

4. Blood appearing at the outlet (will not occur in the event of concealed abruption, as blood loss in this case is trapped behind the placenta).

Any woman with sudden, excruciating, and persistent abdominal pain, whether accompanied by bleeding or not, must be transported at once, and should be given oxygen and treated for shock.

If a woman complains of sharp but sporadic pain, apply heat to the affected area of the uterus and keep a close check on the FHT. The pain may be due to incoordinate uterine action, but transport immediately if it becomes persistent or acute.

Uterine rupture. In spontaneous labor this is extremely rare, particularly if the uterus is unscarred. It occurs when the normal process of retraction goes on and on until the lower uterine segment becomes so thin that it tears. It is associated with:

1. Improper use of uterine stimulant drugs.

2. Obstructed labor due to true CPD, transverse lie, fetal anomalies, or vaginal tumors.

3. Grand multiparity with prolonged labor or improper uterine stimulation.

4. Uterine abnormalities.

5. Pendulous abdomen with resulting malpresentation.

6. Overdistension of the uterus from polyhydramnios or multiple pregnancy.

Uterine rupture can also be caused by separation of a previous surgical incision in combination with invasive procedures such as version or extraction, fundal pressure, or manual removal of the placenta. If rupture is impending, the mother will be anxious, will complain of pain above the pubic bone, and will have elevated pulse with decreased blood pressure. If the baby has not been born, fetal distress will be noted. When rupture occurs, the mother may cry out or report that something has given way inside her, and will rapidly go into shock due to internal bleeding (face and lips white, thready, erratic pulse, cold sweat). Vaginal bleeding may or may not be evident. This is an extremely urgent condition requiring immediate transport. Treat the mother for shock and give oxygen at ten liters per minute.

Third-stage hemorrhage. This refers to an excess of two cups or 500 cc blood loss after the birth of the baby, but before delivery of the placenta. Estimating blood loss is not easy for beginners; try pouring a measured amount of liquid on an underpad (some midwifery instructors use a mix of liquid starch and red food color) to get an idea of what a loss of one or two cups looks like. Do not forget that clots must be added into the measurement.

There are three major causes of third stage hemorrhage: (1) partial placental separation, (2) cervical lacerations, and (3) vaginal tears. **Partial separation of the placenta** is the most life threatening of these, as blood loss is usually greater than with lacerations and more difficult to control. Why is this so? As long as portions of the placenta remain attached, the uterus will be distended and blood will continue to flow from vessels exposed at areas where the placenta has already separated. The only solution for this problem is delivery of the placenta, which permits uterine muscle fibers to contract fully and close off the bleeding vessels.

Although time is of the essence, always **determine the cause of bleeding** before initiating treatment for postpartum hemorrhage. In third stage, quickly rule out cervical or vaginal lacerations. **Cervical laceration** is unlikely unless pitocin, forceps, or vacuum extraction have been used to force labor. **Vaginal lacerations** occurring with a large or deflexed head, compound or face presentation, or persistent posterior may be deep enough to involve small arterioles, which tend to bleed in gushes not unlike blood loss from partial separation. Check the vaginal floor and vault swiftly but thoroughly, dabbing with sterile gauze at any torn areas. If it appears that an arteriole has ruptured, clamp an artery forceps wherever the blood flow is most concentrated and use tie-off suturing to control bleeding (see "Suturing Technique," later in this chapter). But if blood also appears to be flowing from the uterus, indicating partial separation, treat this condition first as it is more life threatening.

Partial separation of the placenta has several causes. A major one is incoordinate uterine action caused by "fundus fiddling" attendants. If left to itself, the uterus will clamp down uniformly and release the placenta completely in the vast majority of cases. But if it is poked and prodded, it contracts only in certain areas and releases just these portions of the placenta. Other factors in incoordinate uterine action include prolonged or precipitous labors, from which the uterus is too tired to separate the placenta in a single effort. Rarely, portions of the placenta are morbidly adherent and resist separating with uterine retraction, even if contractions are strong and coordinate. This is due to

a condition known as **placenta accreta,** which may involve little or all placental tissue (see "Retained Placenta," later in this chapter).

Bleeding without lengthening of the cord, and no apparent urge on the mother's part to expel the placenta, signal partial separation. To make a diagnosis, put on a fresh, sterile glove and follow the cord to the cervix. If the placenta is at the os, it is indeed separated and can be expelled by the mother's efforts, or you may use controlled cord traction to remove it. But if your fingers trail up through the os and into the uterus, you have diagnosed partial separation and should (1) immediately give the mother tincture of angelica, (2) begin vigorous nipple stimulation (if the baby is already nursing), and (3) administer 10 to 20 units of pitocin by IM injection (or by IV if you are able). These measures serve to contract the uterus, hopefully enough to expel the placenta in the next few minutes. (Do not worry that pitocin will close the cervix. It contracts the longitudinal fibers of the uterus only, not the circular ones at the cervical os.)

How you proceed from this point depends on the amount of blood loss. **If blood comes in small occasional gushes,** only a small portion of the placenta is separated. If you attempt to remove it manually, you might encounter large sections morbidly adherent and impossible to detach, and will cause significant blood loss as you distend the uterus with your hand. Repeat pitocin injection eight minutes after the initial dose (you may also try injecting a mix of 10 cc normal saline solution and 10 units pitocin directly into the cord if it has been cut). After several minutes, follow the cord to the cervix again to see if the placenta is present. If not, **transport.**

Remember that anything over two cups blood loss is considered a hemorrhage—some women will go into shock at the loss of four cups. Figure transport time and make a conservative decision. The paramedics will treat the mother for shock (reclining, feet elevated, warmed with blankets, oxygen by mask), but you must

Giving an Injection

1. Take a moment to steady yourself.

2. Flick the ampule to get all the medication into the base, and break the tip off and away from you, being careful not to touch the edges.

3. Remove the syringe from the package.

4. Remove the needle cover, place the needle into the ampule and pull back the plunger to draw up the solution. See that the tip of the needle is all the way into the ampule, to avoid drawing up any air.

5. Pointing the syringe upward, tap the sides to bring any air bubbles up, then press the plunger to remove air and bring the medication to needle level.

6. Locate the outer, upper quadrant of one hip.

7. Use your left hand to cleanse the injection site with alcohol by starting in the center and circling outward, then hold that area firmly, with the skin spread flat.

8. Plunge the needle in about three-quarters of the way in one quick movement.

9. Draw back on the plunger to see if a vein has been entered. If blood comes up, push the needle in a bit more and check again.

10. If clear, inject *slowly*, pushing the plunger all the way down to the base.

11. Draw the needle out quickly in one smooth movement, and put pressure on the site with a cotton ball until the bleeding stops. You may cover the area with a spot bandage.

12. Dispose of needles and syringes properly—that is, in the sharps box provided by your lab. ■

---

be sure to ride with her to assess blood loss and watch for signs of separation, as paramedics are not trained to handle this complication. You can also repeat pitocin injections at eight-minute intervals to control bleeding and keep her stabilized. If she begins bleeding heavily during transport, your only option is to manually remove the placenta then and there.

If blood loss is torrential from the start, manual removal is your only option. There is no time to transport; the mother could die if you delay. Fortunately, heavy blood loss indicates that a considerable portion of the placenta is separated, so manual removal should not be too difficult. Make sure the placenta is not already separated and lodged just behind the cervix, in which case it can be easily grasped and removed. If it is still attached, have an assistant call the ambulance and notify the hospital as you prepare to remove it.

Manual removal of the placenta can be painful for the mother and may lead to postpartum infection. Thus it should only be performed as a lifesaving measure. The procedure is fairly simple. Don fresh, elbow-length, sterile gloves, pour some antiseptic over your gloved hand and insert through the os, using your other hand at the fundus to prevent the uterus from being forced upward. Slip your hand between the separated portion of the placenta (which will be hanging free) and the uterine wall, then pry the rest off, using the edge of your hand like a spatula. Once you have it removed, quickly skim the uterine wall for any fragments, then grasp the placenta and bring it out. Your assistant should give methergine and/or pitocin at this point, and vigorous uterine massage should be started at once. Assess the mother's blood loss and vital signs. If her blood pressure is low, if she looks pale or feels cold and clammy, or if her pulse is erratic, give oxygen and transport at once, treating for shock. If she is stable, push fluids, keep her warm and quiet, and continue to assess vital signs. The placenta itself should be examined carefully to be sure it is complete. If there is any question, take the mother to the hospital immediately for a consultation (she may need a D & C). Bring the placenta in case evaluation by a pathologist is suggested.

If sections of the placenta cannot be removed manually, remove as much as you can. If the mother continues to bleed heavily, methergine can be given as a last resort. This will cause very strong contractions and may close the cervix, but your priority is to save the mother's life by minimizing blood loss during transport, particularly if she has lost more than three cups of blood and transport time is longer than twenty minutes.

I once had an uncanny experience with partial separation. After the mother called to tell me her labor had started, I lay down to clear my mind and focus on my upcoming tasks when an inner voice said clearly, "There's going to be a partial separation."

"Well," I responded, "that's reasonable, she had a little bleeding in the first trimester. No problem, I'll just go up inside the cervix like I've done before and grab it."

"No," the voice insisted, "you've never handled anything like this before. This time you'll have to go all the way up and really pry it off."

Now I was frightened! But I put it out of my mind and went on to the birth.

But it paid to be prepared. The baby delivered beautifully, then torrential bleeding began. I followed the cord up and felt it meet the placenta just inside the cervix and thought, "Oh good, it's right here," but as I attempted to grasp it, I realized the cord was inserted at the placenta's edge and the upper margins were still attached. Before I knew it, I was manually separating a very sticky placenta. I had my assistant give 20 units of pitocin IM (which we drew up in advance) as blood literally poured down my arm. I felt like I was on "automatic pilot," but the process was quickly and safely completed. The uterus firmed up right away, and the mother was stable with an estimated blood loss (EBL) of 800 cc.

In retrospect, I was very glad for this warning, although it raised concerns about recognizing and trusting my intuition, which led me to further study this subject. Now I consider my intuition to be a great asset to my work and give thanks for this powerful initiation.

Fourth-stage hemorrhage. This refers to blood loss in excess of two cups or 500 cc after the placenta has delivered but within twenty-four hours of the birth.

Most cases (80–90 percent) of fourth-stage hemorrhage are due to a condition called **uterine atony** (meaning lack of tone). Nevertheless, you must rule out other causes of bleeding before proceeding with a remedy, unless blood loss is torrential (covered later in this section).

Begin by ruling out cervical or vaginal lacerations. Also check to see if the mother needs to urinate, as a **full bladder** can cause postpartum hemorrhage by impeding the uterus from descending into the pelvis and contracting fully. Ask the mother if she needs to go to the bathroom or palpate the bladder to see if it is enlarged. A few drops of peppermint oil in the toilet bowl or running tap water nearby may help her let go.

Also rule out **sequestered clots,** which form when the uterus does not clamp down firmly after the placenta delivers. The clots distend the uterus, which causes more bleeding and more clotting, on and on in a vicious cycle. The best way to deal with sequestered clots is to prevent them. Massage the uterus firmly after the placenta delivers or, better still, have the mother birth the placenta in an upright position so her internal organs will compress the uterus automatically. Suspect sequestered clots if the uterus feels slightly enlarged or if a slow trickle bleed begins after the placenta delivers and then gradually increases. Check for clots by doing a sterile exploration at the cervical os, and remove by sweeping them out of the uterus with your fingers. Follow up with the uterine massage.

In managing fourth-stage hemorrhage, it is important to understand that oxytocic drugs, herbs, and homeopathic remedies cannot help a uterus filled with clots, or one prevented from contracting by a distended bladder. But oxytocics are crucial for treating uterine atony, which can otherwise result in considerable blood

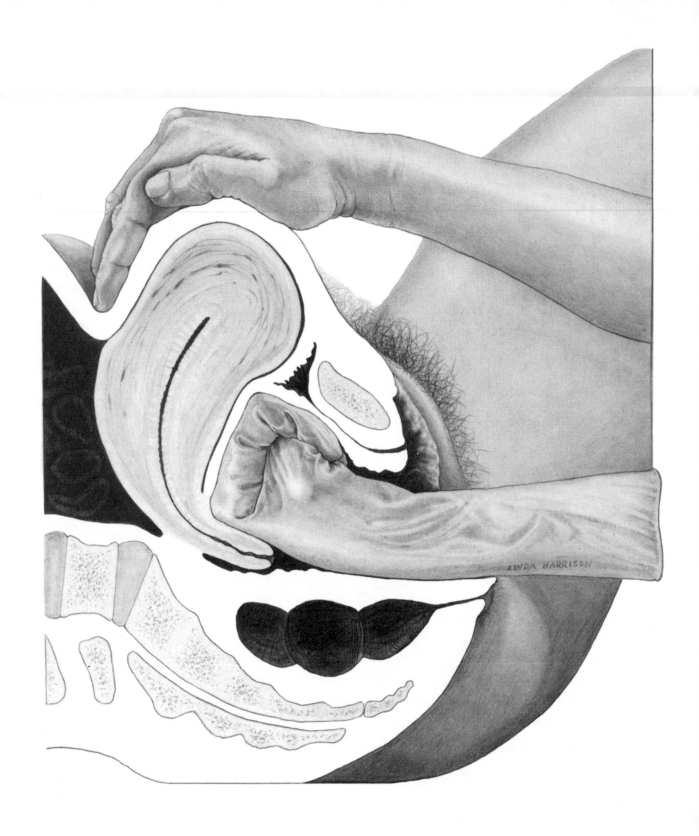

Bimanual Compression

loss. Uterine atony may be caused by long, drawn-out, or precipitous labors, which render the uterus too exhausted to clamp down efficiently. Overdistension of the uterus from polyhydramnios, a large baby, or multiple fetuses may also prevent it from clamping down after delivery. Respond to uterine atony with fundal massage and oxytocic drugs or herbs. This should work, unless a pathological condition inhibits coagulation (which should have been screened out beforehand).

If you are faced with a seemingly uncontrollable fourth-stage bleed—that is, uterine massage and medications do not work—immediately call for help while giving the mother oxygen and **bimanual compression.** In addition to the method pictured in the illustration on page 168, you can perform this maneuver externally by grasping and lifting the uterus firmly with both hands, then pressing them together as hard as possible. Treat the mother for shock and give fluids (by mouth or intravenously).

When dealing with a woman who is hemorrhaging, keep her attention focused on the here and now. This means commanding her to stay present, to look you or her partner in the eyes, or to touch and speak to her baby. In truth, you must call on her to rally her vital force, particularly if she is drifting or fading out. This is one reason why prenatal communication has to be authentic: you must have channels open and ready to be activated in case of this kind of emergency.

To illustrate: My former midwifery partner shared this experience of her second birth. She lived way out in the country up a rough road, and when her husband drove down to get the midwives, she delivered precipitously. After birthing her placenta, she began bleeding heavily and somehow managed to pull out a syringe, load it, and inject herself with pitocin. She later confided, "You know, Liz, I really got how women can just slip away when they bleed like that. I was already so high from the birth, and it would have been really easy just to check out completely. It was the coziest, warmest, most delicious feeling—it just felt so good."

I never forgot this, as only then did I fully appreciate how firmly and passionately the midwife must tell the hemorrhaging mother to stay present.

This links to an experience I had with a young Venezuelan mother who had just given birth precipitously. During pregnancy, she and her adoring partner told me repeatedly, "If there is anything wrong, just tell us and we will fix it." I thought them a bit naive but delighted in their devotion to one another. Soon after giving birth and delivering her placenta, the mother began to bleed quite heavily. My partner and I massaged her uterus, and felt her bladder, but could find no obvious cause, at which point we encouraged her to nurse, gave her some tinctures, and began to prepare the pitocin. Her partner turned to look at us and asked, "What is wrong?"

"She's bleeding too much," we said, "and we'll have to give her an injection."

"Wait a minute," he said. And as though it were scripted, they joined hands, looked into each other's eyes, and began to chant, "No mas sangre, no mas sangre" (*sangre* is Spanish for "blood"). In less than a minute, the bleeding stopped as abruptly and completely as if someone had turned off a faucet. And that was that!

Sometimes you have a case of **slow trickle bleeding**—a lazy, sporadic flow, which, barring other factors, may reflect the mother's emotional state. Brazilian home-birth physician Ricardo Herbert Jones advises, "Postpartum trickles are like tears from the uterus— you can help the mother stop bleeding by asking her how she is feeling."[19] But if the birth has been exhausting, or for some reason the mother is not glad to see her baby, she may withdraw into a state of emotional shock and simply "let it bleed." If so, take a strong stance and tell her firmly to stop. Have her touch and talk to her baby, kiss her partner, and stay involved with her support team. Give her something sweet to drink, with plenty of praise and encouragement. Tinctures of blue cohosh and shepherd's purse may help—give a large dose, a dropperful of each under the tongue.

Watch the slow trickle bleed very carefully. It may start and stop repeatedly, so blood loss must be reassessed continuously. If in excess of 750 cc (three cups), you must transport, even though the situation may not appear critical. You may need to give pitocin or methergine as much as forty-five minutes after delivery if blood loss has accumulated to 500 cc and the mother shows no signs of stabilizing. Experts on the subject repeatedly advise, "It's rarely the torrential hemorrhage, but the slow trickle bleed that kills." Stay alert, and do not leave the mother until blood loss has been fully controlled for at least an hour—longer if it has exceeded 600 cc.

RETAINED PLACENTA

The placenta usually comes away from the uterine wall with the first strong contractions following the birth. This may take ten, twenty, thirty, or more minutes, as the uterus must recover its strength and reduce in size sufficiently to shear the placenta away. Absence of the characteristic "separation gush" is a definite sign to wait and see.

Nevertheless, bring the mother's attention to her sensations as soon as you notice that contractions have resumed. She may not feel much of anything at first, but may suddenly become distracted from her baby or throw you a questioning look. If physical signs concur, advise her that it is time to birth the placenta, and assist her into an upright position. If you stick to this routine, you'll find the placenta usually delivers within the first half hour postpartum.

Certain circumstances may interfere. One is prolonged labor, which may leave the uterus so exhausted that it can't quite finish its job. If the mother is tired and the baby not yet nursing, offer tinctures of cohosh and angelica. After an hour or so, you may wish to administer pitocin IM or by IV. If none of these works, there may be a problem of abnormal implantation.

The rare condition of **placenta accreta,** in which the placenta implants in the myometrium, argues against cord traction under any circumstance. There is an unforgettable picture in *Williams Obstetrics* showing a fatal case of inverted uterus, pulled completely out of the vagina with placenta still attached. Upon transport, a D & C may be sufficient to remove the placenta depending on the amount of tissue affected, or hysterotomy (opening the uterus for surgical removal of the placenta) may be required.

Rarely, the placenta invades the myometrium, or muscle layer of the uterus. This condition, known as **placenta percreta,** is associated with single-layer repair of the cesarean incision. Thus, a midwife assisting a VBAC may request that the mother have an ultrasound to make sure the placenta is not imbedded at this site. Placenta percreta may necessitate hysterectomy if there is no other way to facilitate removal and is associated with a 50 percent maternal mortality rate.[20]

Typically, though, it is maternal inertia that stalls the birth of the placenta. I recall one birth that went quite quickly; we arrived when the mother was 9 cm dilated. She had established deep intimacy with her partner and her own coping routine, and regardless of our closeness to her prenatally, we felt like intruders. She birthed with very little assistance, then we waited for the placenta. Two hours later, after having nursed her baby and taken tinctures repeatedly, she went into the bathroom to urinate and delivered the placenta herself, in private. She came out and handed it to us, saying good naturedly, "Here's what you wanted!"

Some women resist letting go of the placenta because it represents the last remnant of pregnancy, or the last barrier to full-fledged motherhood. Focusing the mother on the beauty of her baby will often bring the placenta. Sometimes a bit of encouragement, "Let's just get the placenta out now and you'll feel so relieved," will provide the necessary prompt to let go.

How long is it safe to wait? As long as there is no bleeding, the uterus remains firm, and fundal height is stable, you can afford to wait for several hours. Beyond that, extended watch may cause anxiety and fatigue for

For Parents: In Case of Transport

1. **For the mother: don't panic!** It is easy to feel despair and lose control upon arriving at the hospital. But you have a better chance for a good outcome if you stay open and relaxed.

2. **For the partner or father:** If your partner is exhausted or nearly so, don't expect her to make complex decisions about hospital routine or physician recommendations. Here is where all your study and investigation during pregnancy really pays off. The better you know your stuff, the easier it is to respond to suggested procedures. And you can always ask your midwife for ideas or support.

3. **For both of you:** Ask for what you want, or enlist your midwives' assistance in doing so. You have only one birth of this baby; don't hold back! The hospital can be an intimidating place, but just because the routine runs a certain way doesn't mean it can't be altered. For example, you can definitely refuse (1) to wear a hospital gown, (2) to have people running in and out of your room continually, (3) to have attendants talking during contractions, (4) to endure bright lights in the labor or delivery room, (5) to have a routine IV, (6) to have a routine episiotomy, (7) to use stirrups for delivery, or (8) to have the baby taken away from you immediately (barring emergency complications).

4. **In the event the baby is temporarily stable but requires care in the nursery,** keep the baby with you as long as possible. Your partner should go with the baby to the nursery and should maintain physical and verbal contact with the baby (the isolettes have holes you can put your hand through) until you are able to join them.

5. **If you are unsure about any recommended test for your newborn,** ask your midwives or pediatrician. Don't be railroaded into a package treatment; let them convince you that each test is truly necessary for the baby's welfare.

6. **If you must stay in the hospital,** activate your postpartum support system immediately. Don't think you can wait until you get home—you need it now! Have fresh fruit, vegetables, bread, cheese, water, and so on brought in daily, as hospital fare is inadequate in quality and quantity for a breastfeeding mother.

7. **Don't hesitate to ask for privacy,** or to be left alone for a while. Routine checks on mother and baby occur on a regular schedule, but unless they are truly necessary because of some specific concern, refuse this constant monitoring or you will never get any rest! You may also find that as shifts change and new nurses appear, each will have some suggestion about wrapping, feeding, or caring for the baby. Offer your thanks but explain that you prefer to figure things out yourself. If they press you, reassure them that you are fine, and they need not worry. Otherwise, you can go crazy with input, and may lose confidence in your natural mothering abilities.

8. **If you have been in the hospital for a few days** due to some complication, be prepared to be absolutely exhausted when you get home. You don't get much sleep in the hospital anyway, but combine this with the stress of transport and the adjustments to your newborn, and imagine how tired you will be! Arrange it so no one is there when you first get home, except siblings and their caretaker.

9. **Take it easy on the processing;** it may take some time before the whys and the wherefores of transport become evident. If you start to feel emotionally overwhelmed, call on your midwives. ■

both the mother and her attendants. Also, the cervix begins to close after several hours, presenting an obstacle to placental delivery. Infection is another potential danger, as cord extending from the vagina may permit germs to migrate to the uterus. After two hours, talk about going to the hospital, and after another twenty minutes or so, transport.

ASSESSMENT AND REPAIR OF LACERATIONS AND EPISIOTOMY

One of the most interesting facets of my apprenticeship was observing the unique ways in which different midwives did suturing. Also interesting were decisions as to when, and when not, to repair. After observing the healing time and relative discomfort caused by various techniques, I developed a personal preference. This method is presented in the following section, along with many other critical elements of technique, by my friend and mentor, John Walsh.

Episiotomy is rarely justified, except in cases of fetal distress necessitating immediate delivery. An episiotomy may be easier to suture than a laceration, but one is obliged to cut through muscle, whereas lacerations are usually more superficial. Episiotomy weakens the musculature unless perfectly repaired and causes much greater discomfort and slower recovery.

With the vast majority of births, the perineum is intact. Otherwise, there may be a few minor abrasions (my midwife friend Tina calls them "skid marks"), none of which require stitches. These are most likely to occur on the labia and look rather like torn chicken skin with smooth and intact flesh underneath. Suturing these is contraindicated, because stitches will not hold unless imbedded in the flesh.

Sometimes a minor internal split of the bulbocavernosus muscle occurs, even though the perineum remains intact. If bleeding can be controlled with a bit of pressure (using sterile gauze), I usually do no suturing at all. Internal tear edges will usually meet and join together as long as the split is no more than halfway through the muscle. First-degree perineal tears also heal nicely by themselves if the mother takes good care of them.

But be sure to make a thorough and honest assessment of each and every laceration. Unfortunately, there is a strange status quest among midwives regarding the ability to do tear-free births; do not let this prevent you from suturing when it is clearly necessary. Sometimes the mother will be more comfortable if sutured, especially if tear edges do not approximate (fit together by themselves). See John Walsh's discussion of suturing technique on the opposite page. (More on aftercare of the perineum in chapter 6.)

INFANT RESUSCITATION

This topic should be discussed with the mother and her partner before the birth. To explain your procedures for resuscitation, you must cite primary causes of neonatal depression. Make clear that some occurrences—placental abruption or cord accidents due to prolapse, true knot, or velameutous insertion—can result in fetal demise despite your best efforts, and that the presence of resuscitation equipment is no guarantee of absolute security. Beyond that, resuscitation procedures should be described in enough detail so that in the event they become necessary, the mother and her partner will have a sense of what is taking place and can work to support your efforts.

Much has been said already about monitoring during labor so that fetal distress is not allowed to persist and deepen into depression. The most common cause of last-minute distress is severe head compression, which seldom presents a problem if the baby is born promptly. However, the baby's ability to tolerate this is based on many factors, including its health status and that of the mother, and whether labor has been prolonged. Remember that the baby of a clinically exhausted mother may react suddenly and severely to head compression in the

Suturing Technique

by John Walsh, MD, midwife

Unlike most obstetricians who prefer to make an episiotomy (with endless rationalizations), midwives take great pride in maintaining an intact perineum. This is the hallmark of a good midwife and is genuine proof of her patience and loving touch. Nevertheless, tears occur commonly and sometimes surprisingly. A nine-pounder slides out without a nick, while a five-pounder creates a second-degree laceration unexpectedly. Often the head is guided out exquisitely, only to have the shoulders do damage because of some urgency. And what does it gain a woman to have a wonderful birth at home only to have to pack up, drive to the hospital, and be sutured by strangers who may receive her with rudeness or even hostility?

Every midwife should learn to suture and do it without recoiling. It is one of those skills with a great aura of mystery about it. This is probably because suturing is considered to fall within the scope of surgery, with firsthand experience not easy to come by. Although it is a skill acquired by seeing and doing under the guidance of a teacher, it requires understanding and rehearsal before actual practice.

It is essential to set up properly for the procedure, or you will not be able to do a good job. The mother should be made comfortable on the bed's edge. She should have a clean, dry underpad beneath her. You must have excellent lighting; carry your own lamp and extension cord or forehead-mounted system to eliminate this worry. Also, you must get in a comfortable position as you begin—your back will definitely begin to ache, and sweat will pour down your nose. This is really hard work.

The first step in repair is careful examination. Wear sterile gloves for this. It may be necessary to place several gauze pads in the vagina to aid exposure and sop up the oozing that can obscure your landmarks. Roll up the gauze and insert like a tampon. Just don't forget to remove it when you are done—it will be practically invisible because it will be blood-soaked. Take your time to be certain you see the full extent of any tears or bleeding sites. Don't assume that everything is okay—you must look.

If the mother is uncomfortable during the exam, give local anesthetic now, starting with lidocaine spray or gel, then subcutaneous injections of lidocaine (1 or 2 percent). Wait a few minutes for it to take effect. Meanwhile, see that the mother is well supported with pillows, holding her new baby and not paying much attention to what you are doing.

Let the mother know that lidocaine does not completely anesthetize tissue, and she may feel moderate pressure or pulling sensations, although these should not be painful. This worries some women, as they are afraid your next movement will hurt a lot. Avoid doing anything suddenly, and the mother will begin to relax and stop anticipating pain.

The basic suture kit needs to contain:

1. **Two needle holders.** Five-inch Baumgartners are probably the best. The tips are small and serrated to hold the needle tightly without slipping. Hemostats should not be substituted, because the balance and the grip as the needle is driven through tissue make a subtle but important difference in doing a good job.

2. **A tissue forceps.** These look somewhat like tweezers but are called forceps. Semkin-Taylor or Addsons are good choices, as they are very delicate. Tiny, interlocking "rats teeth" at their tips enable you to hold and lift tissue very nicely without pinching or destroying membranes. Thumb forceps or dressing forceps are not suitable for handling skin, and the usual tissue forceps found in medical supply houses are too large and clumsy to do precise and careful work.

3. **Two or three mosquito hemostats.** As their name implies, these are hemostats with small tips used for clamping small "bleeders." They should never be used for anything else.

4. **Scissors.** A pair with sharp/sharp tips is used for cutting suture material precisely. This should not be the scissors used during delivery or for cutting the cord.

5. **Four-by-four sterile gauze pads or sponges.**

6. **Betadine solution.**

continued →

7. **Suture material.** Generally, 3-0 chromic gut on a round half-circle needle is most useful. The designation 3-0 refers to the diameter and tensile strength of the suture. 5-0 is smaller, weaker; 1-0 is thicker and stronger. A 4-0, 3/8 circle is best for more superficial tears; it pops through skin easily but can bend if used for deep muscle sewing. The needle is swaged onto the suture material so there is no "eye" or bump of thread to pull through tissue. By the way, catgut really comes from the submucous, connective tissue of sheep intestine. It dissolves in five to seven days, unless impregnated with chromic oxide, which prevents it from decomposing so readily. A new suture material, Vicryl, is increasingly preferred to catgut as it is less likely to irritate tissue.

Your instruments should be kept wrapped until the local anesthetic has been given. Suturing must be done by **sterile technique.** This may seem complicated and difficult to organize at first, but practice makes perfect. It is essential to have an assistant, and you both must know exactly what to do. In the following explanation, the one doing the suturing will be "A" and her assistant will be "B."

1. A opens her pair of sterile gloves and puts them on, then places the sterile inner wrapper down to serve as the sterile field.

2. B (ungloved) opens the outer suture wrapper and drops the sterile suture packet on the sterile field, then does the same with the sterile gauze pads and the syringe (this should be 10 cc, 23 gauge, three-quarters-inch needle).

3. A takes the sterile instruments (needle holder, scissors, mosquito hemostats, and tissue forceps) and places them on the sterile field.

4. B applies lidocaine gel or spray to the wound (without touching it), then wipes the lidocaine top with an alcohol pad.

5. A picks up the syringe and draws up an amount of air equivalent to the amount of lidocaine she wishes to inject—5–10 cc. B holds up the bottle, A injects the air through the rubber stopper and then draws up the lidocaine. A and B must be careful not to touch each other's hands or tools; this requires a delicate choreography between them.

6. A now begins injecting lidocaine around the edges of the wound and prepares to suture.

7. B puts on sterile gloves and assists by holding the labia open while A does the suturing. She can also reach for gauze and dab while A is stitching.

A word now about injections. Always begin by ruling out an allergy to lidocaine by reviewing the mother's medical history. And read the package literature that comes with lidocaine, especially the part about side effects. If the mother says she feels peculiar after you have injected, stop everything and assess the situation carefully. Every now and then, a woman may have a reaction that is simply one of distaste for shots and needles. True drug reactions are rare but emotional reactions common. Make sure that is all it is. If she is feeling faint, suddenly says she feels hot and shaky, or has a metallic taste in her mouth, watch for signs of shock. Take blood pressure and pulse, monitor skin color, check the uterus for firmness, and so on.

Injecting is easiest if you start at the top of the tear (inside the vagina) and work downward. Inject directly into the sides of the laceration, parallel to the skin. Try not to plunge the needle all the way to the hilt, as that is its weakest point. Inject no more than 1 cc at a time, pulling the plunger back each time to make sure you are not in a vein. It takes a surprising amount of force to squirt medication into tissue. Be patient; if you inject too quickly it will sting. The tissue may become somewhat distorted by the anesthetic, so when you are finished injecting, reassess your landmarks.

Now clamp your needle so it is perpendicular to the needle holder and curves away from you. If you are right-handed, the point should be to the left. Once the lidocaine has taken effect, start a row of continuous sutures at the apex of the tear inside the vagina. Your tissue forceps grasps the left side, the point of the needle is placed about a quarter inch from the right edge, and a bite of tissue is taken, moving right to left. The needle pops through the other side to be clamped in the middle by the second needle holder. Unclamp the first needle holder, then pull the suture until you have a short end of about three inches. Reclamp the needle with the first needle holder, set all down on your sterile field, and triple-knot your first stitch, trimming the short end to a quarter inch.

Now make a series of stitches, as above, about three-eighth of an inch below one another. Pull

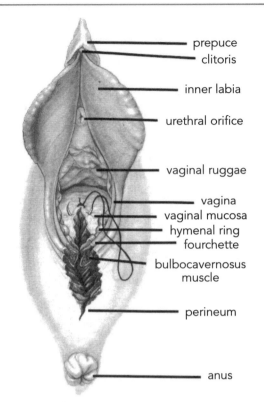

prepuce
clitoris
inner labia
urethral orifice
vaginal ruggae
vagina
vaginal mucosa
hymenal ring
fourchette
bulbocavernosus muscle
perineum
anus

Anatomical Landmarks

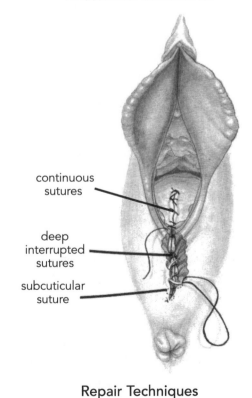

continuous sutures
deep interrupted sutures
subcuticular suture

Repair Techniques

slightly on the strand as each stitch is placed, so the edges to be closed next will come into view easily. It also helps to reapproximate edges (hold them together) every stitch or two, to make sure they are matching up correctly. The last stitch should be placed just inside the hymenal ring. Cut the suture to leave an end of about four inches (you will later tie this to the strand used to repair the perineum).

Next, join the deep muscle tissue with a series of two or three interrupted sutures. These will bring the edges of the skin closer together, evenly distributing tension and eliminating dead space. Start at the top and work your way down. The first of these, where the tear is the deepest, should be done in two parts, one bite on each side (like halves of a circle). These stitches should be parallel to the vaginal floor; be sure to keep your needle holder vertical to avoid entering rectal tissue. The first stitches are triple-knotted, with both ends cut. Your final stitch should be triple-knotted too, but do not cut both ends— *leave the suture string attached.*

Now close the superficial layer just under the perineal skin with subcuticular stitches. Your first stitch goes on the right, parallel to the skin, from the level of the last internal stitch down to the bottom of the tear. Run a second stitch upward on the left side (again, like halves of a circle). To continue to go upward, you must *reverse the needle position in your needle holder,* that is, the point of the needle should be on the opposite side of how it has been thus far. Make your stitch on the right, then switch the needle again to move up the left, and so on. Place your final stitch so the point comes up just inside the hymenal ring, opposite the loose end. Pull each end separately until snug, then triple-tie together, and trim.

Here are some basic principles to keep in mind for any type of suture job:

1. **Close lacerations (no matter where they are) in layers—muscle, fascia, skin.** The basic idea is to eliminate tension in any one spot.

2. **Eliminate dead spaces between layers.** Otherwise, oozing can occur and a small (or large) hematoma can form. These terribly painful swellings can cause the repair to fail. Dead, empty spaces are weak and prone to infection.

continued →

3. **Don't suture too tightly or you will impair circulation.** Anticipate slight tissue swelling after you complete the repair, and compensate by not sewing too tightly. Do not use too many stitches either, as each interferes with circulation to some extent. Vaginal tissue is highly vascular and good at healing itself.

4. **Check your landmarks very carefully and repeatedly.** If you have waited several hours to do a repair, edema may confuse the picture. Double-check what goes with what. Go slowly. The bulbocavernosus muscle at the mouth of the vagina is an important landmark; it should be united very meticulously. Also, if the tear is deep, make certain that the levator ani muscle encircling the anus has not been torn either partially or completely. Repair of a third-degree laceration is strictly a job for the experienced.

5. **Sutures should be placed so that the depth is greater than the width.** This fundamental principle of suturing produces a closure where the edges meet correctly, and it is important to figure out why this is so.

6. **Be careful never to clamp the suture with the needle holder,** as it may break at this site. Suturing is easier if you wet the suture with Betadine before beginning, and as needed as you work. This keeps the string from sticking to itself (and to your gloves).

7. **An assistant can be very helpful by cutting sutures as they are placed.** This saves you the movements of laying down the needle holder and forceps to pick up the scissors. Hold both strands tautly as your assistant prepares to cut. She takes the scissors and then, with the index finger pointing down the blades, opens the scissors tops just slightly, places them slowly on the strands a quarter inch from the knot, and quickly snips. If the tails are cut too short they may slip, whereas long ends cause irritation by poking adjacent tissue.

If there is swelling after the repair, give the mother arnica and have her apply alternating warm and cool compresses to stimulate circulation. Ice packs should only be used if swelling is extreme. Make sure to tell the mother to rinse the area each time she uses the toilet, using warm water with a squirt of Betadine. It is also a good idea to expose the perineum to sunlight, a light bulb, or a hairdryer to keep it dry. The mother should avoid applying vitamin E or other oils to the wound, as this retards the healing process. If you have done a good job, the majority of the healing will take place in a few days. (More on aftercare of the perineum in chapter 6.) ■

---

final stages of labor. As stated earlier, moderate bradycardia or early decels to 60 BPM or less are definite indications for immediate delivery.

When a baby is born in compromised condition, the top priorities for stabilizing it are **warmth** and a **clear airway.** Regarding the latter, it is crucial to appreciate the folly of trying to resuscitate a baby if it is chilled. Naked and wet, the newborn loses body heat rapidly unless placed on the mother's belly and covered, head to toe, with two or three flannel blankets (preferably oven-warmed). Suction as indicated, but be careful not to stimulate the gag reflex by placing the bulb syringe too far back in the throat. The American Heart Association and the American Academy of Pediatrics have developed a course on neonatal advanced life support (NALS), which is more comprehensive than basic CPR. For information, call 800-242-8721, or contact the nearest branch of the American Heart Association.

Unless at risk due to stressful labor, postmaturity, prematurity, or intrauterine growth restriction, a baby with a hypoxic phase of fewer than ten minutes will usually come around quickly if given stimulation and warmth. Minor, last-minute depression causes no significant change in blood pH (acidosis) that might hinder spontaneous recovery. Remember that the baby will continue to receive oxygen from the mother as long as the cord is left pulsing—this allows time for complex internal changes that establish respiration. This transition takes longer for some babies; it is not abnormal for twenty seconds to elapse before significant respiratory efforts are made.

Neonatal depression falls into two basic categories. **Primary apnea** (*apnea* means without breath) describes the baby who has not been hypoxic for long, but has already made gasping/respiratory efforts while in utero in an attempt to compensate. Stimulation, blow-by oxygen (holding tube by the nose), or a few rescue breaths should bring this baby around. But the baby who has suffered a greater degree of hypoxia and has made a second round of gasping/respiratory attempts is in **secondary apnea.** It will not attempt to breathe on its own again, so waste no time with stimulation. This baby needs ventilation, via mouth-to-mouth or bag-mask resuscitation, sufficient to reverse the acidosis caused by severe hypoxia.

Determine appropriate resuscitation techniques by taking your cues from the baby's color, muscle tone, and respiratory efforts. Although Apgar scoring is not officially performed until one minute, a baby rating 6 at birth—blue, a bit floppy, minimal respiratory efforts but definitely present—needs suction, warmth, and stimulation via immediate, firm massage at the base of the spine and up the back. Make this an outpouring of positive energy through your hands. Keep the baby against the mother's skin for continued warmth and contact—you can reach under the blankets to stimulate. Gentle words of encouragement, for example, "Come on, baby," help the mother and her partner stay connected and focused on the baby's well-being. Better yet, *get the mother to talk to her baby.* Neonatal intensive care nurses report that babies' oxygen levels surge upon hearing the sound of their mother's voice.

With these techniques, response should occur within fifteen seconds to twenty seconds; if not, try

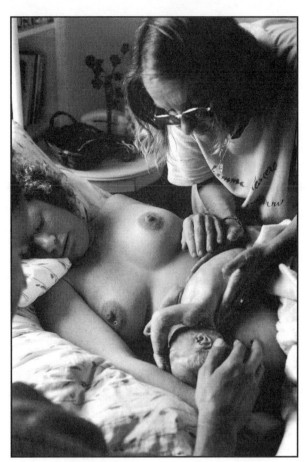

The midwife stimulates a baby making a slow transition, keeping the baby warm against the mother.

using a seesaw motion of rocking the baby from head to toe. This affects diaphragmatic pressure and can stimulate respiration. Remember to keep the baby warm too—change dampened blankets promptly.

Hospital management of the slightly depressed baby is often quite different. Duties are sharply divided between obstetrician and neonatologist, according to their respective liabilities. It is simply not within the obstetrician's scope of practice to stimulate the newborn; it must be passed immediately to the neonatal team. This requires premature cord clamping, which further compromises the baby. The neonatologist then places it in a resuscitation unit, applies mechanical suction to its nose and throat, and, more often than not, bag-masks it even though it is already breathing. Time and again, I have watched babies deteriorate rapidly with this treatment. It is noteworthy that in all this, stimulation is usually overlooked—no one touches the baby. Sometimes I simply do it myself, while encouraging the mother to talk to the baby from across the room.

The baby born in secondary apnea, with an Apgar of 2 or less, is easily recognizable by its shocking white and completely limp appearance. Wrap it immediately in warm blankets, and as soon as suction is complete, administer mouth-to-mouth or bag-mask resuscitation with oxygen. If the heart rate is less than 60 BPM, begin cardiac massage. A friend or the father/partner should call the ambulance at once.

Mouth-to-mouth resuscitation is usually sufficient for all but the most severe cases. Although the "kiss of life" is no longer administered directly, you should begin resuscitation immediately with your pocket mask while the oxygen is being readied. Often the baby will open its eyes and look straight into yours before it begins to breathe, which opens your heart and greatly boosts your concentration.

Sometimes babies make gurgling noises as you resuscitate them. Depending on degree, you may need to suction again (use a DeLee for best results). Rarely, globs of thick mucus are lodged in the throat and must be quickly removed with a fingertip. But don't fuss too much with this—securing ventilation is your top priority. If the Apgar at five minutes is less than 7, keep working to get the baby stimulated and engaged, and redo Apgar readings every five minutes until you have two in a row of 8 or higher.

Circumstances of newborn stabilization are not always black and white. I have seen a few babies birth in fine condition and then rapidly deteriorate due to a lukewarm reception from the parents. Sometimes the mother is so exhausted that she cannot muster welcome for the baby. Or perhaps the baby is of undesired or unexpected gender. You use your heart in moments like these: "What a gorgeous girl (or boy) you have!" Or

to the sibling standing by, say enthusiastically, "You have a sister (or brother)!" Love kindles life—it is just that simple—and it is the midwife's task to bring this to bear if need be.

I had an experience along these lines that bears repeating. The baby was born after an hour-long second stage and trouble-free labor. Heart tones were good throughout crowning, the scalp tone was pink. No meconium in the waters, but there was a tight cord around the neck, which I clamped and cut at once. The shoulders then birthed without delay, so there was no reason to expect what happened next.

Although the Apgar was 6 at birth, the baby failed to make respiratory efforts and lost what little muscle tone and color it had. Stimulation seemed to help, and the baby pinked up a bit with DeLee suction (it actually sucked the tubing). I thought the baby had made it then, but instead it proceeded to go pale and flaccid. I tried a few breaths mouth-to-mouth, to which the baby responded mildly (although it had never really stopped breathing after initial stimulation). The one-minute Apgar was 4. I tried more stimulation, but the moment I stopped, the baby began to fade away again.

Several minutes had gone by, so I decided that I would take the baby and give it all the energy I could muster (I also had my apprentice call 911). As I took the baby in my hands and instinctively began the diaphragmatic seesaw, someone in the room observed that the baby had not yet opened its eyes. At that it winked its lids, and I began to swing its body slowly from side to side, hoping to prompt it to take a peek. Not much of anything, and I was beginning to panic. Then I recalled that its strongest response had been sucking on the DeLee, so I put my little finger in its mouth. I felt a wave of desperation and tenderness sweep through me as I began to speak, "Come on in, baby, it's not so bad here, come on, please come in." At that, it started sucking, opened its eyes, and looked right at me, and then turned nice and pink. Meanwhile, the paramedics arrived, but soon realized that nothing but observation was needed and left shortly thereafter.

How to explain the baby's in-and-out behavior? Likely causes, such as prematurity, infection, or maternal drug use, did not apply. There was, however, severe emotional tension between the parents regarding their relationship and the baby. The father had been unfaithful repeatedly during pregnancy and had made no adjustment whatsoever to his new responsibilities. Just moments after the birth, he literally moved to the far side of the room, and the mother froze up completely. I think the baby simply felt unwanted. The father would not connect with it at all; the mother would not speak to it when I prompted her. No wonder it was tentative! This was why, when I gave it my finger to suck, I instinctively said, "It's not so bad here . . . come on in."

This experience overwhelmed me, as I realized that the baby's life was entirely in my hands—that I alone would make the difference in its decision to live. I had never been in this position before and still recall the confusion of searching for the baby's soul, while hoping to give enough of myself and my love that it would want to stay. And I definitely learned the importance of clearing up chaotic personal issues between parents in advance. As it turned out, the parents separated shortly after the birth, and the woman moved out of the area. But she kept in touch and proved to be a loving and devoted mother.

In any marginal situation like this, be sure to maintain an extra-long postpartum watch. Check the baby carefully and repeatedly (especially the heart and reflexes). Do not leave until the mother is warmly attentive and the baby is glowing. Contact the pediatrician and arrange to have the baby seen as soon as possible.

Principles of Infant Resuscitation

If the baby is born limp and floppy, with white body:

1. **Have your assistant or a family member call 911.**

2. **Provide warmth.** Wrap the baby with blankets and cover the head.

3. **Clear the airway.** Suction mouth with bulb syringe or DeLee if necessary.

4. **Move the baby to a flat surface and position so the chin is up but not overextended.** Otherwise, the airway will be occluded.

5. **Begin ventilation.** Place a mask unit over the baby's nose and mouth, and give two slow breaths, allowing for exhale in between. Watch the baby's chest—it should rise and fall as you work. If not, make sure you have a good seal over the nose and throat.

6. **If necessary, do full CPR.** Have your assistant take the baby's pulse, and if below 60, begin cycles of three chest compressions to one breath, with approximately 120 compressions per minute (or as close to that as possible). Give compressions by placing two fingers on the lower half of the sternum (just below the nipple line), pressing in about a third the depth of the chest. Switch to your ambu-bag (hooked to oxygen) as soon as possible.

7. **After thirty seconds, briefly stop and recheck pulse.** Discontinue chest compressions once the heart rate reaches 60 BPM. ■

FETAL ANOMALIES

Fetal anomalies can be genetic in origin or may be caused by certain viruses, chemicals in the environment or workplace, radiation, street drugs, or pharmaceuticals. Use a current issue of the *Physician's Desk Reference* to identify teratogenic effects of over-the-counter and prescription medications. The Organization of Teratology Information Services (OTIS) is an excellent resource on teratogens of every kind; reach them at (866) 626-6847 or at www.OTISpregnancy.org. Information on parent support organizations can be obtained toll-free from the March of Dimes Birth Defects Foundation at (888) 663-4637.

The most common fetal anomaly is heart defect. Minor defects like cleft palate or clubfoot are undetectable until birth, whereas more serious ones like spina bifida (exposed spinal meninges) may be discovered by blood tests and ultrasound in early pregnancy (see chapter 2). Although generally detected by (AFP) screening, palpation in late pregnancy may disclose hydrocephaly (enlarged cranium) or anencephaly (little or no cranial vault, with extremely large, long limbs).

Whenever a baby is born with anomalies, parents need to see, touch, and bond, regardless. Most mothers readily embrace their babies regardless of defects, often noting the beauty of other features. Just be sure to stay in close proximity to the mother and her partner until you are certain they have noticed the anomalies. Avoid pointing these out unless they are clearly in denial; in which case, do so simply and gently, without discourses on causes, treatment, outcome, and so on. This information will surely be requested later; let the parents set the pace.

Occasionally, a mother totally rejects a severely deformed infant upon its arrival. If so, comment on the many perfect features of the baby. This provides a foundation for bonding without forcing her to confront the anomalies immediately.

Some midwives feel an odd sense of shame when assisting the birth of a baby with anomalies. This is probably a carryover from the medieval days, when midwives were accused of practicing witchcraft and causing fetal deformity. But it is also possible to feel all the joy and wonder of assisting a normal baby—maybe more so. As one midwife colleague reports: "I had always been afraid of assisting a baby with deformities, but when it finally happened I felt thrilled by his beautiful spirit, and very welcoming. He had lots of anomalies, but his body was secondary. I was shocked at how open I was to him, almost as if his imperfections made him more perfect in some way. This touched my heart profoundly."

It is also normal to feel disappointment or sadness, but your most crucial task is to open your heart and stay in the moment. You have plenty of time later to find your own support, but your initial reaction sets the tone for parents to begin making an adjustment.

Most anomalies require no immediate treatment, except for heart defects (indicated by cyanosis and respiratory distress) or spina bifida. In both cases, the pediatrician should be contacted and the baby transported to the hospital at once. With heart problems, keep the baby warm and give blow-by oxygen; with spina bifida, cover sinuses or exposed meninges with sterile gauze soaked in warm saline solution. Although not urgent, a baby with other anomalies should be seen as soon as possible, as there may be other internal defects not readily detected by cursory examination.

Stay in close contact with the parents—not just for weeks, but for months. Do whatever you can to connect them with resources for information and support. This is certainly one area where the Internet has been a boon, as those who once suffered in isolation can now go online and find chat groups of others in the same situation. As mentioned earlier, there are also numerous national and international support organizations dealing with specific anomalies (see appendix B).

If anomalies are so severe as to be incompatible with life, take your cues from the mother and her partner. They may or may not want to transport; you are obligated by professional ethics to respect their wishes. On the other hand, you must also give life support and call the paramedics if the baby appears to be viable. (See the next section on "Stillbirth and Neonatal Death" for more information.)

STILLBIRTH AND NEONATAL DEATH

Often death is caused by severe deformity, and it is clear that there are only moments of time for greeting, acknowledgment, and letting go. It is a blessing that birth generally leaves us refreshed and exhilarated, so if death occurs soon after, it is in a positive, open framework.

It is different when a baby is stillborn, especially with no apparent defect. Depending on when the baby died, the mother will be either in shock or already grieving as she gives birth.

Many women considering becoming a midwife hesitate at the thought of losing a baby. Is it the tangle of emotions, fear of accusation, or confrontation with death itself that is so terrifying? It helps to remember that birth and death are both high-energy, transitional states, and guidelines for moving through them are virtually identical. It is incomprehensibly tragic to lose a baby, but easier if everyone stays emotionally present and connected. Help the mother touch and claim her baby; encourage both parents to look and caress. They may want to save a lock of hair, take foot and handprints or photographs. If they have a name for the baby, encourage them to use it. Bear witness to this rite of passage. Don't give consolation; there will be time for that later on.

The coroner must be notified of any stillborn infant weighing 500 grams or more. Autopsy is at the discretion of the coroner. But if it can be established that the baby has been dead for some time, autopsy is optional. The coroner releases the body to a funeral home of the mother's/parents' choosing. With hospital stillbirth, the physician signs the death certificate; out of hospital, this is the coroner's task.

It is very difficult for the mother in the first few days postpartum. Her hormones fluctuate dramatically, and her milk begins to flow. Lactation can be suppressed with sage tea or by binding the breasts. But the grief is something else. Plan to spend time with the parents daily for the first few weeks. Friends and family will stop by and will look to you for reassurance and support (and they will have lots of questions). Take care of yourself and get plenty of rest, even as you see to the mother's recovery by guarding her privacy, if need be. Just being there as a witness and friend, ready to listen if she or someone close to her needs to talk, is your most important task right now.

After assisting her first stillbirth, a local midwife shared being both surprised and honored that at the memorial, each guest made a point of speaking not only to the parents and the reverend but to her as well. Be prepared to play an important role in this event. And at some point, encourage the parents to make a scrapbook or write a chronicle of the birth and death. Expect to be in touch with them for many months, and make it a point to call regularly, meet them for lunch, and so on. Contrary to popular belief, grieving is often a lengthy, drawn-out process. It does not resolve in an orderly, predictable fashion, but is comprised of rounds—some more vivid and painful than others—that may continue for a lifetime. Know the basic phases of grieving—shock, denial, anger, and resolution—and be ready to share this knowledge with the mother and her intimates as appropriate.

And be sure to have referrals to support groups readily available, as well as written materials on how to talk to children and siblings about death.

Notes

1. E. A. Friedman, and B. H. Kroll, "Computer Analysis of Labor Progression," *Journal of Obstetrics and Gynecology* (British commonwealth) 76 (1969): 1,075–79.

2. E. A. Friedman, and B. H. Kroll, "Computer analysis of labor progression II, distribution of data and limits of normal," *Journal of Reproductive Medicine* 6 (1971): 20–25.

3. Leah Albers, "The Duration of Labor in Healthy Women," *Journal of Perinatology* 19 (2): 114–19, 1999.

4. Margaret Myles, *Textbook for Midwives,* 8th ed. (London, England: Churchill Livingstone, 1975), 111.

5. Anne Frye, *Holistic Midwifery (Volume II)* (Portland, Oreg.: Labrys Press), manuscript pages.

6. Pauline Scott and Jean Sutton, *Optimal Fetal Positioning* (New Zealand: Birth Concepts, 1996), 40.

7. Ruth Ancheta and Penny Simkin, *The Labor Progress Handbook* (Oxford, England: Blackwell Science 2000), 154–56.

8. Frye, *Holistic Midwifery (Volume II).*

9. Frye, *Holistic Midwifery (Volume II).*

10. Jean Sutton, "Occipito-posterior position and some ideas of how to change it!" *Midwifery: Best Practice,* ed. Sara Wickham (London, England: Elsevier Science Limited, 2003), 97.

11. Doña Queta Contreras and Dona Irene Sotelo, lecture notes, Midwifery Today conference, Oaxaca, Mexico, October 2003.

12. H. Hamlin, *Stepping Stones to Labor Ward Diagnosis* (Adelaide, Australia: Rigby, 1959).

13. Henci Goer, *The Thinking Woman's Guide to a Better Birth* (New York: Berkley Publishing, 1999), 210.

14. M. E. Hannah, A. Ohlsson, and others, "Induction of labor compared with expectant management for prelabor rupture of the membranes at term," *New England Journal of Medicine,* April 1996.

15. M. F. Schutte, P. E. Treffers, G. J. Kloosterman, and S. Soepatmi, "Management of premature rupture of membranes: the risk of vaginal examination to the infant," *American Journal of Obstetrics and Gynecology* 146 (4): 395–400, June 1983.

16. Scott and Sutton, *Optimal Fetal Positioning,* 40.

17. Marsden Wagner, lecture notes, Midwifery Today conference, Eugene, Oregon, March 2003.

18. Frye, *Holistic Midwifery (Volume II).*

19. Ricardo Herbert Jones, lecture notes, Midwifery Today conference, Oaxaca, Mexico, October 2003.

20. Frye, *Holistic Midwifery (Volume II).*

Liam Andrew

by Shannon Anton, CPM

We watched the moon rise slowly from inside the jeep. The moon rose slowly, and slowly I watched every detail of her round, white fullness so pronounced. The speed of my life, every movement and interaction, has been altered to reflect the slow pace of grief. Next to the moon I can see a few people leaving the church. I wonder why they don't notice the moon right there, only then I realize she is behind them—concealed yet right there on the horizon, suspended silently in front of me, looking me right in the eye. I am familiar with this feeling in my heart. It is what I feel for an old, old friend that I have loved well but have not thought of for too long. Nostalgic and strange, because someone else now has died and that sadness is again permeating my days, slowing them until I can see the beauty in everything. Sometimes I must be slowed so very much before I can see it clearly; then there it is and the moment can pass to the next.

A few days ago I walked in the park, and crossed the land bridge between the ponds. On the sand were the usual folks, plus ducks and turtles, which always skitter into the water as I approach with my dogs by my side. A single turtle stayed on the sand, making no move toward the water. I was quite close before I realized she was still there, looking at me, unwavering. Her eyes found my gaze and held it. I stopped. It was a long moment of slow stillness. The scent of the pond, the sand, the lush green on the banks became like a fog around me and mixed with the heat of hiking. I took a step forward to steady myself in her gaze. Once there I continued on, walking fast away from her because, I told myself, the dogs would bother her. Uh huh. And now I think of her stare and know that today I could meet her gaze completely.

What I remember most from Susan's pregnancy is her smiling face above her growing belly. We laughed easily during our visits. Her baby moved in response to our feeling his knees, his back, kicking us while we listened to his heartbeat. We guessed sometimes he was a boy, sometimes a girl. The Blessingway brought my assistant Jane and I into the circle of loving closeness that surrounds Susan and Mark.

Susan called me at 6 A.M. On the phone she was nervous and giggly, contractions woke her around 4 A.M. after not much sleep. We talked, and I planned to come when she called me back, or if I hadn't heard from her by 10 A.M., I would come by and check in. I arrived at their house around 11 A.M., and Susan was in early labor. She was kneeling on the floor with her elbows on the bed, beginning to be uncomfortable during her contractions. I worked to help her stay relaxed during them, to breathe deeply and loosely. She moved into the ease of that without struggle, and as she did, the contractions became longer. I took her blood pressure and we agreed to listen to the baby's heartbeat after the next contraction.

Susan leaned back on the bed and I pressed the fetascope to her belly. I heard nothing, and seeing from the shape of her belly that the baby was still posterior, continued to listen in other places, guessing how the sound of the heartbeat might travel around folded arms and legs. I sat back to stretch and saw with some surprise that the bottom half of her belly was covered in the small ring-shaped indentations left by my fetascope. I had still heard nothing.

I grabbed my Doppler from my bag and explained that I wanted to use it to try and hear the baby; Susan agreed. I listened. I heard nothing. I asked Susan if she'd been feeling the baby move and she said she thought so, though as the contractions became stronger it might have been the start of each contraction that she had thought was movement. I jiggled her belly, rubbing the baby's knees, hoping for a kick to let me know all was well. Nothing. I put my Doppler on the charger, thinking maybe it wasn't working properly, and sent Susan downstairs for a glass of juice to try to wake the baby up.

A few minutes later we tried to find the heartbeat again, this time downstairs on the couch where we had always done prenatals together. I told myself that she hadn't been flat enough upstairs to hear easily. With the fetascope I again heard nothing, covering her lower belly once more with round indentations.

I went upstairs to get my Doppler again, and while I was in the bedroom I felt that same unsteadiness I'd felt with the turtle. I told myself I'd been on my knees too long and now I'd run up the stairs, no wonder. But once downstairs again with the Doppler, still I could hear nothing of the baby's heartbeat. Out of frustration both with the technology in my hands, and the feeling that at this point, I might not know the heartbeat if it bit me, I held the Doppler to my own heart and heard it clearly: boom . . . boom . . . boom.

Satisfied the Doppler was working, I held it again to Susan's belly. The words "silent uterus" rose up from somewhere deep in my mind. I thought how strangely accurate they were: I could hear no sound at all. Susan had felt nothing of movement yet, and was beginning to believe she might not have felt the baby move since the night before; she and Mark had spent time together, feeling the baby kick.

We went back upstairs so I could do an internal exam. I thought if I could stimulate the baby's head, he might give us a kick. We worked between contractions, Susan lying back while I reached with my fingers to find her cervix opened three centimeters and a bulging bag of water in front of her baby's head. The baby's head itself was slightly overlapping at the sagittal suture, and I thought the edge of the suture line had a jagged, shard-like quality to it. The baby's head was still high in her pelvis, high enough it seemed odd that there would be molding now, already. When I pressed against the head, I could feel a wrinkly, loose scalp over the crown. Thinking back now, things seem obvious, but then it seemed that nothing made sense.

I tried one more time to hear the baby's heartbeat and when I could not, I said to Susan and Mark, "This has never happened to me before, it's just never taken me this long to hear heart tones. We haven't felt the baby move and I don't know what else to try. I think we need to go to the hospital and try to get the baby on the monitor."

continued →

Susan and Mark agreed. I added, "We'll probably get there and find the heartbeat right away and I'll feel like an idiot, but I don't care. I'll go call now while you get things together."

I went downstairs and phoned labor and delivery. The voice on the other end was familiar, and when I identified myself, she said, "Shannon, it's Jan Randall. How are you?"

In a moment's passing my mind flashed through my experiences with Jan; she'd apprenticed with me for a short time. I recalled the sense of her at my shoulder as a young, single mom pushed her baby out after a few short hours of labor, the mom's laboring sounds and then the baby's cries echoing off the high ceiling of her Victorian apartment, grayish morning light filtering through tall windows. I also remembered her very pregnant body just a few months ago: she'd given birth at home herself, to a healthy baby boy.

Realizing time was doing that amorphous thing it does around birth (and death), I came back to the present, to Jan, and in the same breath I laid out everything that had happened so far. When I came to not having any other ideas except coming in, she agreed. She said it was a slow day there and she could take care of us herself; she wanted to keep things low key for Susan and Mark.

I called my apprentice and gave her a brief version of what was happening. She would meet us at the hospital.

We drove on the freeway. I followed Mark and as we drove, I thought to myself how good it was that we were staying in the exit lane, since we were going so slowly. I glanced at my speedometer and was surprised to find it at 60 mph. I looked around—even knowing this I would have guessed our speed at around 30 mph. I backed off Mark's bumper to a reasonable distance, vaguely aware that something was definitely up. I was in an altered state now and felt a sense of something important to come.

On arrival, we made our way to labor and delivery. The ward was quiet. No one was willing to meet my eye directly, and while one nurse handed us a clipboard with admission forms on it, she turned abruptly on her heel and retreated behind the desk. I felt as if everyone there had heard of our concern and no one was quite sure how to respond to us in

this limbo time of not knowing. So to be respectful, no one engaged with us. I stayed by Susan and Mark while they wrote down the few lines of information needed.

Jane arrived. Then Jan came over to us and greeted us warmly, showing us all into a room. She made explanation of the technology at hand, reminding Susan that it takes a while sometimes to find the heartbeat with the monitor. Jan swept slowly across Susan's lower belly. She paused at intervals, waiting, looking at the monitor, listening for the familiar and reassuring blip of heartbeat. Nothing. She told Susan and Mark that she liked to have a second person try before being convinced that we couldn't get anything on the monitor. Jan looked at me and asked if I'd like to give it a try. I took the sensor in hand and repeated the search. My sense of the baby was obscure, not like usual when I have an idea where to try and hear heart tones. I knew I was in the right area but it still felt off, like I only thought I knew where to listen.

After searching across her belly again, I asked Jan, "What's next?" She recommended a sonogram; Susan and Mark agreed. Jan went to get a doctor, and we waited. The room was quiet. I didn't know what to say to fill the space, so I said nothing. We waited together quietly. Inside myself I was feeling a dread certainty; I hoped I was wrong and I hoped I wasn't too transparent.

The door squeaked open and Jan returned with a doctor following. The doctor came directly to look Susan in the eye and introduce herself. "I'm Dr. Frazier. I've brought a sonogram machine with me so we can have a better look at your baby. Is that all right with you?" Her voice had the kind steadiness that I knew from other transports when we'd worked together. I felt relieved to see her on duty, a friendly and familiar face. I felt like we were being buffered by a soundness of community that surprised and comforted me.

As Dr. Frazier moved the sono probe across Susan's belly, I held my breath. She was quiet, looking hard all around. Then she swept over the baby's ribcage and I could see clearly the brightly lit ribs in silhouette around the heart. There was only stillness. No movement, no heartbeat.

In a tone of voice that was kind but left no room for possibility, Dr. Frazier said, "I'm looking right now at your baby's lungs and heart and I don't see any movement. The baby's heart is not beating. Your baby has died."

Susan and Mark were stunned, my eyes were already tearing and I felt no breath in my own body.

After a brief pause, Dr. Frazier asked Susan, "Have you been laboring a long time?"

Susan's reply was like a reflex, "No! It's just really started."

"When did you last feel the baby move?"

"Well, I thought I was feeling movement with every contraction, but as the contractions got a little stronger, I think I was feeling the beginning of them, maybe not movement. But the baby was moving a lot last night, we both felt it." Susan looked at Mark and they held hands a little tighter.

"This is intense news I'm giving you, and I have to tell you I've been up all night. So before I say for certain, I'd like another doctor to have a look, just to be sure. Is that all right with you?" I knew that Dr. Frazier was willing, hoping to be wrong. But I also knew what I saw on the sono screen, what I sensed as time went on. I could appreciate her wanting to be wrong. Knowing but not wanting to believe. But still, knowing.

For the next hour we hung in a limbo that felt like days. Susan couldn't really let labor go on, she couldn't quite begin grieving, she couldn't feel all was well. The sono machine sat blindly against the wall, waiting with us. At one point Susan said, "Second opinions are good. We'll wait."

At long last, three doctors entered the room together. Dr. Frazier introduced Drs. Jones and Irwin. It was Dr. Irwin who repeated the sonogram and at 3 P.M. confirmed the baby was dead. There was a long moment of shocked silence, and then we all began to cry. The doctors excused themselves, saying softly that we could have all the time we needed and to come get them when we were ready to talk about a plan.

The door swung shut and Susan and Mark, holding each other, began to wail. I felt the wall against my back. Cool, solid, I slid down to sit at its base, the floor rising up to meet me. I could not look at Jane for a long time. My face was wet but I wasn't sure if I was crying. Jane caught my eye and crawled over to put her arms around me. We both sobbed.

I remember thinking how empty I could still feel with someone's arms around me like that. It wasn't Jane's embrace that was empty: it was the emptiness

of loss that I remembered couldn't feel any better no matter who held me. That is the forlorn truth about grief. It's just in you until its not anymore. It seemed tragic to have it fill me again, to know the hard path of its eventual leaving, that path stretching out long and lonely before us all, especially before Susan and Mark.

We mourned hard for the first hour after the news of their baby's death. At the end of that time, Susan's labor was beginning to pick up; she was getting practical. She looked at me squarely and, not asking for confirmation, said, "I still have to birth this baby, right?"

I was standing close to her and Mark. I forced my voice out of my body, "Yes."

Susan looked first at Mark and then at me again and nodded, "Okay."

"Should I go and get Dr. Frazier now?"

"Yes."

I moved through the door and down the hall. The lights were too bright, the skin on my cheeks and around my eyes was strangely tender; coming to the nurses' station I felt my eyes squint. Dr. Frazier was reading my chart on Susan. I sat down next to her and waited for her attention to turn to me. Another of those long moments passed.

"Hi, how're you doing?" she asked. I could only inhale and nod my head a little. She spoke directly, this time to me, "You gave her good care. There isn't anything you should have done that you didn't."

At this I had tears on my face, "Well, something like this happens, I have to wonder . . ."

Dr. Frazier took my hand and said, "She received excellent care from you. I'll tell her the same thing. If she'd been our patient she wouldn't even be here yet. She's forty-one weeks, but that isn't enough for our postdates protocol to set in. You did a good job." She paused and added, "And we're not gonna do anything about this." I realized she was referring to having me investigated or arrested, and I couldn't believe how far that was from my mind. The thought of having to protect myself right now was too much. I just could do what I was doing. I felt so still inside, like movement or speech required incredible intention.

I sniffed and thanked her, "It's really nice of you to say that."

continued →

She nodded, "One of the docs here had a daughter getting top OB care at Stanford; at thirty-nine weeks her baby died. They don't know why. We may not find out either." She turned back to the chart and asked, "Is she ready to talk?"

"Yes, I came to get you."

We walked into Susan's room and all attention turned toward the doctor. She spoke in soft tones and laid a hand on Susan's arm. The contractions were getting stronger. Dr. Frazier and Susan briefly discussed the options: staying here to have her baby or having her baby back at home. Then I heard Dr. Frazier tell Susan that there wasn't anything she should have done that she didn't do, that she had gotten excellent care with her midwives. Then she left us to the decision-making.

The door closed and Susan asked me if I would still help her have her baby at home. I said, "Of course. We'll be wherever you are. If you stay here, we'll stay. Whatever you want to do is really okay." She asked if she could have her friends come to the hospital. Her contractions continued to get stronger. It seemed too difficult to return home at that point. I went to call Peg and Jackie.

For the next twenty-four hours, the labor of birthing and grieving coexisted. Alternately each would fill the room—laughter and tears. Friends and family came to call, more like after a death than in preparation for a birth. None of it felt wrong.

Susan worked with her contractions, breathing, moaning, sighing, until the last bit of cervix was dissolved around her baby's head. She felt pressure enough to make her want to push, and as she bore down she felt the need to be more upright. She pushed well that first time, very vertical using the squatting bar and coming a bit onto her feet at the end of the bed. After that contraction, I felt inside to check on the baby's descent and position.

Another contraction came quickly, and as I was removing my fingers from Susan's vagina, I could feel the bones of the baby's head shifting suddenly and sharply beneath the scalp. The molding was extreme and the scalp loose over it. The edges of bone felt sharp and shard-like, as I remembered from before.

I thought of a squirrel I'd skinned after a road kill and how the skull was fractured into a hundred tiny sharp pieces. The sound those pieces made when I shifted the squirrel in my hands, it traveled not through the air to my ears but instead vibrated through my fingers and up my arms. Like broken glass but denser, like stoneware, but hydrated and suffused with the stuff of living. It was a sensation of sound in my body. The baby's head bones made a similar clicking and grinding.

For one frightening moment I could imagine the baby's head coming apart, the bones tearing through the scalp and compressing together flatly. I motioned to Jane to help me position Susan in a more reclining posture, allowing more space toward her sacrum for the baby's head to descend, removing direct pressure from the pubic bone.

She pushed again in this new reclining position, and I felt the need to check once more to assure myself that the worst was not happening. The baby's head then felt normal, still sharpish around the edges but molding in a reasonable way.

Susan pushed a bit more. Suddenly we could see the baby's head through her labia! I brought Mark down on the floor with me; on our knees we watched as more of the head gradually appeared. This baby had a good amount of dark hair, wavy and wet.

I felt inside again to see how the head was molding, how it was moving the bands of muscle out of the way toward crowning. I was afraid again of what might happen to the baby's head if I wasn't careful. I began pressing evenly on the muscle bands at Susan's vaginal opening. All I could think was, "I don't want the baby's head to come apart." I thought then, "Wow, I wonder if all bottoms feel this tight before the baby's really pressing more toward crowning? I never ever do this. Why am I doing this?" I stood up and stood back, thinking, "Geez, girl, get a grip!" I looked around and saw Anne, our nurse, standing nearby. I whispered in her ear, "Have you been to a stillbirth before?" She nodded yes.

"How careful of the head do I have to be?"

"Oh, not very."

I looked at her with my heart and so completely trusted her that I just moved back to the floor, beside Mark, and knew I'd be all right, the baby would be born without damage, and Susan could see and hold her baby without ugliness or horror. I felt a huge worry leave my body. I was warm and relaxed all at once. The world around me slowed again.

I looked at Mark and said, "We'll do this together so neither one of us will be alone." He nodded and smiled a little.

Susan continued to push. Each time, the baby moved a little bit. I was glad to see the gradual movement; her bottom was stretching perfectly with the gentle pressure of the baby's head. Even though the head had begun to come around the pubic bone with her pushes, between contractions it would slip back up again. Susan could feel this and felt at first like she was losing ground. I assured her that with the next contraction, the baby would move right back down again. A bit of a running start. Susan laughed at my joke and I realized what joy and expectation filled the room.

When the baby stayed in view between pushes, I kept pressure on the occiput of the baby's head to help keep it flexed, and to protect Susan's urethra and inner labia. There was a lot of give in her perineum; she was stretching around the baby's head beautifully. She reached down around my hands and felt the bulge of baby's head and smiled like when you just can't believe something so wonderful is happening.

Susan slowly crowned her baby's head. Little by little, the baby was born to his forehead. Mark's forehead, the baby had Mark's forehead! A long pause for the next contraction, and then the baby's nose and finally mouth and chin were born. Dark fluid drained from the baby's nose and mouth. I said to Mark, "The airway is getting squeezed clear now, this is really normal." Mark, not taking his eyes off the baby, nodded.

I felt along the baby's neck and found the cord, loosely there. I pulled an easy loop but it wasn't enough to go over the head. I reached for the first cord clamp and said, "The cord's around the neck and we need to cut it. Mark, do you want to cut it?"

"No, no, go ahead," he said. A little more time went by as I reached for the second clamp and then the scissors and said, "Okay, Mark, you wanna cut it?"

"Oh . . . sure, why not."

I held the cord by the clamps and he slid the scissors under, along the baby's neck. My fingers protected Susan and the baby. Mark cut the cord and helped me unwrap it from the baby's neck.

The next contraction and push didn't change anything. I carefully reached inside along the baby's back to find the shoulders completely unflexed. The usual sweep that brings unflexed shoulders together only moved loose bones in their joints; the baby had no real form. Utter lack of muscle tone allowed movement away from my hands rather than my hands shaping the baby's movement. With two hands I gently rotated the shoulders, and ever so slowly the baby restituted to face the right.

I heard Dr. Irwin ask me if I wanted suprapubic pressure, and heard my reply, no, the shoulder was right here. Concentration consumed me. I had to support every bit of the baby's birthed body or it would fall loosely to the bed. Susan continued to push and slowly, slowly the baby's body was born completely.

Mark helped me hand the baby up to Susan's belly. We all stood around the edges of the bed, around Susan and the baby. I don't know what we expected; no one was prepared for such a beautiful baby. We all just stared with awe for a moment before tears began to fall. We cried hard in those first minutes. Mark lifted the baby's leg to see, boy or girl? He was a boy. Susan and Mark said his name right away: Liam Andrew. He was named. He was their son.

I looked down as I cried, and tears splashed on my left breast. I'd been in the same dress for two days; the weight of the cotton had the neckline plunging, my bosom quite exposed. The sensation of Liam's birth was so much on the surface of my body, the sensation of the tears on my breast filled and startled me. It somehow echoed on my skin, the sadness in my heart. I was transfixed with the moment: I could see birth and death, the cycle of life before me. I was filled with a deep and abiding trust in life. It was a moment when everything came together vividly to make sense, to make a whole; it was also a moment of blinding grief. Susan was glowing, triumphant in her birth, ravaged and grieving in her son's death. So much all at once. It was a sacred and perfect time. I hope never to experience it again; I pray never to forget its influence.

We stayed together for five hours after Liam's birth. We held him, prayed for him, bathed and dressed him. We took photographs. We even laughed.

After having seen Susan and Mark the next day, I stopped on my way home to get food for my dog. When I returned to my car, it wouldn't start. It was

continued →

→ Liam Andrew, *continued*

a hot day and everything remained in slow, vivid motion. Moment by moment passed as I stared at the brightness in the air around me. The last thing I wanted to do was deal with a towing company. I just wanted not to talk to anyone. I left my car and began the two-mile walk home. I headed for Golden Gate Park, for home on the other side.

Walking felt heavy but good. Everything was blindingly bright. I think I walked with my eyes closed, the heat searing through my eyelids in a swirling red density. I'm sure I was not alone.

I strayed from the present just as I crossed the polo field. By the time I skirted the ponds and was overcome with the moist smell of the mud, the tall grasses and their whispering shuffle, I was back in Iowa, following another dirt path, and headed for the short track. I recalled that bright day well. Skeater wore no helmet; he rounded a corner on his cycle and met Roger head on. Literally. Skeater collided with Roger's bike and then his helmet and landed finally in the soft grass of the field. It was my first true loss. Grief held my hand as I crested the sandy bank of the pond. Today the turtles won't meet my eye; they skitter into the water and are gone. That rich muddy smell, all heady and ripe: I recognize the scent of decay, of loss and turning under. I am relieved to name it. I am comforted by the familiarity of it. I give a nod of greeting to my old dead friends and see Liam among them. All those nice boys together.

As I broke through the line of grass and found my feet on asphalt, I was at once confused. I spun around, reeling, really, and the foreground popped back into focus. It is 1995. I am a midwife. I have a place on my left breast that is ablaze. That is where the grief leaks out, where it exactly meets the light of day. Darkness to light, inside to out. It is a small opening, like for a pinhole camera, and the view is incredibly sharp.

A few days later, in the chair with Natasha leaning over me, needle buzzing in hand, I read the sign on the wall that says "Yes, it hurts," and I think, "But not that bad." She asks me something and I don't know how to reply; it was a simple question I can't recall now, but what I did say was, "I'm a midwife and I had a stillbirth in my practice. Liam Andrew Brooks O'Donnel." She paused and looked at me closely. She didn't look away, but she went back to my breast, back to her work. It's a beautiful tattoo. Tending it was both painful and validating. Something physical hurt, but I could put salve on it and it felt better. At least on the surface. ■

Chapter 6

POSTPARTUM CARE

The postpartum period is the last frontier for midwives and those concerned with maternal well-being. Far too many mothers find themselves virtually abandoned after a day or two of the most rudimentary care. We now refer to the first three months following birth as the fourth trimester, with the understanding that pregnancy and birth are transformative experiences culminating in this crucial phase of reintegration. Important information is emerging with increased research on the physical and psychological challenges of this period.

Preparation for the fourth trimester should begin prenatally. There is nothing more important than connecting pregnant women with one another, or better still, with those who have recently given birth. Prenatal classes or support groups may serve to accomplish this, but however it happens, it is not optional. This is particularly crucial for the self-contained, independent woman, for once the baby is born and helpers have resumed their normal lives, she may be overwhelmed by the intensity of daily mothering, with nothing to break the monotony. If she is used to choosing her friends carefully, insisting on intellectual common ground, suggest a more practical approach for the time being. Mothering in the first few months is made up of many mundane concerns, and contacts with others in the same phase, even if not the most profound intimacies, will serve a great purpose.

For all its sweetness, this is one of the most challenging times of a woman's life. It has wisely been said that struggles in pregnancy and birth are but preparation for the enormous adjustments required postpartum. I often tell women that the first six weeks of caring for a newborn is the hardest work they will ever do. Sometimes an expectant mother is unwilling to consider this, in which case, tune her in to what is impending by suggesting books on breastfeeding, mothering, and so on. Also provide a comprehensive resource list, including local chapters of La Leche League. Bottom line—you simply cannot give your full attention to every new mother with problems or your current clients will suffer. Besides, a new mother is embarking on a new stage of life; better for her to launch herself with a sense of self-reliance than dependency. Remember that midwifery is an art of facilitating passage! The midwife plays a guiding role for a while, but after the baby is born, the mother needs her own mechanisms of support.

A former client presented this intriguing vision of postpartum outreach. She wanted to connect expectant mothers with those who had recently given birth and were willing to help with baby care and light chores in the early weeks. The bonus of this arrangement is that it taps the helper's growing expertise in breastfeeding, infant sleep patterns, family integration, and other matters. This frees the midwife to concentrate on the physical aspects of postpartum care, rather than trying to address the myriad emotional and physical concerns so common at this stage.

These issues are pressing because postpartum support is almost nonexistent in the United States. That we treat new mothers as if nothing has changed, expecting them to be back on their feet and in charge of their affairs in a matter of days, is the height of denial. In nearly every society but ours, continuous care is provided at this time; the mother's only obligation is to stay in bed and focus on the baby.

Mothering the mother leads to her complete recovery. The better she feels, the more easily she will integrate her new role and learn to distinguish the needs of her child from her own. Good care frees her to develop as an individual and gives her a healthy foundation on which to base her social interactions, present and future. Her child reaps the benefits of her security and respect for its own rate of growth. Care of new mothers assures survival of the species, but more than that, it positively affects the quality of life for all of us.

Postpartum customs of Native American and Indonesian cultures literally make sure that the new mother is not left out in the cold. Providing adequate heat is the centerpiece of care, as new mothers are con-

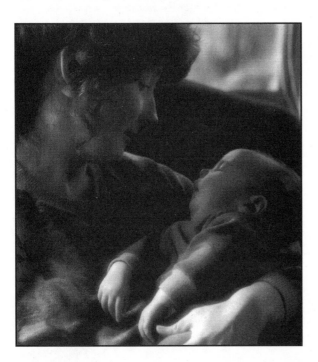

sidered to be opened by birth and thus greatly susceptible to chill and loss of energy. A fire may be built near or even under the mother's bed so she may nurse spontaneously, remain unclothed, and feel fully at ease. In Mexico and Guatemala, she is treated to a **temescal** (steam bath with herbs) just days after giving birth. In contrast to the numbing isolation endured by most mothers in our society, women of these cultures are surrounded by female peers and relatives who feed and counsel them, joking and marveling at the miracle of their newborn. In the Philippines, a new mother is believed to be in such a state of grace that if she dies in the first forty days postpartum, her soul will automatically be in heaven.

When a woman is not well cared for at this time, there are complex, often long-term effects on her body, personality, and sexuality. If she is forced out of bed or back to work too soon, overproduction of adrenaline will derail her recovery. Thus the "Amazon" concept of postpartum recovery is mostly myth: women never did give birth in the bush and jump back on their horse, unless their survival depended on it. Without sufficient rest, postpartum recovery is grueling and prolonged, and frequently incomplete.

To put it another way, the scandalously high incidence of postpartum depression in the United States has frustrated biological needs at its root. But there are emotional factors too. Consider that all new mothers invariably experience loss, some of it quite painful. Single friends may lose interest, and the primary relationship, rather than reverting to the way it used to be, is likely to be strained by stress and fatigue. Old routines and ways of handling the most basic tasks must be altered, and privacy becomes a thing of the past. If a mother extends her maternity leave, she may also experience a loss of income and change in her standard of living. When chronic fatigue compounds this, the ground for depression is laid.

More than anything else, giving birth makes clear that control in life is just an illusion. Ideally, a woman's experience of making this discovery is exhilarating; if not, her self-esteem may be negatively affected. Perhaps the midwife's most critical task in the immediate postpartum is to help the new mother debrief her birth experience. She may express anxiety about her behavior in labor as early as day one and may need additional opportunities over the next few months for more discussion and reassurance. This is particularly true if the birth was difficult or disappointing. Certainly the course will be rocky if there are problems with the baby's health, but even if the baby is perfect, the mother may still be devastated if things did not go as she planned. She has the right to grieve, and you, the responsibility to support her in this.

New mothers are fragile, vulnerable, and impressionable. Well-meaning but misguided advice sinks deep; criticism is not easily forgotten. Keep this ever in mind, and do all you can to provide your clients as much physical and emotional warmth and protection as possible.

DAY-ONE VISIT

When you come back the day after the birth, begin by appraising the environment for order and cleanliness. If laundry or dishes have piled up, or the refrigerator is bare, lend a hand as necessary. Also see what the mother has been eating and drinking (there should be a jug of water at her bedside). The room should be comfortably warm, and baby things readily available. She may not have had a chance to shower yet, so help with this if need be. Ask how she has been feeling in

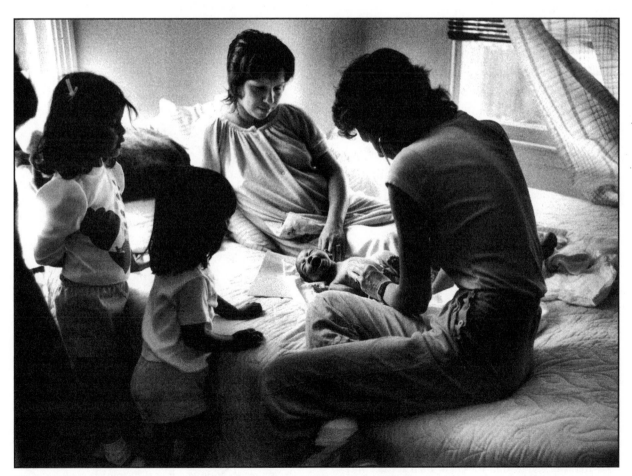

The midwife gives care to the entire family during the postpartum period.

general: any dizzy spells, extreme exhaustion, or emotional upsets? Her report will depend largely on what her labor was like, and on what kind of help she is receiving from her partner or friends.

It is critical at this point to stress her need for a full ten days of absolute rest. Tell her to follow her body's signals for sleep and nourishment just as she did while pregnant. Explain how high levels of oxytocin released with breastfeeding prompt **uterine involution,** the return of the uterus to its prepregnant size, and further contract vaginal muscles to restore tone. But she is overactive or stressed out, she will release adrenaline instead, which inhibits this process. In other words, the more she rests and lets her body recover, the sooner she will look and feel her best. This message bears repeating, as it is critical to her recuperation.

That said, also suggest that she walk several times daily, even if just up and down the hallway or stairs. This stimulates circulation in her legs, which helps prevent thrombophlebitis (see "Thrombophlebitis and Pulmonary Embolism" later in this chapter).

Always wash your hands thoroughly upon arrival and before examining the mother. Use aseptic technique when handling the baby and universal precautions when in contact with any secretions. Things to check include:

1. **The nipple, for soreness or cracking.** If soreness is developing, evaluate the way the baby is taking the breast. The vast majority of breastfeeding problems result from improper positioning. See that the mother is lifting the baby to the breast, and that it is not hanging from the nipple. Although you may have demonstrated this to her already, she may have forgotten or has received conflicting advice from friends or relatives. Reassure her that she need not limit how long the baby sucks, but must always make sure that it is taking the nipple correctly, with an **asymmetric latch** (more areola drawn in at its lower jaw than at the upper). If the nipples are cracked, suggest applying a bit

of vitamin E between nursing sessions. Stress how important it is that she continue to breastfeed. Have her begin with the least affected breast, then switch to the sorer side once she has had let-down.

2. **The uterus, for normal involution.** It should be just below the mother's umbilicus, and should feel firm, not tender. Massage it briefly to expel any clots, and have her sit up for a few minutes before checking her flow.

3. **The lochia, for color, amount, and odor.** Lochia is postpartum shedding of excess endometrium. On day one, expect **lochia rubra,** or red-brown flow in amounts like a heavy menstrual period. The odor should be fleshy, like menstrual blood.

4. **The perineum, especially if there has been swelling, tearing, or suturing.** All the swelling should be gone; if not, suggest that she continue alternating warm and cool compresses, but also make certain she is rinsing her perineum twice a day with warm water and a bit of Betadine. If swelling has increased and she complains of pain, check for a hematoma (see "Hematoma" later in this chapter).

This is also a good time to assess for **cystocele** or **rectocele.** With these, vaginal tissue will pooch forward at the opening of the vagina. If the bulge appears at the perineum, it is a rectocele, due to weakening or straining of pelvic floor muscles. If the bulge appears near the urethra, it is a cystocele, due to weakening and straining of the muscles in the vaginal vault. In either case, suggest that she gradually resume the elevator exercise (see chapter 2, page 57), and reassess at seven days.

If she has had stitches, check to be sure they have held. The edges should be pulling together, and should be clean and dry (if not, have her apply fresh aloe vera or bottled gel). Signs of infection include inflammation, pain, and discharge; consult a physician if these are noted. If the mother complains of tenderness but the area looks healthy, recommend sitz baths three or four times daily. Plain hot water is fine, although a ginger solution will increase circulation and relieve itching. Use an entire root for a large pot of water, slice thin, then simmer twenty minutes, strain, and divide into several portions, which can be diluted with plain hot water in a sitz basin.

Also check to see if she has had any pain with urination. If so, remind her to pour warm water over her vaginal area as she urinates. (Check her temperature, too, to rule out urinary tract infection, below). See if she has had a bowel movement, and if not, recommend fiber-rich foods. Sometimes the fear that stitches could come out with bearing down can cause the mother to hold back—if so, suggest a bit of counterpressure with a folded tissue.

5. **The mother's temperature record.** If elevated, she may be dehydrated, may have a systemic, urinary tract, or uterine infection. Rule these out one by one. If there is perineal pain, check for a hematoma.

6. **The mother's pulse.** If elevated, see above.

7. **The mother's blood pressure.** This is particularly important if it rose during or immediately after labor. If elevated, check for signs of preeclampsia and consult with backup as indicated.

8. **The baby's cord stump.** It should look clean around the base, not red or swollen. Be sure that whoever is diapering the baby is folding the top edge back so urine won't irritate this area and is swabbing the cord regularly with alcohol or hydrogen peroxide. Remove the cord clamp only if the stump is completely dry.

9. **The baby's skin color, inspecting for jaundice.** Depress the flesh on the baby's chest and extremities, checking for yellow undertone. Jaundice is unusual on day one and should be immediately referred to a pediatrician. Depending on degree, the baby may need a bilirubin count (see "Jaundice," page 203).

10. **The baby's skin consistency, for dehydration.** If the baby's wrists and ankles look cracked and wrinkly, it needs to nurse more often. Dehydration can develop rapidly in very hot weather and is more apt to be a problem with postmature or IUGR babies who have very little subcutaneous fat. Also note the temperature of the skin—if overwarm, see that the baby is not overdressed, and take its temperature.

11. **The baby's elimination pattern.** It should have passed meconium by now and should be urinating frequently. If it has not had a bowel movement by forty-eight hours, consult a pediatrician.

12. **The baby's nursing pattern and behavior.** Sleepiness (especially after a long labor) is normal for the first day. Lethargy (characterized by drowsiness, disinterest in nursing, and lack of muscle tone) is of concern. The lethargic baby should be checked by a pediatrician immediately, particularly if the mother's temperature is elevated or if neonatal jaundice is noted.

Also ask parents about the baby's cry. If they report a high-pitched, catlike wail, jaundice, neurological problems, or hypoglycemia (see "Hypoglycemia" in the next section) may be at fault. Evaluate the cry yourself, and if questionable, refer to a pediatrician.

13. **Anything unusual in the newborn exam.** Reevaluate if parents have not yet seen a pediatrician.

The main purpose of the day-one visit is to see that the mother is off to a good start: relaxed, happy, comfy with her baby and well cared for. If she looks frazzled or unhappy, you must try to find out why, as most women are in bliss at this point. On the other hand, her partner may be exhausted, finally registering the strain of lengthy labor support and loss of sleep. If so, suggest they send out for dinner (if this has not been covered already), spend time in bed with the baby, and take the phone off the hook until they feel a bit more stable. Also suggest they place a message on the answering machine or note on the front door, "We had the baby, it's a ____, we're fine but tired, please call in a few days so we can plan to have you over."

The mother may also wish to talk about the birth, particularly if it was difficult. Make yourself fully available for this discussion, wherever it may lead.

And you may want to give the mother this special **rebozo treatment,** as suggested by traditional Guatemalan and Mexican midwives. Have her lie on her back on a flat surface (like a carpeted floor) in a warm room.

Place the center of the rebozo under her head, making sure it is folded neatly (not bunched up). Kneel on the floor facing her head, with an assistant on the other side. Cross the rebozo over her forehead and, with each of you taking one end, pull firmly and hold for at least a minute.

Then move the rebozo down to her shoulders, lower ribs, waist (gently), hips, thighs just above the knees, calves, and ankles. Each time, cross the rebozo, pull taught, and hold. When she is ready to get up, instruct her to turn to her side and push herself up with her hands, to help keep her ribs closed.[1]

Oh, how mothers love this! It feels like a full body massage and yet is intended to serve a specific function, which the traditional midwives call "bringing the bones back together." Both physically and emotionally, the mother feels held and hugged by the rebozo; the treatment is soothing and helps counter the propensity to chill. Advice varies as to how often this should be performed, but there is no harm in doing this at every postpartum visit.

If anything unusual is noted on day one, visit again on day two. Do not try to reassess by phone, as even minor physical concerns can exacerbate emotional breakdown in this fragile period. Specific indications for prompt reexamination at forty-eight hours include problems with perineal repair, elevated maternal pulse or temperature, excessive blood loss, difficulties with breastfeeding, or signs of neonatal jaundice or dehydration. If everything is normal on day one, a follow-up phone call on day two is sufficient.

DAY-THREE VISIT

By day three, the challenge of integrating newborn care with daily life has become evident, and emotional meltdown is common. At the same time, hormone surges that initiate lactation may increase the mother's instability, causing tears to flow just as her milk comes in. The baby must make its own adjustment to breast milk and so may experience fussiness or crying spells. All of this plus deepening fatigue can greatly exacerbate emotional distress in both parents. Day three is truly the point of reckoning: the birth is over, the baby is here, and nothing is the same. Particularly if the mother's partner has been handling all household responsibilities, he or she may be at the point of collapse. This may leave the mother feeling stranded; if so, see that her postpartum support system is fully activated.

This is an excellent time to give the mother a ritual bath. See the herbal recipe and instructions suggested by Janice Kalman and the Chico midwives in the "Herbs and Homeopathy Postpartum" sidebar, on page 199. As an alternative, disinfect the tub, run plain warm water and float rose petals on the surface, light candles, and put on music (mother's choice—perhaps something she listened to during the birth) to create a beautiful ceremonial moment of honoring the mother in her new role. With this, discussion of the birth may begin (or resume).

To best facilitate the mother's processing of her birth, you might pose the question, "Are you happy with your birth, or is there anything you wish had been different?" Of course, you must be entirely relaxed and receptive if you expect her to be fully honest with you. If she doesn't have much to say, be patient—there will be plenty of time later on to talk things through. For now, just encourage her to express whatever she is feeling—this is prime time for emotional release.

Be sure to check:

1. **The breasts.** Check for engorgement by feeling for lumps at the sides of the breasts and in the armpits, looking for reddened areas. If engorgement is a problem, make sure the mother is nursing on demand and with proper positioning. Have her soak her breasts (or whole body) in warm water, as this will stimulate the release of any backed-up milk. Then show her how to express milk it.

Many women find this easier if they oil the entire breast and, using long strokes toward the nipple, work down from the collar bone with one hand and up from the base of the breast with the other. If specific lumps are noted, have the mother work from behind these areas. This may hurt a bit at first and she may need to go slowly, but make sure she applies enough pressure to bring the milk out. Up to ten sweeps may be necessary before milk appears at the nipple. Demonstrate the proper way to get the flow started by grasping the edges of the areola, pressing inward, squeezing together, and then pulling toward the nipple.

Another tried and true remedy for engorgement is the application of cold cabbage leaves, or steamed comfrey leaves, left in place for twenty minutes. Repeat periodically throughout the day. For lingering engorgement, try hot ginger compresses under the arms or in the upper, outer quadrants of the breasts.

If the nipples are cracked, check positioning and the baby's latch. Also rule out a short frenulum, which could compound the problem. Recommend vitamin E on the nipples between nursing sessions. Cold cabbage leaves tucked against the nipples may also provide relief.

2. **The uterus, the lochia, the perineum, and so on.** Recheck the perineum thoroughly, using guidelines from day one. Ask the mother if her flow has been consistent—any clots, heavy bleeding, or dark-red blood? By day three, her flow should be a bit lighter than before, beginning to change from rubra to a pinker **lochia serosa.** Palpate the uterus for enlargement, and note any tenderness that might indicate infection. Check the odor on her pad to be sure it is normal. Recheck for cystocele or rectocele, and if evident, remind her to do the elevator exercise. Ask if she feels any vaginal pressure or dragging sensation when out of bed to emphasize the importance of this.

3. **The mother's temperature.** Elevation to 101 degrees is normal at the time the milk comes in. Nevertheless, rule out urinary tract or uterine infection by checking for symptoms (see page 207).

4. **The cord stump.** You can definitely remove the cord clamp by now, or if it has been a lotus birth, the cord should have come away cleanly by this time.

5. **The baby, for jaundice.** A bit of a yellow tinge is normal in the face and down to the nipple line, but unusual in the extremities. Ordinarily, excess bilirubin is diluted and flushed from the system by breast milk. If the baby is very yellow, have the mother place him or her in a sunny window, as sunlight helps the liver conjugate and eliminate bilirubin. Make sure the baby is nursing long and frequently, and check again the following day (also see "Jaundice" later in this chapter).

6. **The baby, for dehydration.** This is particularly important if jaundice is present or if noted on day one.

7. **Baby's behavior, nursing pattern, crying pattern, and so on.** See 5 and 6, above, and section 8 below.

8. **Mom's relationship to nursing.** This is crucial. Make certain that she is not trying to get the baby on a schedule or limit time at the breast. In other words, replace any notion of structuring the baby's need for food with a sensual, loving approach based on trusting its instincts. The sensation of letdown varies from mild tingling to a sexual sort of release, and some women experience orgasm while nursing. Try to promote a positive feeling around letting go with the baby.

9. **Sleeping arrangements.** Check to see what has evolved. If the baby is in bed with the couple, how does the mother's partner feel about this? If the baby is in a basket or crib, how does the mother feel about getting up to nurse? Is she getting enough sleep? Is her partner willing to get up and bring the baby to her?

You may receive a phone call from the mother after this visit, especially with regard to the last three points. Amazingly enough, concerns and conflicts about discipline may already have arisen between the mother and her partner (or relatives). Men in particularly often worry that the baby will be spoiled by too much attention, too much contact, too much love. Some respond by setting limits on how much time the baby spends with the mother or insist that it be left to "cry it out" when it fusses, which exacerbates the problem. Whether due to cultural conditioning, anxiety, or simple jealousy, this misguided approach to parenting should be set aside as soon as possible. Explain that the baby has literally been enveloped by the mother for nine months, its every need immediately met. It has no experience of waiting to be fed or held, and when upset, cannot know that its mother (or father) is close by in the next room. Babies need all the security they can get; there is no such thing as too much love for a newborn!

Help the mother and her partner see that by surrendering to the sensitivity and vulnerability engendered by love, they will be stronger and wiser in the end, and their baby will grow to be a loving, secure child. Encourage them to relax and get to know the baby through touch, play, and gentle massage. (Infant massage is also an antidote for colic.) Advise them to set aside a time each day when they can share their feelings, concerns, and frustrations, and suggest they conclude this time with cuddling. Do all you can to generate a container of protection for the burgeoning family. Let them know that you care, that they are doing fine, and that they are safe.

On the basis of your findings at this visit, check in for the next few days. As with the day-one checkup, anything unusual is best followed up by a house call, rather than by phone. Otherwise, if everything is normal, a phone chat each day is sufficient.

DAY-SEVEN VISIT

By day seven, the mother's partner will probably be back at work, and friends and relatives may be busy once again with their own concerns. No wonder the new mother may suddenly feel depressed and forgotten—her emotions remain volatile, and her energy is nowhere

near prepregnant levels. And if, on top of her own physiological adjustments, she has been entertaining well-wishers or doing more around the house than she should, she will be even more deeply exhausted. A definite sign of overactivity is increased lochia flow, or change from serosa back to rubra. A mother in these straits needs help—a close friend or relative should help with cleaning, laundry, shopping, and running errands, or someone must be hired for this purpose.

Once again, the mother may wish to discuss her birth. This may in fact be instrumental to her recuperation and ability to relax and enjoy her baby. Graciously accept any feelings of resentment, frustration, or sadness she may express, and try to respond *without being defensive*. Pay tribute to her strengths, and downplay her shortcomings, if any.

And listen carefully to the scope of her personal difficulties. Most women have no idea how relentless the responsibility of mothering is until it is upon them. Under the circumstances, it is hardly surprising that many new mothers suffer from postpartum blues. It is important to differentiate this from depression, though. The blues diminish as time goes by, but depression—characterized by increasing withdrawal and inability to cope—may develop at this point or not for several months. It is important that the midwife be able to distinguish these states, and acknowledge that there are times when professional intervention is indicated (see "Postpartum Depression," page 210).

By day seven, signs of physical recovery should be clearly evident. If the mother had perineal repair, the skin should be closed by now. Lochia flow should have decreased. If the mother has been exercising her pelvic muscles, cystocele or rectocele should be diminishing. Breastfeeding should be fairly well established. Besides these landmarks of physical recovery, assess the mother's emotional condition and provide referrals if indicated. Do your best to help her with any difficulties, as you will not see her for several weeks unless she calls for help.

But do not forget to bring up the topic of sex. Advise the mother to have nothing in her vagina until her lochia flow has stopped completely. Suggest that she wait to see you before going ahead, particularly if she had stitches. Encourage her to listen to her body (as always) in making decisions on when she is ready.

Over the next few weeks, if she calls to report extreme fatigue, exhaustion, continued bleeding, or sensations of pressure or dragging in her vagina when she is up and about, see her at once, as these are symptoms of poor healing that must be addressed promptly if she is to recover.

THREE–SIX WEEKS CHECKUP

The timing of this visit depends on the mother's rate of recovery. If her flow ceased at least a week prior to contacting you, you can assume her uterus is well involuted, her cervix firmed up, and that she is ready for her final checkup.

One important reason for this checkup is to give the okay for sexual activities involving penetration, along with suggestions on how to make these as pleasurable as possible. Tell the mother to use plenty of lubrication, as breastfeeding causes dryness and fragility of the tissues no matter how intense her desire. If appropriate, you should also raise the issue of birth control. Although rare, ovulation can occur as early as six weeks after giving birth. I have known of several nursing mothers who conceived in the first two months postpartum, in spite of breastfeeding exclusively.

If the mother had stitches, the timing of this checkup is also determined by the condition of her perineum. Before she comes in (and if she is willing), ask her to wash her hands and gently insert two fingers to see if the area is still sensitive to pressure; if so, she is probably not ready for sex (or barrier method contraceptive fittings). Wait no longer than six weeks to see her, though, for if adequate healing has not taken place by then, you must determine the reason. Sometimes

second-degree tears take a while to heal, and provided her lochia flow has stopped and she is feeling fine, you need not worry.

Emotional conditions may also precipitate scheduling this visit sooner than later. For example, if a woman calls at three weeks to report feeling depressed or emotionally incapacitated, see her at once, even though her physical recovery may still be weeks away.

Depending on the size of your community, this may be the last time you will see the new mother for a while. Under these circumstances, it is also your last chance to fully assess her recovery before she makes her way back into the world. Look closely, noting her color, energy level, and general demeanor. Is she happy, content, in love with her baby, and most important, at peace with herself? If she seems weak or ailing in any respect, speak to her directly about your concern.

Energetically, she should be drawn back together by now, self-contained, whole, and radiant. If you have any doubt of this, offer a final rebozo wrap and continue to keep in touch.

Things to check at the final exam include:

1. **The uterus.** It should be out of range of palpation, except by bimanual exam. If it is enlarged, she is probably still bleeding, indicating poor recovery. Prescribe rest, long relaxed nursing sessions to allow oxytocin to do its work, optimal nutrition with plenty of calories, supplements as indicated, and involuting tea or tincture of black haw and shepherd's purse.

2. **The cervix.** It should feel firm, closed, and situated high in the vaginal vault as with initial pelvic assessment. However, some women do not regain their prepregnant cervical position and tone until cutting back significantly on breastfeeding (when introducing solid foods to the baby).

3. **Internal muscle tone.** This should almost be back to normal by now if the mother has been doing vaginal exercises. If not, explain the importance of strengthening the pelvic muscles to keep the uterus and other internal organs in their proper

positions, not to mention enhancing sexual desire and sensitivity. Check for tone in two areas: high in the vault and just inside the vaginal opening. Often a woman has good tone in one area but little in the other. Review vaginal exercise techniques (described in chapter 2).

4. **Lacerations or episiotomy.** Healing should be complete, although there may still be tenderness with labial skin splits as newly formed skin takes time to toughen up. This may cause some discomfort with sex, but adequate lubrication and creative positioning can help.

   If the perineum feels rigid with scar tissue, encourage the mother to do perineal massage to soften the area, using evening primrose oil. This procedure can be emotionally and physically reassuring for any woman nervous about having sex again.

5. **The abdominal muscle tone.** Have the woman lie down, place your fingertips along the juncture of abdominal muscles running from the umbilicus to pubic bone, and then have her lift her head and shoulders. Check for gaping; women typically have about a half-inch separation at this point. If the separation is greater, suggest abdominal exercises, starting with single leg lifts and progressing slowly to full sit-ups (with knees bent). You might also refer the mother to postpartum exercise or yoga classes, or suggest she meet informally with other new mothers for exercise interspersed with baby massage and conversation.

6. **The breasts, for tenderness or lumps.** It is said that the hormones of pregnancy can accelerate abnormal cell growth if any is preexisting. Even if the mother has seen a physician since the birth, she may not have had a thorough breast exam, so do it yourself. This is also a good time to review self-exam with her.

7. **The cervix, by Pap smear.** For reasons stated earlier, do a repeat Pap even if the mother was screened in early pregnancy.

8. **The hemoglobin or hematocrit.** This is especially crucial if the mother appears weak or exhausted, or if she has a history of hemorrhage either with the birth or during the postpartum period.

9. **The diet.** A new mother often forgoes her physical needs in deference to the baby's. She hardly has time to eat, let alone cook. Her partner may offer to take on meal preparation, but may not be aware of the nutritional demands of breastfeeding. If the mother complains of chronic fatigue, nervous irritability, or upper respiratory infection, prescribe more protein, more calories, good sources of vitamins B and C, and trace mineral supplements. If her hematocrit is less than 37 or hemoglobin below 12 (nonpregnant standards), treat her for anemia with nutritional recommendations, herbal tinctures or teas, and supplements.

10. **Adjustment to parenting.** This is a broad category of evaluation, but a few well-chosen questions will reveal any disturbing trends. Ask the mother how well she has been sleeping, how she and her partner are getting along, and how she is coping with the frustrations of mothering. It is wise to have the mother's partner present as you discuss these important issues, unless you have reason to believe that the mother needs privacy to express herself candidly.

The Baby: Complications and Concerns

HYPOGLYCEMIA

Hypoglycemia refers to abnormally low blood sugar levels. Fifty to 60 mg glucose per 1 ml blood is normal for a newborn; anything below 30 is of serious concern. Infants at risk include those large for gestational age, small for gestational age, premature, postmature, or whose mothers are diabetic. Otherwise healthy babies who suffered hypoxia during labor or were depressed at birth are also at risk. Symptoms include apathy, irregular respirations, inability to regulate body temperature (hypothermia), refusal to nurse, and a high-pitched cry.

If the baby is at risk, do a dextrostix to check glucose levels. This is done by heel stick; a drop of baby's

Herbs and Homeopathy Postpartum

by Shannon Anton, CPM

Keep the room warm immediately following the birth, and do not give a postpartum woman cold drinks. If a newly postpartum woman has to warm her body after a chill, or if she has to warm up the contents of her stomach, she is wasting vital energy. Her entire course of postpartum recovery can be greatly affected by these factors. Her energy at this time is precious. Respect and conserve it.

Postpartum Bath

If a woman has been consistently stable in the immediate postpartum hours, I offer her a healing postpartum bath. Here is a recipe, contributed by midwife Janice Kalman and originated by the Chico midwives:

Boil one large bulb of **Garlic** in a big pot of water for twenty minutes. Turn off the flame and add dried herbs: one handful **Comfrey** leaves, one handful **Witch Hazel,** half a handful **Uva Ursi** leaves, several slices of dried or fresh **Ginger** root, half a handful **Yarrow** flowers, a large pinch of **Rosemary,** and steep covered for at least twenty minutes. In the meantime, scrub the tub thoroughly and rinse carefully. Paint the entire surface with Betadine and let stand twenty minutes. Rinse tub completely. Run warm (not hot) water to fill, include a large handful of sea salt, and strain the herbal concoction into the tub. The mother and baby may both get in the bath, provided someone stays with them constantly.

Afterpains

These can be very painful and distracting for the new mother. Strongly brewed **ginger** tea brings relief from afterpains. Pour one cup boiling water over three to five slices of fresh ginger and steep five to ten minutes. **Motherwort** tincture also eases afterpains—begin dosage at half a dropperful and increase as needed.

Herb Pharm makes an excellent herbal compound tincture called **Hellonias Viburnum** that greatly relieves afterpains. Take one dropperful as needed.

Prolapsed Uterus or Cervix

Sometimes a woman's cervix comes down to her introitus after giving birth. If so, reglove and gently push the cervix back up to its usual position. Instruct the woman to stay in bed as much as possible and to begin exercising the pelvic muscles. In addition, homeopathic **Sepia** 200C offers vital support.

Homeopathic Sepia 200C is also indicated when a woman reports feeling her insides dropping or sagging when she walks or stands. Have her take several times a day, and continue to rest in bed.

When there is uterine, bladder, or hemorrhoid prolapse, or when a woman seems especially exhausted and compromised in the weeks postpartum, this indicates compromised liver chi. Refer her to a skilled practitioner of Traditional Chinese Medicine (TCM). It is worth noting that uterine prolapse at any age can usually be corrected with TCM. Recurrent yeast infections also indicate weakened liver chi.

Healing after Cesarean Section

Homeopathic **Staphysagria** promotes healing after a cesarean, or any surgical procedure. Staphysagria 30C taken several times a day will support full recovery. When painful symptoms ease, discontinue use.

Nipple Soreness

Expressing a few drops of milk and rubbing it into the areola will help sore nipples heal. Also allow nipples to air-dry after nursing, or expose them to sunlight. If nipples are cracking and bleeding, try homeopathic **Graphites** 30C, taken several times a day.

Milk Fever and Mastitis

Because most engorgement and milk fevers occur during night time hours, I ask my clients to include in their birth supplies four homeopathic remedies: **Arnica, Bryonia, Phytolacca,** and **Belladonna,** all

continued ➔

in the over-the-counter potencies of 6x or 30C. Timely treatment demands that these be already on hand.

When the breasts are full, tender, and hot to the touch, getting the baby to nurse or expressing a bit of milk so she or he can latch on is crucial. In addition, try homeopathic **Bryonia** 30C and **Phyto-lacca** 30C, alternating every twenty minutes until engorgement symptoms resolve, usually in a few hours. **Echinacea** tincture—half a drop per pound of body weight—can be taken several times a day when the breasts are engorged to prevent the onset of mastitis.

Compresses

Compresses can stimulate the flow of milk, preventing it from backing up and becoming infected. Warm water may be used, but steamed, fresh **Comfrey** leaves or strong Comfrey tea compresses are more therapeutic. Keep compresses on for twenty minutes. Whole, raw **Cabbage leaves** (which steam on the breast) may also be used and should be left until they soften. During this time, the mother may cry and express concerns, disappointments, or fears. Be present and ready to listen. Also have something warm available for her to drink.

Fever with Engorgement

Engorgement or lumpy soreness in the breast accompanied by a rising fever can be resolved with homeopathic **Belladonna** 30C, taken every twenty to thirty minutes. Fever should reduce to normal in the next few hours, and the homeopathic remedy can be discontinued.

Meanwhile, she must also nurse or express milk from congested areas. Coating the breasts with **Aloe Vera** helps reduce the risk of secondary infection. Doses of **Echinacea** tincture also support the body in healing mastitis. Make sure she is well hydrated, well nourished, and getting complete rest.

Building the Milk Supply

Galactagogues help women maintain an abundant supply of breast milk. They may be helpful to any mother having a difficult time recovering from birth.

A classic galactagogue is **dark beer;** have the mother drink one a day, with a raw egg mixed in. **Hops** in tincture form can also stimulate milk production.

Another old remedy is **Fennel/Barley** water. Boil half a cup pearled barley in three cups water for twenty-five minutes. Save the barley water, and reheat it (do not boil) to make fennel tea, one cup barley water to one teaspoon fennel. Do not steep longer than thirty minutes.

Drying up the Milk Supply

As midwives, we sometimes help women who have miscarriages or stillbirths, or for some reason choose not to nurse their babies. Still, they will have milk. To help ease engorgement, follow the instructions above. In addition, help her bind her breasts with a long, stretchy wrap. Cold compresses also act to dry up the milk (though cold in any form undermines postpartum healing). Drinking **Sage** tea is a dependable method for reducing milk production, and two drops daily of **Pokeroot** tincture minimizes engorgement.

Extended Postpartum Bleeding

Some women continue bright-red spotting after six weeks postpartum. To remedy this, try **Shepherd's Purse** tincture, half a dropperful twice a day for up to a week. **Moxa** therapy applied midline between pubic bone and umbilicus (known as the "conception vessel") and over the sacroiliac joints supports uterine involution. Referral for TCM is appropriate.

Umbilical Cord Care

A few drops of **Echinacea** tincture on the newly cut cord stump is a reliable way to treat the umbilical cord. You may also use **Goldenseal** tincture or **breast milk.** Treat the cord several times a day until the stump falls off.

Jaundice

Traditional Chinese Medicine offers a very effective remedy for newborn jaundice, which parents can obtain from a Chinese apothecary or herbalist. Simmer this root and swab the liquid inside the baby's mouth. One or two applications will usually clear jaundice.

Colic

A few teaspoons of crushed **Fennel** or **Caraway** seed tea can greatly relieve the discomfort of colic. Try light pressure and warm compresses on baby's belly, or bringing its feet slowly up to its ears several times. Clockwise massage in a sweeping motion above the belly button may also be effective.

Homeopathic remedies are fairly specific. Most common is homeopathic **Chamomilla,** followed closely by **Nux Vomica** and **Mag Phos.** Highland makes a colic formula, available at most natural foods stores (their teething remedy is also excellent).

Misalignment of the skull or spine may also be implicated in colic. Have the baby see a chiropractor with pediatric expertise (newborn adjustments are more like massage than manipulations).

Some babies find great relief in this simple exercise. With the baby on its back, grasp the thighs and lift the feet toward its head, like during a diaper change. Continue to roll upward and raise the baby until it is hanging upside down. Really! Now wait and watch it move; it will rotate its back this way and that, and when it seems finished, gently let it down. First touch its head down, then roll down shoulders, back, butt, and let its legs uncurl. Babies particularly benefit from this exercise when it is offered daily. ■

blood is then collected on a special strip and tested for glucose levels. If at or just above 45, have the mother nurse the baby as often as possible, and give water with a little molasses (1 teaspoon per cup) every few hours, preferably after a nursing. Rather than introducing a bottle, have her use an eyedropper or the tip end of a small spoon.

Central nervous system damage can result if blood glucose levels are insufficient, so recheck daily until levels are normal. Some babies require more aggressive treatment than fluids by mouth, such as IV therapy with hospital surveillance. Consult with a pediatrician if blood glucose levels dip below 45.

MECONIUM ASPIRATION

Any infant with moderate to heavy meconium at birth is at risk for serious respiratory problems. If you are unsure that suction was sufficient to clear all the meconium from the baby's respiratory passages before it began to breathe, listen carefully for any sign of lung obstruction. If the baby is breathing rapidly, be alert to other signs of **respiratory distress syndrome.** These include nasal flaring, grunting with exhale, retractions of the chest and abdomen, and cyanosis. If any of these symptoms are present, give blow-by oxygen (holding an oxygen tube to the baby's nose) and immediately contact a pediatrician to arrange for transport.

If the baby seems congested but not otherwise compromised, help it breathe more easily by providing steam. The easiest way to accomplish this is to turn on the shower full-force, then take the baby into the bathroom. You may also wish to apply percussion to release meconium from the lungs. To do this, place the baby on your lap with its head down, back exposed. Tap sharply with two or three fingertips in each quadrant of the lungs, particularly in any area you know to be obstructed.

If the baby resumes a normal breathing rhythm and is stable for several hours, and the mother and her partner understand warning signs of further trouble, check back again the next day. But if the baby remains congested despite the use of steam and percussion, contact a pediatrician immediately.

TRANSIENT TACHYPNEA

This is a temporary condition of the newborn involving abnormally rapid respirations. Normal rates are 40–60 breaths per minute; with tachypnea, rates may increase to 120 breaths per minute. Transient tachypnea is caused by delayed absorption of fetal lung fluid. By itself, it is not a significant problem.

However, tachypnea is associated with several serious conditions: respiratory distress syndrome, meconium aspiration, and sepsis. In the absence of these, it will resolve spontaneously with a bit of time. But if there are predisposing factors for the above conditions, or if tachypnea is accompanied by any sign of respiratory distress, you must take the baby promptly to the pediatrician. In any case, you cannot leave the baby until the problem is resolved. Once in the hospital, X-rays will be performed, and the baby will be carefully monitored until it is back to normal.

NEONATAL INFECTION

If the mother had fever or foul-smelling fluid during labor at a point too late to transport, or if fever or uterine tenderness develops postpartum, the baby should immediately see a pediatrician to be screened for sepsis. This is particularly crucial if the mother is group B streptococcus (GBS) positive and declined antibiotics. Cultures will be performed on the baby, and because some of these take up to seventy-two hours to return, prophylactic antibiotic treatment is recommended. Considering that one of the first symptoms of GBS infection is apnea (cessation of breathing), hospitalization may also be advisable.

The septic baby may show a variety of symptoms: lethargy, irritability, jitteriness, fever, dehydration. Tachypnea is a sign of sepsis, as is cyanosis. If the baby appears to be infected, cultures of the spinal fluid may be recommended to rule out meningitis.

In the event of continued hospitalization, it is important to help parents stay as close to the baby as possible. Your support and reassurance can enable the mother to establish a good milk supply and experience continued bonding with the baby. It is more than over-

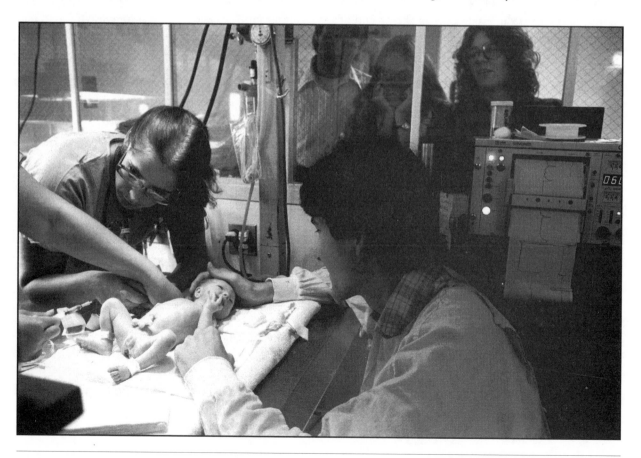

whelming for new parents to face the fact that their baby may be ill or to watch painful tests be administered repeatedly. They will need the expertise of a good pediatrician, as well as your continued presence, advice, and encouragement.

JAUNDICE

Neonatal jaundice is no longer the blind concern it was a decade ago. We now recognize the vast majority of cases to be **physiologic jaundice,** unassociated with the dangerous rise in bilirubin characteristic of pathological types.

What causes physiologic jaundice? While in utero, the baby's need for oxygen is met by a high percentage of red cells in its bloodstream, higher than in most adults. Once the baby is born and breathing, it no longer needs all these red cells, so the excess are broken down for elimination. A by-product of this breakdown is bilirubin, which imparts a yellow tinge to the baby's skin. Physiologic jaundice usually manifests on the second or third day postpartum and is remedied when the mother's milk comes in and flushes the baby's system clean.

One factor in increased physiologic jaundice is altitude—babies at 10, 000 feet are four times more likely to have excess bilirubin than infants at sea level. It is also more common in premature infants, infants with bowel obstructions, or those with infection.

Another kind of jaundice that seldom requires treatment results from **ABO incompatibility.** This phenomenon is similar to RH sensitization: if blood from an O type mother transfers to her A or B type baby during the birth, the baby will have more trouble eliminating excess red cells and so will have excess bilirubin. **Breast milk jaundice** is yet another non-threatening condition caused by a hormone in the mother's milk that can interfere with the baby's ability to process bilirubin. Unlike most other varieties of jaundice, it manifests after the milk comes in.

In contrast to the above, **pathological jaundice** may be caused by liver disease, an obstructed bile duct, infection, or RH hemolytic disease. This is easy to differentiate from physiologic jaundice in that it generally manifests within the first twenty-four hours. However, jaundice from ABO incompatibility may also appear early. To be on the safe side, refer any jaundice on day one to a pediatrician. If the jaundice is pathological, high levels of bilirubin may be nearly impossible for the baby to eliminate and may seep into the basal ganglia of the brain, which leads to **kernicterus,** or permanent brain damage.

Depending on the degree and type of jaundice, the baby may be hospitalized for treatment—placed under bili-lights, with periodic blood draws to assess bilirubin levels. If bili-lights are used, it is crucial that

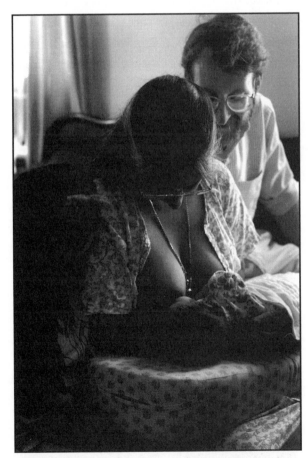

Nurse the baby frequently to help flush bilirubin from the system (note pillow support for positioning).

the baby's treatment is properly supervised, as dehydration, burning, and possible genetic damage can occur with excessive exposure. Jaundiced babies are also at risk for infection.

Although physiologic, ABO and breast milk jaundice are essentially normal and self-correcting, they can occasionally cause the baby to become lethargic and disinterested in nursing. If the characteristic yellow tinge is noted on the baby's face and neck but runs no lower than the nipple line, encourage the mother to nurse often and to expose the baby to sunlight (with its body naked and eyes protected) for thirty minutes twice daily. It has been my experience that babies kept in dark rooms for the first few days of life have higher bilirubin levels than those liberally exposed to sunlight. Contrary to medical opinion, physiologic jaundice appears to be unrelated to late cord clamping. Unless there is an emergency, I never cut the cord until it has completely ceased pulsing (or not at all with a lotus birth), and in all my years of practice, only two babies have become heavily jaundiced. In each case, lack of light was the primary factor.

Babies born to mothers whose labors have been induced or augmented with pitocin must be watched carefully. Pitocin competes with bilirubin for binding sites, rendering elimination difficult. The same is true of vitamin K, and certain drugs like diazepam, sulphonamides, steroids, and salicylates. If the baby's extremities appear jaundiced, consult a pediatrician.

CIRCUMCISION

Circumcision is a controversial procedure. It is no longer routine; in fact, the American Academy of Pediatrics now states that circumcision cannot be justified on medical grounds. Nevertheless, the practice is ancient—it is portrayed in Egyptian murals and has long been a central rite in Jewish tradition. Circumcision has mostly been practiced by cultures living in hot, dry climates, with water for bathing at a premium. But today, and particularly in the West, it is a custom perpetuated chiefly by fathers wishing their sons to look as they do. If the mother and her partner are considering circumcision, they should carefully weigh the pros and cons before making a decision.

Circumcision is a surgical procedure. It is often done without local anesthetic, so the baby must be strapped spread-eagled in restraints. The skin adherent to the tip of the penis is severed and cut back to completely expose the glans, and then clamps are placed to control bleeding. Sometimes a Plastibell device is used instead, which clamps and cuts off blood flow to the foreskin, causing gradual tissue necrosis. In either case, the pain is severe. Babies generally cry so hard with this procedure that they can scarcely breathe. Possible physical side effects include infection (several deaths have been documented), and penile sloughing necessitating reconstructive surgery.

Knowledge of the procedure is enough to persuade most parents of its dangerous and emotionally traumatic nature. Opponents of the procedure, many of whom are prominent nurses and physicians, deem it a form of sexual mutilation or even child abuse. But what about the alternative—the uncircumcised penis? What about the supposed dangers of infection, and how about basics of good care?

The foreskin covers and adheres to the glans for the first year or two, at which point the boy will pull it back as he becomes aware of his genitals. Parents should not pull back the foreskin for any reason, as this can trigger a vicious cycle of bleeding and infection. Once the foreskin is moveable, teach the boy to pull it back in the tub or shower to clean beneath it—this is as simple as cleaning under the fingernails or cleaning secretions from the folds of the female labia.

There is continuing debate regarding the effect of circumcision on sexuality. On an uncircumcised male, the foreskin captures the first drops of moisture secreted with arousal; then, as the erection increases, the foreskin pulls back and the glans is automatically lubricated.

Empirical evidence shows that circumcised men require more stimulation to become and remain sexually aroused.[2] This makes sense, as the foreskin preserves the sensitivity of the glans, which may be dulled on the circumcised penis due to constant friction with clothing.

Returning to some fathers' concerns about their sons appearing different from them or from other boys, it comes down to this: if we agree that circumcision is a violent and potentially harmful procedure, we simply must break the cycle. In all fairness, we should really leave the choice to the boy himself—it is his body, and he can decide in the future if he wants the procedure done. My personal feeling is this: if nature had intended man to be without foreskin, baby boys would be born that way.

NERVOUS IRRITABILITY/COLIC

Dealing with a colicky baby demands the same patience, focus, and endurance as does giving birth. However, if labor has been unusually difficult or postpartum assistance minimal, the mother and her partner may feel overwhelmed if the baby is frequently fussy. Above all else, help parents maintain their objectivity, so they will not project feelings of guilt or resentment onto every anxious cry the baby utters. Suggest that they use familiar labor-coping tools when their patience is at an end, such as deep relaxation, deep breathing, and touch/massage. Reassure them that it takes a while to get to know the baby's signals, but they will soon be able to differentiate fatigue-based cries of overstimulation from those demanding food, diaper changing, or simple contact.

A useful approach is for parents to notice when crying spells most often occur and see if there is any correlation with their own tense times during the day. In many cases, crying and fretting reach a peak around 6 P.M., when the mother is busy making dinner and trying to share the day's events with her partner, who has just come home from work. The baby feels the excitement, the confusion, the stress of it all, and reacts by crying excitedly. If such is the case, perhaps evening transitions can be made more gradually, with conversation between partners saved for later in the evening. Dinner hassles

For Parents: What to Do If the Baby Cries

1. If the birth was complicated by malpresentation or shoulder dystocia, or if manual manipulations of the head were performed or molding was extreme, consider cranial-sacral therapy. This gentle realignment of the baby's head, neck, and spine can work wonders.

2. Try nursing in peace and quiet, without jiggling the baby around.

3. Have the baby's bed in a space that is quiet but still close to the center of activity.

4. If the baby wakes when set down, try nursing lying down and then quietly getting up once the baby is asleep.

5. Let the baby spend lots of time in a baby carrier positioned near your heartbeat.

6. Establish a ritual break period for yourself, when your partner completely takes over for an hour or so (immediately following a nursing is best). Use that time to rest, take a shower, call a friend, or otherwise rejuvenate yourself.

7. If the baby seems to have gas (pulls its legs up sharply, its stomach rumbling), try giving warm catnip tea by bottle or eyedropper (also see massage technique in "Herbs and Homeopathy Postpartum" sidebar, earlier in this chapter).

8. If all else fails and the baby is crying hysterically, try running the shower or turning on the vacuum cleaner. High-frequency sounds may be calming if the baby is very upset. ∎

can also be alleviated by relying on soups, stews, or casseroles made while the baby naps and reheated later.

Sometimes, in spite of every effort, nothing seems to work for the baby. Most of the time, it will rapidly outgrow its initial crankiness, but on the other hand, babies' temperaments differ, running the gamut from high strung and intense to quiet and content. In fact, it is my experience that a baby's nature is fully evident at birth. I can think of numerous occasions when, after not seeing them for many years, I have run into a family whose birth I assisted and sure enough, the personality and energy of the baby I remember are there in the child before me. In other words, babies are what they are! Every baby has its own journey in life, style of coping, strengths, and vulnerabilities. If you are reasonably certain the mother and her partner are doing the best they can, advise them to relax and accept what is. This is especially crucial for the mother, as chronic anxiety or frustration can sap her emotional reserves and hinder her recuperation.

MINOR PROBLEMS

1. **Diaper rash.** After a carefuly cleaning the baby's bottom, a natural oil should be applied with each diaper change. Aloe vera gel (for wet, open sores) and calendula cream (for chafing or inflammation) are also effective. Rural mothers report that Bag Balm (intended for use on livestock to reduce teat inflammation) is a miracle diaper salve. Sometimes diaper rash is the result of improper diaper laundering; ammonia residue can build up and cause repeated episodes of rash unless it is removed by bleaching. To prevent this, soak diapers immediately after rinsing in a bucket of water with bleach added, then wash with plain soap flakes and double-rinse before drying (the double-rinse removes bleach residue, which also can be irritating).

2. **Cradle cap.** Apply a natural oil to the scalp before bed and leave it on all night. The scales can then be removed with a soft toothbrush and natural shampoo.

3. **Heat rash.** The obvious solution is to cool off living areas and have the baby cozily but loosely dressed. Teach the mother to check the baby's temperature by feeling its hands and feet, which should be slightly cool to the touch.

4. **Thrush.** This mild infection can be identified by a white coating on the baby's tongue. Because thrush is caused by the same organism that causes vaginal yeast, screen the mother and treat her if necessary. Remind her to assiduously wash her hands after toileting or any contact with the vaginal area. The baby can be treated with topical applications of acidophilus solution, three times a day by cotton swab. Thrush may take several weeks to go away; be patient. If it is severe enough to interfere with nursing, the baby should see a physician.

In general, try to avoid synthetic, artificial substances for bathing and toileting. Baby powder is blended with talc, a substance known to be dangerous to the lungs, and most baby oils are made with a base of mineral oil that leaches vitamins from the skin. Baby shampoos claim to be mild and gentle, but most are complex chemical preparations rather than simple soaps. Many synthetic products also contain carcinogenic dyes, which can be absorbed through the skin. Suggest simple natural substances like olive or vitamin E oils and liquid castile soap (which can also be used as shampoo).

The Mother: Complications and Concerns

MINOR PROBLEMS

1. **Constipation.** This complaint commonly arises immediately after delivery, particularly if labor has been prolonged. A daily serving of high-fiber bran cereal is probably the most effective and pleasant remedy. Prune juice, taken in modera-

tion, can also be used for its softening effect. *Adequate fluid intake is critical.* Most nursing mothers need about three quarts daily in order to meet their own needs and produce sufficient breast milk.

2. **Hemorrhoids.** Most common immediately after delivery, these respond well to cool compresses and the application of witch hazel. If rupture and bleeding occur, aloe vera gel speeds healing. Both as treatment and as a preventive measure, follow the above recommendations for constipation.

3. **Afterpains.** These commonly occur with a second or subsequent baby, and are generally experienced during nursing or immediately after. Some women say these pains actually hurt more than labor! This may be an exaggeration, but afterpains can be very uncomfortable. They are caused by loss of uterine tone—that is, if the uterus has been overly stretched by successive childbearing, the contractions prompting involution will hurt. Herbs such as cottonwood bark or the cramp bark can help by promoting uterine toning, and black haw tincture is particularly effective. It is also critical that the mother keep her bladder empty, or the uterus cannot fully contract. Suggest she lie face down with a pillow beneath her lower abdomen to force the uterus firmly into place— this should provide some relief. Rarely, Motrin may be necessary for pain relief.

HEMATOMA

Hematoma is an asymmetrical and painful swelling in the perineal area. It is caused by soft tissue trauma in second stage and a faulty repair job whereby homeostasis has not been achieved—that is, bleeding vessels continue to seep below skin or mucosal surfaces. Although these hemorrhages almost always cease spontaneously, the blood takes time to reabsorb. Pooled blood readily permits the growth of bacteria, thus the primary danger of hematoma is infection. This can lead to breakdown of the repair, because surfaces will not adhere and close properly once sepsis develops.

Traction on the sutures from inflammation is another factor in repair dehiscence.

Immediately refer any woman with signs of hematoma to a physician; she should begin antibiotic treatment as soon as possible. To reduce swelling, have her alternate hot and cool soaks, which stimulate circulation and encourage reabsorbtion of pooled blood. Also make sure she pours warm water with a bit of Betadine over the vaginal area each time she uses the toilet, and remind her to dry and air her perineum thoroughly afterward. If the repair does break down, reconstructive surgery may be necessary. Do your best to prevent this!

UTERINE AND PELVIC INFECTIONS

Symptoms of uterine infection—**puerperal infection** or **endometritus**—include fever over 101 degrees, elevated pulse, pelvic pain, and subinvolution of the uterus. Risk factors include anemia, a compromised immune system, prolonged rupture of the membranes (PROM), numerous vaginal exams in labor, manual rotation or other manipulations of the baby during labor, maternal exhaustion, delayed placental delivery, hemorrhage, uterine exploration (as for manual removal of the placenta or sequestered clots), postpartum dehydration, or improper perineal hygiene.

In my experience, a prime cause of uterine infection is overactivity and exhaustion in the first few days postpartum. I have seen only two cases in my practice; both women had other children to care for and resumed normal activities immediately after the birth. And both had notably uncomplicated deliveries, with none of the precipitating factors just cited. One woman actually went to a swap meet the day after the birth, walking around in the heat and dust with nothing to drink for many hours! Take care to warn mothers who had easy deliveries that bed rest is essential postpartum, not only to speed recovery from the birth but from the entire pregnancy. Also reiterate that adequate rest permits oxytocin to involute the uterus, tone the vagina, and facilitate breastfeeding, whereas stress or overactivity cause counter effects of adrenaline to slow recuperation.

Sepsis may not only affect the uterus, but the pelvic ligaments, connective tissue, and the peritoneal cavity. Infection of these areas occurs only if uterine sepsis is untreated and will cause severe symptoms of vomiting, chills, and extreme pain. Rarely, the tubes and ovaries may also be affected, usually by a preexisting gonorrhea infection that has flared up again.

THROMBOPHLEBITIS AND PULMONARY EMBOLISM

Thrombophlebitis is the inflammation of either a superficial or deep leg vein. Women with varicosities are particularly at risk. **Superficial thrombophlebitis** causes leg pain, with heat, tenderness, and redness at the site of inflammation. To confirm, check for **Homan's sign** by having the mother sit in bed with her leg straight, and then gently press on her knee and dorsiflex her foot: if she has pain in her calf, the test is positive. **Deep thrombophlebitis** is indicated by high fever, severe pain, edema, and tenderness along the entire length of the leg. With either condition, contact a physician immediately. Meanwhile, have the mother stay in bed and keep the affected leg elevated. *And hands off the leg—* if you massage it, blood clots may loosen and enter her circulation. Should a clot lodge in her lungs, the life-threatening condition of **pulmonary embolism** will result, characterized by chest pain, shortness of breath, rapid respirations, and elevated pulse. If any of these develop, administer oxygen to the mother immediately and call the paramedics.

DIFFICULTIES WITH BREASTFEEDING

Problems with breastfeeding often spring from distraction. If a mother feels anxious about her primary relationship, worried about money matters, stressed over changes in her lifestyle, frustrated by lack of support, or impatient with her rate of recovery, she may find breastfeeding less than simple and fulfilling.

In order to evaluate breastfeeding difficulties, we must first understand the normal physiology of the process. Each breast has approximately twenty lobes, which consist of **lobules** divided into **alveoli** and **ducts.** The alveoli contain **acini cells,** which produce the milk, and **myo-epithelial cells,** which contract and propel milk from the breast. **Lactiferous ducts** carry milk from the aveoli and empty into one large duct that widens to create a **lactiferous sinus** or **ampulla** near the nipple. **Lactiferous tubules** emerge at the surface of the nipple and release the milk from the breast. The nipple itself is comprised of erectile tissue, which contracts during nursing to control the flow of milk.

It is important to appreciate the role of the baby's latch in terms of how much milk it receives. For many years, standard advice was that it should take the areola symmetrically into its mouth, on the assumption that this would stimulate a complete release of milk. Now we know that an **asymmetric latch**—one with a greater portion of the areola taken in at the lower jaw than at the top of the mouth—positions the nipple more deeply so the sucking reflex can work most effectively. (It also frees the baby's nose for easy breathing.) Prior to this new understanding, any woman who breastfed successfully discovered this more or less instinctively (although she may have worried from time to time that she wasn't doing it exactly right).

The hormone oxytocin plays a critical role in stimulating let-down of milk, but the hormone prolactin is primarily responsible for milk production. Prolactin is inhibited during pregnancy by high levels of estrogen, which fall immediately after the birth to prompt lactation. Continued production of prolactin and oxytocin depends on long, frequent, relaxed nursing sessions. The more relaxed the mother is when she nurses, the greater the release of these crucial hormones.

It is nature's design that by giving birth, a woman learns to let go of her inhibitions and trust her body. This is key to a successful breastfeeding experience. However, disapproving relatives or unsolicited advice may virtually negate maternal instincts. Breastfeeding is an intimate act between mother and baby that requires privacy, especially in the beginning. It is also a physically demanding activity and can be quite exhausting unless there is good physical and emotional support. If a mother is having breastfeeding problems unrelated to the mechanics of proper positioning, see to her needs for rest, good nutrition, privacy, and support.

And by the way—orgasmic breastfeeding is more than just an intriguing concept; it is a fact. This should come as no surprise, since the let-down hormone oxytocin is a precursor to orgasm. "Orgasmic" connotes the ability to engage oneself fully in an endeavor, to let go and respond according to what the situation demands. Thus it is in nursing a baby. In certain circumstances, levels of oxytocin are sufficiently high and the mother is relaxed enough to experience orgasm. It is important that new mothers realize this is possible so they will not worry if it occurs.

Breastfeeding can, in fact, have similar therapeutic value to sexual intimacy in affording a way for mother and baby to reaffirm their connection, stay close, and be of comfort to one another in times of change. It is a gift of tenderness and vitality, with the mother's urge to nurse the perfect complement to her baby's desire. Breastfeeding also provides a invaluable boon to infant/child maturation. In his excellent book, *Evolution's End,* Joseph Chilton Pearce makes clear that for optimal neurological development, the baby must have frequent face-to-face contact with its mother, and suggests that the relatively low protein content of breastmilk prompts the baby to nurse almost continuously in the early weeks so it can receive this crucial growth stimulus.[3] The more we learn about breastfeeding, the less we should be inclined to interfere with this highly personal and richly variegated intimacy between mother and child.

Physical complications of breastfeeding include engorgement and mastitis. **Engorgement** results from an amount of milk beyond what the baby immediately needs; it is normal for it to occur when the milk first comes in or when the baby gives up a feeding. Engorgement may be uncomfortable but will resolve spontaneously as the milk supply adjusts to the baby's demand. To facilitate this, apply heat and massage the breast toward the nipple, hand-express milk to start it flowing,

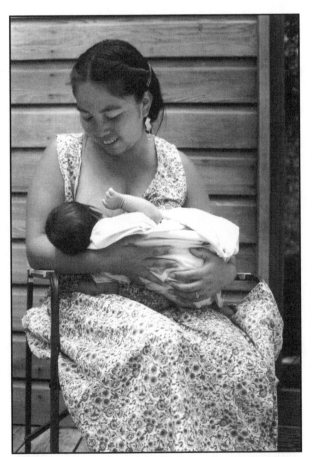

Alleviate sore nipples by lifting the baby to your breast rather than letting him hang from your nipple.

and have the baby nurse. (See additional suggestions earlier in this chapter under "Day-Three Visit" and in the "Herbs and Homeopathy Postpartum" sidebar.)

If milk is left pooled in the sacs, particularly if a residual amount remains time after time, it becomes a breeding ground for bacteria that can enter through the nipple. This is how **mastitis** occurs. Personal cleanliness is important in preventing mastitis, as are proper positioning, proper latch, and relaxed, unhurried, thorough nursing on demand. Naturally, the mother needs adequate fluids, calories, and rest to maintain resistance to infection. Mastitis is characterized by reddening of the breast (either lumpy areas or streaks) and high fever—103 or 104 degrees. Borderline cases are occasionally resolved with heat treatments, herbal or homeopathic remedies, and plenty of rest, but once fever has spiked as above, antibiotics are necessary. Dycloxicillin is generally recommended because it does not destroy intestinal flora and will not hurt the baby, although the mother may suffer indigestion. However, timely treatment is critical to prevent an abscess from developing, which can cause even more trouble with breastfeeding.

Some mothers ask about weaning just days after starting to breastfeed. This may indicate ambivalence about nursing or simple curiosity regarding the end points of the experience. Recommend letting the baby set the course; its need for solid food will be indicated by interest in what others at the table are eating (psychological readiness) and by teething (physiological readiness). Many pediatricians believe that solid foods are unnecessary for up to nine months if the baby is completely breastfed, as it takes about this long for its digestive system to fully mature. A relaxed approach saves the mother a lot of trouble and allows the baby to follow its natural pace of development.

POSTPARTUM DEPRESSION

Postpartum depression must be carefully differentiated from **postpartum blues.** Up to 70 percent of women experience the blues, which usually begin two to three days postpartum and are thought to be associated with hormonal swings, sleep deprivation, and impending lactation.[4] There is also evidence to suggest that the natural suppression of the maternal hypothalamic-pituitary-adrenal axis (HPA) in the immediate postpartum may cause emotional instability until full function resumes in about ten days.[5]

The blues are more likely to occur in women who are not physically up to par, particularly if the birth has been difficult or debilitating. For example, a mother who hemorrhaged at delivery might experience blues off and on for the first few weeks, due to anemia and resulting exhaustion. Particularly if the mother has no history of emotional problems, look to her current health status. Check her hemoglobin, review her diet, and recommend supplements as indicated.

Even with no physical factors, the blues can affect any sensitive, intelligent woman faced with a multiplicity of postpartum adjustments. As mentioned earlier, losses experienced at the onset of this new phase of life are very real. Help the mother identify and address these directly. Sometimes loss engenders grief; other times, anxiety. Here is one mother's description of her postpartum struggle:

Postpartum blues? No, not me! The joy of long-awaited motherhood and the emotional stability I had achieved over the years disqualified me, I thought, as a candidate for the postpartum syndrome. But I was not immune! My "blues," however, did not fit the picture of what I had expected. In fact, I came to feel that nothing I'd read or heard had adequately prepared me, since I was not depressed according to my usual definition.

For me, the experience was one of drowning in a vacuum of mind—consumed with worry, anxiety, and uncertainty. The responsibility seemed overwhelming. In spite of reassurance from my midwives, doubts and questions plagued me . . . was my son becoming jaundiced?. . . was his cord healing properly?. . . why was his skin peeling? . . . how would I bathe and groom him? I longed for the recommended rest and would be famished, yet could not seem to coordinate time for my own needs with

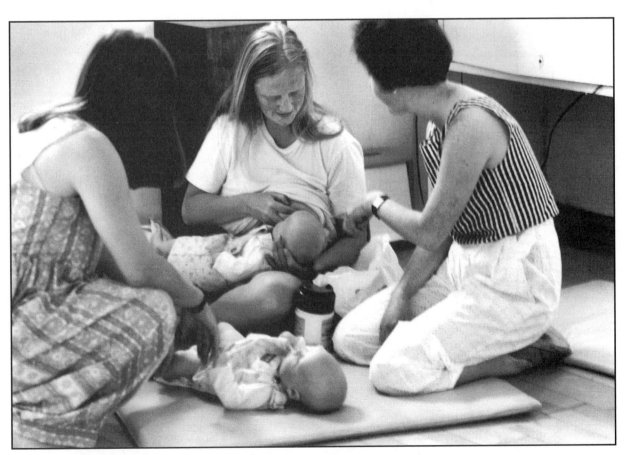

There is just no substitute for sharing concerns and insights with other new mothers.

that of caring for him and feeding him every few hours. Trian was a good, quiet baby, but I didn't have a handle on my end at all. I felt like I was failing miserably at my goal of being a perfect mother.

Trian was several days old when I suddenly realized while nursing him that I had not leisurely touched and explored his whole body. At this moment, I knew I had been in a vacuum for days, functioning but not fully aware.

To my amazement, I just couldn't "organize" my newborn. Fifteen years of pride at being a successful organizer in my career now proved totally useless. I had to learn to simply flow with Trian, emotionally and psychically, and let go of intellectual anticipation, expectations, and planning.

My love for Trian was the grounding cord that held me together as I floundered with anxiety at the enormous task before me. When I learned to recognize my signs of postpartum syndrome—irrational fears overtaking me, heart racing, nausea, excessive perspiration, and shallow breathing—I would relax, do the deep breathing I had been taught for the birth, and concentrate on how much I loved my baby. This allowed me to center myself and deal rationally with my fears, so that I could carry on.

One powerful remedy for postpartum blues is regular outings with family and friends—just doing whatever it takes to get time away from home and the usual routine. Most babies will sleep contentedly during a long car ride, which provides a much-needed break for everyone. Frequently, what the exhausted mother needs most is physical space, a chance to get the baby off her body for a while. To make the most of this, she should use this time to recuperate, letting her mind and body rest completely. If she can get someone to watch the baby so she can be truly alone, she may enjoy a favorite leisure activity.

In contrast to the above, **postpartum depression** develops at ten days after the birth or later, and tends to worsen with time. Occurrence is from 8 to 15 percent.[6] Depression not only affects mothers but has been shown to negatively impact child development.

Depressed mothers do less relating to their infants, who in turn show fewer positive facial expressions and have more eating and sleeping disorders.[7]

Occasionally, what appears to be postpartum depression may be caused by thyroid imbalance. The condition known as **postpartum thyroiditis** leads to hypothyroidism, which is characterized by fatigue and depression. Thus any new mother showing signs of depression should immediately be screened for thyroid problems.

Midwife and author Constance Sinclair has divided predisposing factors for postpartum depression into four categories:

1. **Psychiatric factors,** including negative birth experience, history of psychiatric disorder, low self-esteem, or stressful life events.

2. **Demographic factors,** including age, marriage status, access to medical or social assistance, and economic difficulties.

3. **Relationship factors,** including separation from parents in childhood; poor support in childhood; poor support in pregnancy; history of sexual, emotional, or physical abuse; or poor relationship with partner.

4. **Cultural factors,** including community support, spirituality, and clear role definition in culture.[8]

Extensive research on postpartum depression by midwife Cheryl Tatano Beck has resulted in the Postpartum Depression Predictors Inventory (PDPI), with the following thirteen predictors:

1. Prenatal depression

2. Child-care stress

3. Life stress

4. Lack of social support

5. Prenatal anxiety

6. Marital dissatisfaction

7. History of previous depression

8. Challenging infant temperament

9. Maternity blues

10. Low self-esteem

11. Low socioeconomic status

12. Unmarried

13. Unwanted or unplanned pregnancy.[9]

One relationship dynamic particularly predisposes to postpartum woe. If the father has been indifferent during the pregnancy but becomes compulsively bent on proving himself in the immediate postpartum, the mother may be more than a little disoriented and may have trouble bonding with her baby or trusting her instincts. Typically, she plays passive-dependent to his authoritarian role, and he responds to the demands of fatherhood with a strict set of rules regarding baby care, discipline, breastfeeding, housework, expenditures, sexuality, and so on. He may also use spiritual or political beliefs to judge the mother's performance. No wonder she gets depressed! I have had heated discussions with fathers of this temperament and find it does little good; if the mother has chosen this situation, what is an outsider to do? As a typical passive-dependent, she will ask continually for your help and advice but will seldom use them. Refer the mother to counseling and extract yourself from this configuration as soon as possible.

Postpartum depression resulting from a disappointing birth experience can be difficult to heal, particularly if pain medication was used or bonding was disrupted. Scars from these experiences run deep, and painful memories may be especially overwhelming in the early weeks when intensified by hormones and fatigue. Any mother who has transported unexpectedly should be given opportunity to go over the birth in detail and air all misgivings and regrets. At the root of her depression is grief, so support her in dealing with loss of her birth dream by bearing witness. Let her define the issues and ask the questions she considers important when she is ready. If time goes by and she

becomes increasingly depressed, refer her to counseling or hypnotherapy.

In contrast, the woman convinced perfect birth is her destiny may be embittered by transport and may have trouble caring for herself and the baby once out of the hospital. Keep a close eye on her. She desperately needs contact with more even-tempered and mature mothers, whose flexibility and receptivity she can emulate. Do what you can to facilitate this.

Depression following cesarean birth is in a class by itself. The mother may feel that she failed her partner, the baby, and herself, particularly if she had general anesthesia and missed the actual moments of birth. This is especially hard on the well-prepared mother who, aware of the importance of immediate bonding, may feel that her relationship with the baby is hopelessly damaged. Even if she has made peace with the cesarean, she may still have subconscious yearnings for the climax of birth and may dream vividly of vaginal delivery in the first few weeks postpartum. Acknowledge her loss and share in her feelings. Help her find a cesarean support group. If depression persists, refer her to counseling.

Besides counseling, treatments for postpartum depression include both allopathic and natural remedies. It is important to understand the physiology of depression to appreciate the pros and cons of each. In general, the current rise in depression mirrors increased levels of stress in our lives—estimated to be a hundred times greater than that faced by our grandparents. The more stressed we are, the more catecholamines (adrenalines) we produce. Serotonin balances the effects of these, but overproduction of catecholamines makes it hard for the body to make enough serotonin to keep up. Without adequate serotonin, we become anxious or depressed on an ongoing basis.

Drugs like Prozac and Zoloft, which belong to a class known as SSRIs (or selective serotonin reuptake inhibitors), keep serotonin circulating in the body. But they do not increase levels of serotonin; instead, they cause the body to use up its reserves by pulling them into the nerve synapses. Adverse affects include violent outbursts and suicidal urges. Natural aids to serotonin production include the amino acid tryptophan (concentrated in shrimp, tamari soy sauce, raw crimini mushrooms, cod, snapper, halibut, chicken breast, scallops, turkey breast, and tofu), omega fatty acids, vitamins B-6, B-2 (riboflavin), and B-3 (niacin), folic acid, and magnesium. The supplement 5-HTP (found in most health-food stores) may be especially helpful, as tryptophan converts to this before converting to serotonin. Coffee, alcohol, chocolate, and cigarettes must be strictly avoided.[10, 11]

Then again, an extreme form of depression requiring medication is **postpartum psychosis,** characterized by manic or depressive episodes of confusion or disorientation, delusional thinking, and suicidal or infanticidal behaviors. Sadly, this condition has been brought to the public eye with several horrific examples of new mothers harming or even killing their children. Mothers with a history of bipolar disorder are particularly at risk. The incidence is 2 to 3 percent—doesn't sound like much, but it actually amounts to eighty thousand women in the United States each year.[12] If you are in any way concerned about a mother in your care, secure the advice and support of a family health agency before referring her to a psychiatrist.

SEXUAL ADJUSTMENT

Not enough has been written about postpartum sexuality, aside from the physiological aspects. Maintaining sexual communication after the birth can definitely help a couple surmount the stresses of this period. But if used to making love on the spur of the moment or taking their time, the newborn will undoubtedly get in the way. Like it or not, their intimate relationship must somehow incorporate the baby.

Put simply, love is the key to making this adjustment. If partners can recognize the baby as an extension of their love while continuing to uphold the primacy of their relationship, they will find their way through the frustrations of this time. Eventually, their intimacy will deepen, but meanwhile fatigue, tension, loss of privacy, and a sense of isolation can make getting together difficult. Loss of privacy actually begins in pregnancy, as the mother discovers that society considers her pregnant body to be public property. Perfect strangers feel free to touch, advise, and speculate. Her partner is likewise exhorted to support her appropriately. Once the baby is born, strangers advise and admonish with even greater zeal. These are culturally inculcated behaviors intended to uphold the most basic building block of society—the family. But it is easy to see how a couple might feel personally invaded by all this, and how their sexuality might be affected.

There seems to be a critical point at about six weeks postpartum when expectations and disappointments run high, as this is when the mother is supposed to be physically recovered and ready for sex again. But readiness is often tempered by the hormones of breastfeeding, which tend to repress sexual desire. At six weeks, the mother is still totally absorbed with her baby; the two are almost inseparable. They are also psychically attuned, to the effect that the mother will wake seconds before her baby begins fussing, or the baby will wake crying when its mother has had a bad dream. These powerful bonds are important to the health of the family but may also cause sex to be pushed aside indefinitely.

It is also important to appreciate how a new mother's desire may be dampened by unsettling feelings of dependency. As one bluntly stated, "I realized when I was pregnant that I really needed to depend on this guy, now here I am with a little baby, and I feel so helpless . . . what if he [partner] turns out to be a creep?" On one hand, our culture endorses motherhood; on the other, we worship youth, freedom, and sexual autonomy. No wonder the new mother may feel dowdy, out of place, or invisible as a sexual being, all of which affect her desire for intimacy. If her partner

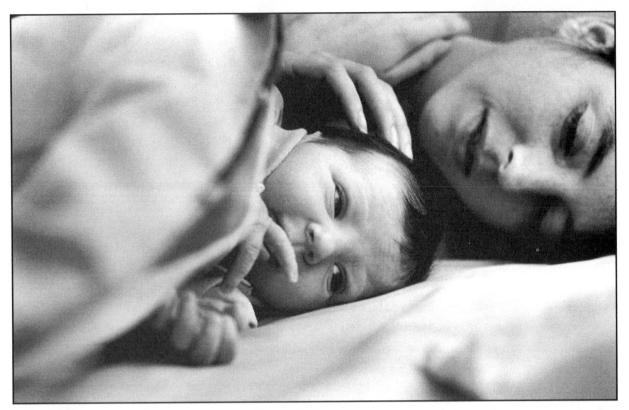

Don't forget to share the tenderness you feel for the baby with your partner.

does little to reassure her, or teases her in any way about her body, the situation goes from bad to worse.

But usually her partner will very much want to help. He or she may also be more desirous of time with the baby than expected and so may resent the distraction of having to be away at work. If her partner is pushing hard to deal with financial responsibilities, and the mother clings for want of companionship and reassurance, her partner will feel torn in two, and she will feel guilty and insecure. These stresses may push both of them to the breaking point. Although sex is a logical way to reunite diverging energies in relationship, chronic fatigue and mounting resentments can definitely interfere.

The best solution is to have a grandmother, another female relative, or a trusted sitter take the baby for an afternoon or evening so the couple can get away for some time alone. Expressed milk can be frozen in a glass bottle, and given to the baby after warming in a bowl of water. Once in privacy, partners should take time to relax and talk a while before diving into sex with overloaded expectations. If getting away is impossible, the second best alternative is to make a weekly date for dinner, a video, and lovemaking in some private part of the house. Older children can spend the night with friends or relatives. And even if the baby interrupts, at least partners know their next date is only a week away.

Although prolactin tends to repress desire, oxytocin serves to increase it. Oxytocin levels have been shown to be exceptionally high in women who nurse for long periods on demand. And if a couple can make it happen, the simple fact is that having sex makes us want more—the more we have, the more we want! This is due in part to the neurotransmitter dopamine, which counteracts prolactin and causes us to perceive and pursue pleasure. Thus sex itself may be a remedy for sexual disinterest. Masturbation works too.

Couples must place a premium on keeping their rites of intimacy. If partners make a point of daily check-in with each other, they can certainly hold their ground and may find new ways of working together. With time, and with intention, sex can become more meaningful, wild, and wonderful than ever before—*but it does take time.*

CONTRACEPTION

Before sexual activity resumes after birth, heterosexual couples must address contraceptive issues. It feels strange to return to birth control after not having to bother for so long, and depending on the method used, it may become just one more barrier to intimacy.

Birth control pills are not really suitable for breast-feeding mothers—estrogen suppresses milk production, and progesterone-only minipills are not as effective as the combination formulas. The Copper 7 IUD is another option, but many women find this less than desirable for a variety of reasons, not the least of which are side effects of chronic bleeding and low-grade infection. The fertility awareness method is difficult to implement postpartum, as the course of lactation causes erratic fluctuations in basal body temperature and cervical mucus. Norplant and Depo-Provera cause heavy bleeding and can delay the resumption of menses when discontinued. This leaves the barrier methods: condom, diaphragm, or cervical cap.

Apart from the difficulty of finding an appropriate birth control method is the difficulty of being diligent in its use. One of the more subtle conflicts affecting couples who have known the thrill of conscious conception and ecstatic childbirth is the desire for the no-barriers sexual intensity that accompanies these events, versus the desire to delay or forgo having more children. This conflict is usually unspoken, but after some time has passed and the family has stabilized, this psycho-erotic desire for conception can rise up and wreak havoc with future plans, as well as compliance with birth control.

Coping with these feelings depends on mutual acknowledgement and communication. A couple may succeed at preventing conception, but unless conflicts regarding the use of birth control are expressed, their intimacy is at risk. Encourage them to consider contraception an open issue, one apt to arise repeatedly for review and worthy of sensitive and candid discussion.

Notes

1. Doña Queta Contreras and Doña Irene Sotelo, lecture notes, Midwifery Today conference, Oaxaca, Mexico, October 2003.
2. M. Mylos and D. Macris, "Circumcision: male—effects upon human sexuality," in *Human Sexuality: An Encyclopedia,* ed. Vern Bullough and Bonnie Bullough. (New York: Garland Publishers, 1994), 119–22.
3. Joseph Chilton Pearce, *Evolution's End: Claiming the Potential of Our Intelligence* (San Francisco: Harper San Francisco, 1992).
4. F. G. Cunningham and others, *Williams Obstetrics,* 20th ed. (Stamford, Conn.: Appleton and Lange, 1997).
5. M. A. Magiakou and others, "Hypothalamic corticotropin-releasing hormone suppression during the postpartum period: implications for the increase of psychiatric manifestations at this time," *Journal of Clinical Endocrinology and Metabolism* 81 (1996): 1,912–17.
6. M. Righetti-Veltema and others, "Risk factors and predictive signs of postpartum depression," *Journal of Affective Disorders* 49 (1998): 167–80.
7. L. Lamberg, "Safety of antidepressant use in pregnant and nursing women," *Journal of the American Medical Association* 282 (1999): 222–23.
8. Constance Sinclair, *A Midwife's Handbook* (St. Louis, Mo.: Saunders, 2004), 239.
9. C. T. Beck, "Revision of the Postpartum Depression Predictors Inventory," *Journal of Obstetric, Gynecologic, and Neonatal Nursing* 31 (2002): 394–402.
10. Dean Rafflock and Virginia Rountree, *A Natural Guide to Pregnancy and Postpartum Health* (New York: Avery Penguin Putnam, 2002).
11. George Mateljan Foundation, "World's Healthiest Foods Nutrient Rating System," available online at www.whfoods.com.
12. Janet Balaskas, *Active Birth* (Boston, Mass.: The Harvard Common Press, 1992), 373.

Chapter 7

BECOMING A MIDWIFE

I f you are considering practicing midwifery some-day, this chapter is for you. It is one thing to decide to become a midwife, though, and another to face the realities of acquiring the necessary training. As mentioned in chapter 1, current educational pathways are often circuitous and may require much determination and endurance on the part of the student. But what more appropriate introduction to the dedication required of the midwife? Although many are attracted by the glamour of midwifery, it remains one of the most challenging professions. Even as a student, one must endure long hours, intense personal interactions, and repeated sacrifice of personal concerns. Thus it is best if midwifery is less a career choice and more a calling.

If you decide to become a nurse-midwife, your course of study will be fairly well mapped out for you. See appendix M for a list of nurse-midwifery programs, or contact the American College of Nurse Midwives (ACNM) for an update. For direct-entry programs, also see list in appendix M.

The respective advantages and disadvantages of nurse and direct-entry midwifery training have been partially articulated in chapter 1. To reiterate, a major advantage of being a nurse-midwife is legal practice anywhere in the country, with reciprocity state to state. Having utilized the political infrastructure of nursing for professional development, nurse-midwifery has been recognized by our health-care system. But some of the perks of being a nurse-midwife are falling away.

As HMOs seek to control costs by using midwives in high-volume clinics or labor units with little or no continuity of care, the midwifery model is subsumed by profit margins and institutional efficiency, and midwives are reduced to obstetrical technicians. Certified nurse-midwives are losing their collective bargaining power as HMOs systematically fire them, only to rehire them for longer hours at less pay, often without benefits.

As for direct-entry midwifery, the fight for legitimacy continues. State by state, physician lobbies continue to throw up roadblocks, so midwives must repeatedly reorganize to meet new challenges to their right to practice. It all comes back to "pick your battleground"; only you can decide where you are most suited to struggle, for if you intend to practice true midwifery, struggle you must.

Meanwhile, we must recognize that at the root of how and what we practice, how we define ourselves both professionally and politically is the manner in which we are educated. Nurse-midwifery programs are usually based in hospital. Most are weighted toward theoretical instruction, with minimal hands-on training, little continuity of care, and limited scope of practice. Instructor and student alike are subject to highly restrictive practice protocols. Consequently, students often suffer overdevelopment of their analytical faculties at the expense of the intuitive, compassionate qualities so necessary to humane caregiving. In my experience, the primary stumbling block for nurse-midwifery graduates is fear—fear of the responsibility of private practice, of being inadequately prepared to work independently.

The challenge to today's midwifery educators is to create a curriculum that develops the student as a human being, combined with supportively supervised clinical experience. All too often, the nurse-midwifery graduate has done countless rotations in clinical settings but has never known primary responsibility for a single client from start to finish. When life-threatening complications of shoulder dystocia or hemorrhage occurred, she was obligated by chain of command to call for help, and then step aside and watch. Predictably, she feels ill equipped to "practice on her own responsibility."

In contrast, the student in an apprenticeship is one-on-one with clients throughout the entire perinatal cycle. She is also one-on-one with her preceptor, requiring that she develop and refine not only technical skills, but equally important abilities to communicate assertively and listen effectively. Learning takes place in context, as the senior midwife debriefs the day's events and suggests sources for further study. Students are more readily able to discern technical and interpersonal shortcomings when involved in cases from start to finish, and when interactions with preceptors are ongoing. In other words, continuity of care and instructor prompt the student to personally engage in her learning process, as in any long-term relationship.

Nurse-midwifery programs may come and go as funding dictates, but apprenticeship will endure because it is community-based, cost-effective, and perfect for women with small children who require training with a flexible time frame. If you are considering the apprenticeship route, check first to see if your state has any provisions for qualifying midwives. Some states require on-site academic programs in conjunction with apprenticeship; others have coursework requirements that can be met at-a-distance (similar to external degree or independent study programs offered by most uni-

versities). Other states have licensing or certifying mechanisms entirely competency-based, with the usual requisites of documented experience, skills verification, and comprehensive exam. Many states have incorporated NARM CPM requirements, and several use the CPM route exclusively. Consult MANA for a list of representatives that can familiarize you with various state educational and practice requirements; consult NARM for an updated list of all states that recognize the CPM. Consult Midwifery Education Accreditation Council (MEAC) for a list of accredited direct-entry programs (see appendix M).

If your state has no mechanism for regulating midwifery, you may wish to investigate the guidelines established by NARM for becoming a CPM, and use these to create your own framework for learning. Once you know what knowledge and skills you must be able to demonstrate, and the clinical experience necessary to acquire these, you will have some idea of how to proceed. Your initial efforts will probably involve (1) studying midwifery texts, (2) participating in a midwifery study group, and (3) attending births as a doula or birth assistant.

TEXTBOOKS AND OTHER REFERENCES

Aspiring midwives unable to be on-call for births can begin with book study. To get your bearings on educational routes, read *Paths to Becoming a Midwife*, edited by Midwifery Today. If you have already read extensively on reproductive politics, prepared childbirth, nutrition, breastfeeding, and parenting, concentrate on beginning midwifery texts. If you have read very little, start with books that feature plenty of birth stories to help you glean the emotional and spiritual aspects of the childbearing experience.

Although there are many fine birth books available, some have become classics. Ina May Gaskin's *Spiritual Midwifery* features exceptional birth stories, as does her latest, *Ina May's Guide to Childbirth*. For the politics and anthropology of birth, don't miss Robbie Davis-Floyd's *Birth: An American Rite of Passage*. *Birth Reborn*, by Michel Odent, and *Let Birth Be Born Again*, by Jean Sutton, show us what is truly natural in human birth. Any book by Sheila Kitzinger is a pleasure to read; for a perceptive overview with extensive illustrations, try *The Complete Book of Pregnancy and Childbirth*. Penny Simkin and Ruth Ancheta's *The Labor Progress Handbook* is a remarkable little text loaded with illustrations that show how best to assist women in labor. These books can give the aspiring midwife a firm foundation from which to pursue other studies in childbirth education, breastfeeding, parenting, and so on.

When ready to move on to midwifery or obstetrical texts, Harry Oxorn and William R. Foote's *Human Labor & Birth* gives basic pregnancy and birth information in a concise outline format perfect for beginners. Diagrams are abundant, clear, and easy to understand. The main drawback of this reference lies in its focus on obstetrical care—for example, there are lengthy sections on the use of forceps and vacuum extraction, and nothing on routine prenatal assessment. However, suggested management of complications is quite moderate, and the tone of the text is fairly respectful of mother and baby.

Another well-known text is *Myles Textbook for Midwives*, edited by Diane Fraser and Margaret Cooper (14th edition). This essential text for British midwives is detailed and complete, with a strong emphasis on caregiving. The format lends itself to study, with diagrams realistic and profuse. A brief but thorough chapter on care of the newborn is yet another positive feature. *Varney's Midwifery*, by Helen Varney, is a newer text, used primarily by nurse-midwifery programs in the United States. An outstanding aspect of this book is its sections on clinical procedures like venipuncture, Pap smear, and IV infiltration, with instructions that are easy to understand and fully detailed.

A new and very useful text is *A Midwife's Handbook*, by Constance Sinclair. Designed to slip into your birth bag, this quick reference guide consolidates essential information for handling complications, including herbal and homeopathic approaches. This book bears the mark of the midwife: practical, diverse, and complete.

And then there are the thoroughly remarkable texts by Anne Frye, *Holistic Midwifery, Volumes I and II*. Frye is an independent midwife through and through, and it shows: her books are grounded in respect for physiology and feature a wide range of approaches and treatments for full scope practice. Her philosophy of care is entirely woman-centered; her presentation of cultural diversity is unmatched by any other text. Absolute beginners may find these books a bit overwhelming, but they are essential. Another excellent book by Frye is *Understanding Diagnostic Tests in the Childbearing Year*.

Although these references are more than adequate for basic practice, you may also need an obstetrics text from time to time for in-depth understanding of any pathological development, or if only to be aware of the medical standard of care. *Williams Obstetrics* is notoriously challenging for beginners, due to its dry, scientific style. Invest in a good medical dictionary, like Tabers, to help you wade through the terminology. A newer text used by many midwifery programs is *Obstetrics*, edited by Gabbe, Niebyl, and Simpson. If possible, compare the two and see which suits you best.

Another groundbreaking work, *Obstetric Myths Versus Research Realities*, by Henci Goer, examines the research on such controversial subjects as gestational diabetes, episiotomy, cesarean delivery of the breech, postdatism, and induction of labor. Her latest book, *The Thinking Woman's Guide to a Better Birth*, is one of the best to recommend to anyone skeptical about out-of-hospital birth. Marsden Wagner's *Pursuing the Birth Machine* covers similar material but focuses primarily on the political underpinnings of the overuse of technology in the perinatal period.

Of course, the list goes on. Another breakthrough book, *Birthing from Within*, by Pam England and Rob Horowitz, is an important read in that it sparked a new, woman-centered approach to childbirth preparation. Other favorites include *Bestfeeding*, by Suzanne Arms, *Your Amazing Newborn*, by Marshall and Phyllis Klaus, and *The Wise Woman Herbal for the Childbearing Year*, by Susun Weed.

Other valuable sources of information are midwifery newsletters or journals. The *MANA News* focuses on political and practice issues of midwives in Canada, Mexico, and the United States. The *Journal of Nurse-Midwifery* (published by the ACNM) presents research articles and an open forum. *Birth* also publishes scientific research, with a focus on humanizing obstetrics. *The Birth Gazette,* edited by Ina May Gaskin, features human-interest articles, practical advice, and political updates for midwives and their supporters. And then there is *Midwifery Today,* possibly the most comprehensive and inspiring newsletter for aspiring and experienced midwives alike. *Midwifery Today* has an active website with a monthly e-zine and organizes regular conferences on the East and West Coasts, as well as internationally.

Also check to see if your state midwifery association publishes a newsletter, or you may wish to subscribe to newsletters from other states. Write or email MANA for contact information (see address in appendix B).

DOULA WORK, OR BIRTH ASSISTING

Attending births as an assistant is an important step in midwifery training. Absolute beginners benefit immensely from discovering the extent to which birth is nonintellectual and transformative. Women who have already had children have opportunity to refine their understanding of the adage, "It's not my birth," as they help those who lack support have the best possible experience.

Aspiring midwives who have not had children may encounter skepticism regarding their suitability for this work, or may wonder about this themselves. I must admit that I once thought it nearly impossible for anyone who had not given birth to be truly effective as an assistant. But through exposure to many exceptional students, I came to appreciate that the most important qualification is knowledge of one's inner resources as gained by some experience of being on the edge, facing or meeting one's demons, or enduring grief through personal loss. Nevertheless, any aspiring midwife who has not given birth should attend births as early in training as possible, so her text-acquired knowledge will not overwhelm her instinct, intuition, or common sense.

Whether assisting births at home or in a hospital, there is a lot to learn. If the mother's partner or other helpers are present, you must find ways to work respectfully with her intimate circle. As you suggest comfort measures, massage techniques or certain labor positions, you will discover the relative effects of each. And if the mother is by herself, you will quickly begin to appreciate the dedication and endurance that will one day be required of you as a midwife. Most beginning birth assistants have worries about making mistakes, saying or doing the wrong thing, or being rebuffed by the laboring woman. But rest assured—as long as you surrender your own fear of birth's intensity and keep pace with the mother's rhythms and needs, *you will know what to do in the moment.* Learning to speak and act spontaneously may be unnerving at first, but every student midwife must find her own voice in order to encourage laboring women to express themselves freely.

Regardless of your role, the first few births you attend will be profoundly affecting. Reverence for the power of birth, and willingness to feel it on a visceral level, are the best possible start for any aspiring midwife. But as patterns of labor and the intensity of birth become familiar, you may begin to turn your attention to the skills and style of the midwife or physician in attendance. It is easy to be critical at this stage, to focus on the flaws of more experienced practitioners rather than on their strengths. But keep these observations to yourself—there is no point in alienating those with whom you work, as you never know what special favor you may require from them some time in the future. Keep the channels of communication open, and above all, *learn* from your seniors, don't merely react to them.

BIRTH ASSISTING AT HOME

Most birth assistants work in the hospital, as that is where women are least likely to have support. So if you have an opportunity to attend a home birth, count your blessings! Home births generally involve minimal intervention and provide the student opportunities to learn the natural rhythms of labor through pure obser-

vation. *Observe, observe, observe*—notice how different women respond to labor, which positions work best in each stage, which breathing patterns seem most effective, and how best to involve and integrate the rest of the family.

The latter is one of the subtler aspects of effective coaching, that is, wisely assessing how to focus the efforts of everyone on the birth team. A competent doula discreetly directs the mother's supporters into effective participation, based on the limit of what each can handle. Primary relationships can be greatly strengthened in labor; old wounds can be healed. Thus the birth assistant's task is to inspire enough confidence in the mother so that she can let go and enjoy intimacy with her partner and other supporters if she so desires. This contributes to bonding among all involved, which in turn can ease challenging postpartum transitions.

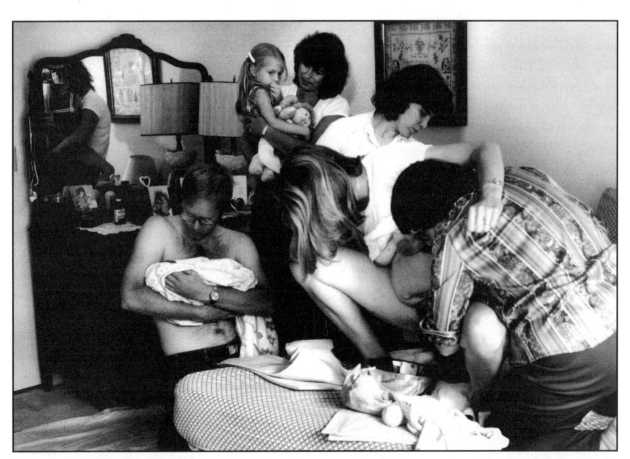

Assisting at home births affords the chance to share in a team effort and to experience birth as normal.

Sometimes a midwife will use the doula's "extra pair of hands" for some routine task and, sensing enthusiasm, will do a bit of teaching. I recall one midwife calling me to attention while she was suturing, telling me to "watch and learn." I had been holding a flashlight at the perineum for what seemed like forever; my arm was aching and my interest was wavering. But because of what I witnessed, I acquired a better understanding of the repair process. Never pass up an opportunity to assist a primary care provider, especially at home births, where there is more time to ask questions and more opportunity to follow up later.

BIRTH ASSISTING IN HOSPITAL

Hospital doula work affords the opportunity to serve a diverse group of women while learning about current obstetrical practice. It also provides a potentially shocking introduction to the political aspects of medicalized childbirth. For this reason, many women shun birth attendance in hospital, believing their personal discomfort level to be ample indication that home-birth assistance is their destiny. This may result in a very long wait to attend births—a very long wait indeed.

Apart from all that is offensive about hospital births, they do provide opportunities to see complications that seldom occur at home, and to observe medical management of preexisting pathology. A student seeking apprenticeship (or admission to a formal program) can use her birth attendance in hospital to show potential preceptors that she has this background, and further, that she can handle being on-call and will support women in labor no matter what the circumstances.

I began doing hospital doula work to augment sporadic home-birth attendance early in my apprenticeship. I registered as a volunteer birth assistant by calling labor and delivery at the local general hospital, and was well received because of problems with understaffing. I agreed to be available on-call several nights a week, and over a ten-month period, attended nearly sixty births. On-call coaching is a boon to mothers unprepared for labor, and definitely tests the mettle of the aspiring midwife.

One very unappealing aspect of working in hospital is the environment itself. Hospital rooms are typically overheated, lack adequate ventilation, and have nothing but overhead lighting. And there is the standard package of obstetrical procedures to contend with—IV, fetal monitoring, and continuous vaginal exams. This predisposes the mother to pain medication and cesarean birth, and will thus be deeply disturbing to any birth assistant who has seen the alternative in home birth. Just as the mother can be undermined by tension, so may the birth assistant, who must overcome her own stress before she can hope to reassure her client. One of my students who is also a doula confided that she takes nice pieces of cloth, flowers, and small birthing goddess statues with her to births, and with the mother's consent, transforms the hospital room as much as possible.

Always remember when doing on-the-spot assisting that an unprepared mother must contend not only with pain, but also with fear. If confronted with a woman who is writhing or screaming, first calm yourself, then make eye contact and explain that you are there to help. Women who are panicked or terrified of their sensations often breathe too rapidly, which can lead to hyperventilation. Avoid this by having her breathe lightly, or better yet, by slowing her breathing down. You can help by breathing with her, starting at her rhythm, then asking her to breathe with you as you make each breath a fraction slower and deeper than the one before. Place a hand on her belly and as you look into her eyes, ask her to bring her breath down to the baby. It may take some time to win her trust, but don't give up!

Once her breathing is regular, relaxation can be initiated by using touch, massage, and verbal cues. Ask her between contractions if you can rub her back, whether she would like to sit up or lean forward, and

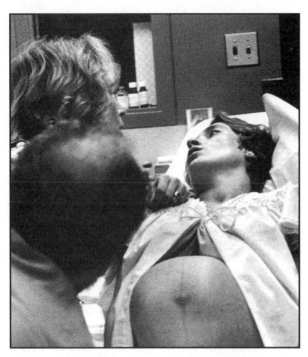
Often you are the mother's only support in hospital situations.

so on. If she is tightening her hips or legs, a foot massage may help her let go. She may also respond to phrases like, "Let your legs feel heavy," or "Let your bottom melt into the bed." Several times I have assisted Asian and Hispanic women who spoke no English and had to rely entirely on touch and sign—and things went well.

Even in the best of circumstances, though, unprepared mothers tend to progress very slowly. More than anything else, hospital doula work will try your patience. This quotation from Grantly Dick-Read says it perfectly: "At the bedside of a woman in labor we have to await the will of intangible forces. The emotional conflicts and physical reactions of women present a constant stream of problems. Initiative, clear thinking and honest exposition must be at hand to control the fearful, encourage the failing and support the tired. No force of mind or body can drive a woman in labor; by patience only can the smooth course of nature be followed."[1]

Basic to finding patience is validation of your own needs, both physical and emotional. If the mother you

are to assist is alone, perhaps you can bring another doula with whom you can alternate break times and compare notes. If not, hospitals usually have a nearby coffee room for staff, and while one of the nurses is checking on the mother, you may be able to take a quick break. Because hospital rooms are often overheated, wear something light, cool, and loose. You might want to bring an extra change of clothes, in case you are in the way when the mother vomits or her water breaks. As a precaution against HIV and hepatitis, you may wish to wear protective glasses, and you should bring your own gloves for handling underpads, and so on. If you have long hair, tie or clip it out of the way. Bring lozenges to keep your mouth moist, and lip balm too, as breathing with the mother may chap you. Also bring enough food and bottled water to see you through twenty-four hours.

The main difficulty in assisting mothers birthing in hospital is that no one is directly accountable for their care. Even if a woman has engaged a private physician, her labor may be managed by nurses or residents she has never met, and then, as shifts change, new faces appear. Thus a doula must repeatedly reassert her client's wishes. And despite the growing demand for compassionate care, women are still systematically disempowered and sometimes treated brutally in birth, which is the opposite of your intent. Much of what you see will disgust you, but hopefully you will persist in your efforts and vow to do better in your own practice someday.

Lest you think your work as a doula is futile, though, rest assured that women never forget an act of kindness in labor, whether a simple touch, an encouraging word, or a compassionate look. I know this from my own experience with my first birth in 1972; I was overwhelmed by a pitocin-induced labor of only two-and-a-half hours. My Lamaze preparation was useless; the contractions peaked immediately and I never had more than ten seconds' rest between them. Basically, I screamed my way through labor. For the most part, the nurses shunned me because I wanted a natural birth. But then, one came in and sat at the edge of my bed, touched my arm, and said quietly, "Let's try to slow your breathing down a little," showing me what to do and letting me squeeze her arm so hard I am sure she had fingernail marks the next day. I can't say she made everything better, but I will never forget her sweet face, her kind intent, and her caring spirit.

In other words, women in labor are highly aware of what those around them are feeling—what they believe, and what they fear. You can't hide anything from a laboring woman, so don't bother to try. By the same token, whatever you give from the heart will be deeply appreciated and always remembered.

On-call assisting is also good preparation for the midwifery lifestyle. You will learn to give your intimate relationships special attention before leaving for a birth, and as much energy as you can muster upon your return, to compensate for your abrupt and frequently prolonged absences. You will experience the frustration of doing hard work for minimal compensation, particularly if you are out-of-pocket for gas and babysitting expenses. As you become aware of the time and energy commitment you will make as a midwife, you will get a better idea of the kind of support you will need in your personal life.

What are other ways to keep up your birth attendance? Women who have had some exposure to birth and have specific techniques and insights to share may find teaching childbirth classes to be the answer. Most locations have pregnancy resource centers where you can register your course. You might also consider volunteering at one of these centers to gain exposure and make contacts. Or you might offer prenatal exercise or yoga classes. Community hospitals may be particularly open to having you teach "early bird" classes on health and nutrition. Educators are often asked to births as support persons; thus teaching is a potent avenue into the birthing community.

MIDWIFERY STUDY GROUPS

Participating in a study group with other students and instructors is a most exciting and integrating aspect of learning. Texts have their value, and assisting at births is crucial preparation for apprenticeship, but listening to experienced midwives discuss case histories and management of complications is a practical education that can't be beat. Study groups also afford golden opportunities for students to get extra help in troublesome subject areas, thus tailoring studies to their needs.

I participated in a study group for more than a year, and during that period went from student to primary caregiver. We had two midwives and a physician working with us, and were therefore able to practice skills like giving injections (we practiced by injecting oranges with water) and drawing blood (which we did on each other). We also learned intubation from a guest pediatrician. Discussion of our recent birth experiences usually determined our next topic. During the time our group met, we practiced working in teams at prenatals, births, and postpartum visits under the guidance of our midwife instructors. Several of us formed liaisons that later blossomed into midwifery partnerships.

Starting a study group can be as easy as posting signs in birth resource centers or any other location where new mothers or women likely to be interested in midwifery might gather. A variation of the study group learning situation can be found by attending state midwifery meetings as well as regional or national midwifery conferences. Contact MANA for the name of a regional representative in your area, or email *Midwifery Today* or *The Birth Gazette* for conference schedules (see appendix B for contact information).

APPRENTICESHIP

Ideally, contacts made in the study phase enable a student to find a senior midwife with whom she is comfortable and vice versa, so that apprenticeship is a

Core Areas of Study

General Subjects

Aseptic Technique
Human Reproduction
Anatomy of Pregnancy, Birth, and Postpartum
Physiology of Pregnancy, Birth, and Postpartum
Applied Microbiology of Pregnancy, Birth, and Postpartum
Embryology/Fetal Growth and Development
Pharmacology of Pregnancy, Birth, and Postpartum
Nutrition for Pregnancy and Lactation
Obstetrical Procedures for Complicated Pregnancy and Birth
Well-Woman Gynecology and Contraceptive Care
Childbirth Education, Theory
Childbirth Education, Instruction
Infant and Child Development

Provision of Care: Prenatal Period

Risk Assessment
Comprehensive Prenatal Care
Communication and Counseling Techniques

Management of Common Complaints in Pregnancy
Charting
Interpretation of Medical History, Lab Work, and Diagnostic Testing
Complications of Pregnancy
Contraindications for Out-of-Hospital Birth

Provision of Care: Intrapartum Period

Management of Normal Labor and Birth
Complications of Labor and Birth
Emergency Care
Immediate Care of Mother and Newborn
Assessment of Lacerations and Appropriate Action
Newborn Exam

Provision of Care: Postpartum Period

Management of Normal Postpartum and Lactation
Newborn Care
Management of Common Postpartum Problems
Newborn Complications and Appropriate Action
Maternal Complications and Appropriate Action

---

natural extension of an already established relationship. Many students worry about finding an apprenticeship, and it is true that political and legal difficulties have caused the ranks of practicing midwives to be somewhat erratic. Nevertheless, maintaining a high profile in your local midwifery community is always a step in the right direction.

How will a student know when she is ready to apprentice? She will reach a certain level of confidence after mastering basic midwifery knowledge and attending a number of births. Her personal life and finances will be sufficiently in order to take on the responsibility of 24/7 call. She will understand that she is making a long-term commitment, and that the midwife who trains her will count on her to provide as much assistance as possible in exchange for training. And she will show deference to the style and experience of the midwife from whom she is soliciting instruction.

If she is chosen, the apprentice will not only help at births, but will also share the weighty responsibility of managing (and debriefing) emergency complications and transports. It stands to reason that the senior midwife should choose a student with whom she feels fully comfortable and compatible. Conversely, the apprentice must have respect for her senior midwife's style and philosophy of practice. This requires tact and reserve at times but does not preclude asserting new ideas or conflicting beliefs at appropriate moments and in a respectful way.

Apprenticeship usually begins with assisting at prenatal visits and acquiring rudimentary skills of uterine palpation, fetal heart auscultation, and maternal blood pressure assessment. If a midwife is training several apprentices, she will probably rotate their attendance at prenatals to establish which mothers and students work best together and will then arrange for those combinations at births. Depending on the size of her practice, apprenticeship can last for several years or more.

Sometimes students have difficulty forging agreements with their senior midwife regarding the rate at which they will acquire skills and primary care experiences. In this respect, participation in a formal program can provide some structure to apprenticeship. As an example, the **National Midwifery Institute** (of which Shannon Anton and myself are codirectors) combines distance course work with apprenticeship. Our mission is to provide students with a solid theoretical foundation in midwifery, while helping them find apprenticeships in their own locale. Apprenticeship is structured in that student and midwife make an agreement on their working relationship and have regular opportunities to give feedback to each other and to the program on how the agreement is working out. This program is also MEAC accredited, which assures the student of its ethical and fiscal integrity. For a complete listing of midwifery programs, including those that are MEAC accredited, see appendix M.

In self-directed situations, the backbone of apprenticeship training is skills acquisition and evaluation. In 1995, NARM conducted a survey of midwives to determine entry-level skills for direct-entry practice. The resulting practical skills list is utilized by NARM in its certification process. These skills are outlined step-by-step in the handbook *Practical Skills Guide for Midwifery*, by Sharon Evans and Pam Weaver.[2] Using the list and handbook, an apprentice and her senior midwife may be able to formulate a plan so that the skills and experience necessary for certification or licensure are acquired in a reasonable amount of time.

What about educational costs? Apprenticeship is traditionally a relationship of exchange, whereby a master of a given trade exchanges knowledge for labor. But if part of a formal program leading directly to licensure or certification, the student should expect to pay for apprenticeship. In less structured situations, the apprentice may receive a nominal sum to cover trans-

portation and child care, and if the midwife intends to incorporate the apprentice as a partner, she may increase her pay over time to full partnership level.

How can an apprentice best contribute to the midwife's practice? She can offer assistance with housekeeping, bookkeeping, filing, stocking supplies, public relations outreach, errand running, and so on. She can provide emotional support to clients at births when the midwife is occupied with technical duties. She can field the basic concerns and questions of new mothers. As she becomes increasingly skilled and self-confident, her responsibilities will increase to include labor sitting and checks on mother and baby until the midwife arrives, and finally, to catching babies herself.

How will an apprentice know when she is ready to practice independently? Meeting state or national standards for skills and experience is only one aspect of

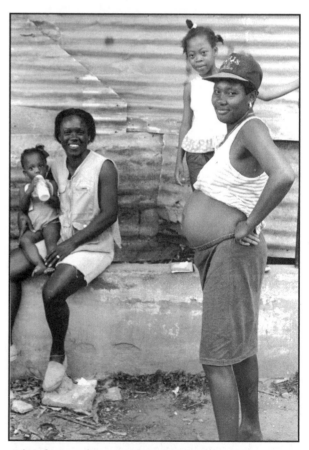

A brief internship outside the United States can greatly expand the student's horizons.

preparedness. Some students are by nature overeager and need extra time to integrate the fine art of caregiving. Others are timid and must be given unexpected and challenging responsibilities to help them appreciate their competence. If their relationship is good, an apprentice can trust her teacher's judgment regarding her readiness to practice. Apart from this, some students feel a need to work with an additional teacher or in a different practice setting—perhaps with a high-volume midwifery practice or out-of-hospital birth center.

OTHER DIRECT-ENTRY OPTIONS

In addition to the **National Midwifery Institute,** there are numerous programs available for students without a nursing background who wish to pursue midwifery training. **Maternidad La Luz** is a birth center and teaching facility serving the larger community of El Paso, Texas, as well as women from Mexico who cross the border so their children may have U.S. citizenship. The great strength of this program is that it offers academic preparation concurrent with clinical training.

The **Florida School of Traditional Midwifery** offers a three-year, holistic curriculum incorporating the apprenticeship model. Also in Florida, the **Miami-Dade College, Midwifery Sciences Department** offers a three-year program located in a community college, with theoretical instruction prior to clinical training. The **Seattle Midwifery School** is a private school with much the same structure but also has a distance-learning option. For a bachelor's degree in midwifery, contact the **Birthingway School of Midwifery** in Portland, Oregon, or the **Midwives College of Utah.** For both bachelor's and master's degrees with a distance-learning option, contact the **National College of Midwifery** in Taos, New Mexico. All of these programs are MEAC accredited.

Perhaps the best guideline for the student unsure of what kind of program to choose is to consider her learning style. Ask yourself if you need lots of structure in order to master academic material—that is, a classroom setting with quizzes, tests, and assignment due dates. If so, look for an on-site program. Or, if you are a self-starter, quite capable of working autonomously and without a need for deadlines to keep you on track, you may be better suited to distance learning. Most students need a program that provides both structure and freedom. If you are the type of person hesitant to begin hands-on work for fear you don't "know enough," you may need a school that provides theoretical preparation prior to clinical training. On the other hand, if you feel you learn best by doing, look for a program that will integrate theory and practice right from the start.

Investigate the distinction of MEAC accreditation to learn how it safeguards student interests. Make sure the programs you consider have ample opportunity for student input, and mechanisms for providing student feedback to potential enrollees. Also take every opportunity to query recent graduates for their opinions of their training.

NURSE-MIDWIFERY PROGRAMS

Nurse-midwifery programs also vary greatly in terms of their structure, especially concerning prerequisites. Some require a BSN to be admitted; others, an RN certificate only. Several master's level programs that incorporate nursing into midwifery training accept students with BA or BS degrees in any subject; in three years, the student earns an RN, MSN, and CNM. (These are considered by the ACNM to be direct-entry programs.)

Unfortunately, many CNM programs are focused more on efficiency than on the art of midwifery. One way to identify a program's philosophy is to see what type of clinical settings are involved. If most or all are tertiary, high-tech medical centers, you will get more active-management, interventive training than woman-centered birth experiences. Programs with training in birth centers or hospitals known for expectant management teach more of the art of midwifery.

The Community-Based Nurse Midwifery Education Program (CNEP) and the Institute of Midwifery at Philadelphia University have on-site theoretical portions but allow students to do the majority of their course work and clinical work at a distance. I know from personal experience that the program at the University of California, San Francisco, emphasizes holistic, woman-centered midwifery, as does the Women's Health Care Studies Program at the University of Pennsylvania. When applying to a program, always ask to speak to a current student or recent graduate to get a better sense of what is offered.

A ray of hope for those planning on the nursing route to practice: the Bridge Club, a wonderful organization residing within the ACNM, represents midwives who do out-of-hospital birth or otherwise strive to provide independent, woman-centered care. All nurse-midwifery students intent on upholding the midwifery model would do well to attend a Bridge Club meeting at the annual ACNM convention.

Notes

1. Grantly Dick-Read, *Childbirth without Fear* (Harper & Row: New York, 1959).

2. Sharon Evans and Pam Weaver, *Practical Skills Guide for Midwifery,* 2nd ed. (Bend, Oregon: Morningstar Publishing: 1999).

Chapter 8

THE MIDWIFE'S PRACTICE

As a midwife's status changes from apprentice to primary caregiver, her focus shifts from the thrill of catching babies to her burgeoning professional responsibilities. In order to practice successfully, she must effectively combine the demands of work with those of her personal life. Putting together a cohesive and comfortable practice can be challenging for a beginner.

The best way to get started is to clearly articulate your intention, which readily translates to your philosophy of care. This is the linchpin on which many of your practice decisions will be based. Your philosophy should incorporate your beliefs regarding optimal care and responsibility in childbearing. If your philosophy is clearly stated, it will define your purpose. For example, if your philosophy states that midwifery must serve the needs and desires of childbearing women, your purpose is clearly to support women in choosing how they wish to give birth. From this point forward, the structure of your practice should at all times and in all ways uphold your philosophy and express your purpose.

It might seem that all midwives share a similar philosophy. But one has only to look at the services and clientele of several different practices to see that this is not the case. If you are unclear on your philosophy or intention, you may wish to try this simple exercise I give my midwifery students.

Choose one of the following statements: "A pregnant woman should . . ." or, "A pregnant woman should never . . ." or, "A pregnant woman's partner should . . ." or, "A pregnant woman's partner should never . . ." or, "A new mother should . . ." Now write a response as spontaneously and exhaustively as possible, not censoring anything, just jotting down your thoughts. You may have quite a list when you finish but will probably find that one "should" or "shouldn't" really stands out and is highly charged for you. Then, in the same way as before, write down all possible reasons why this matters to you, based on your personal history. To conclude, recognize this "should" or "shouldn't" for the bias it is, and look closely at how it might impact a mother or partner's experience of receiving care from you.

Were you to do this exercise in a group, you might be surprised to discover that other participants hold biases in direct contrast to your own. The same is true of practicing midwives—they all have their biases, and on that basis, make decisions of whom they will and will not care for. Smart midwives readily refer prospective clients they find trying or difficult to other midwives who might work better with them. The point is that our biases determine, to large extent, our motivation for, and philosophy of, caregiving.

As regards getting your practice to match your philosophy of care, there is much to consider. You must figure out backup arrangements, define your working relationship with partners or other assistants, choose an office location, name your business, establish a financial structure, create promotional materials and marketing strategies, and so on, all based on the needs and desires of your anticipated clientele.

It can be challenging to find your footing in the beginning, particularly in terms of finances. Will your initial client volume be adequate to pay the bills? Would it be better to have an office in your home for a while, to keep overhead low until things get going? Is your personal life stable enough to withstand these startup stresses? Your first clients seem to take all of your energy as you work hard to make the best impression, agonizing over every detail lest anything be overlooked. Your family life may begin to show some strain, which puts an extra burden on you.

Just remember to take one challenge (and one day) at a time. Step back periodically to reflect on your progress. Most established midwives schedule regular weekly meetings with their associates to go over client issues, to attend to business matters, and to otherwise clear the air. Especially in the beginning, consider having these meetings in casual or retreat settings, which are more conducive to the visioning needed to get off to a good start.

LOCATION: URBAN OR RURAL PRACTICE?

Urban practice has benefits in the ready availability of medical facilities, support from other midwives, and easy access to consultation. These serve to make home birth quite workable in an urban setting. However, close contact with the medical community demands good working relationships.

Difficulties with urban practice depend largely on the midwife's legal status. If practicing illegally or in a hostile environment, she will eventually find herself in the untenable position of having to transport and face the consequences of inadequate or nonexistent backup. On the one hand, the safety of mother and baby may require that she relay details that necessitated transport; on the other, she knows if she provides this information she incriminates herself. Thus she must be discreet, keep her practice quiet, get plenty of support from her peers, and gain clear agreements with her clients as to her limits. Urban midwives often have more difficulty in this respect than their rural sisters, whose home-birth practices may be tolerated in that not one else is caring for mothers far from hospital.

If political oppression is not an issue, urban practice may be hindered more by urban lifestyle than anything else. A common problem is finding the time to really get to know your clients, as well as making them aware of their need to slow down and let pregnancy determine lifestyle, rather than the other way around. The stresses of noise, air pollution, and harried pace are hardly conducive to good health. Urban midwives have the challenging task of calming their clients down enough to show them what is really essential in preparing for birth.

Sometimes a city or town has several competitive midwifery practices. In the past, midwives have succumbed to factionalism and slander of one another's work. But the more organized midwives have become, the more they recognize the need for cooperation. Only by sharing resources, exchanging information, and passing clients along freely can they generate the strength needed to cope with limited scope of practice, lack of autonomy, and unhappy outcomes.

The real competition for city midwives is in hospital-based alternatives. Women who might otherwise investigate home birth are often impressed with the "home-like atmosphere" of nicely furnished, decorator birthing suites (an undeniable improvement over the stark white of standard labor rooms). What they don't realize is that, regardless of which room they occupy, they will still be subject to standard obstetrical guidelines and procedures. Unfortunately, a woman may be aware of this and yet be bound by financial considerations to choose hospital birth. Although insurance coverage for home birth is increasingly available, it all too often depends on physician backup.

An alternative to this dilemma may be found in the freestanding birth center. Although backup may still be difficult to obtain, it is certainly easier to secure than for home birth. Midwives working in freestanding birth centers are generally subject to more stringent practice guidelines than are home-birth midwives. However, they are ultimately accountable to accreditation standards for out-of-hospital, not hospital birth. Working in a freestanding birth center can also provide the midwife some relief from the woes of private practice, particularly that of being continuously on-call.

Thus the urban midwife's practice situation is complex, and yet, with good standing in her community and supportive backup, opportunities for professional growth are tremendous. Working in the city takes a midwife across class and cultural boundaries, fostering adaptability in the joy of serving diverse populations.

As regards **rural practice,** the main benefits are environment and pace. Open space, clean air, and a relaxed lifestyle are obvious perks for the rural midwife and her clientele. Living in conjunction with nature and the seasons can be a source of strength for expectant mothers. They also tend to feel more connected to their community, which makes it easier to find support. Birth in a rural setting is often an extended family event, in contrast to the couple-only style of birthing endemic of urban woman's social isolation.

Problems with rural practice typically result from a large practice radius. Although it makes sense in urban areas to do prenatals on certain days at a central location, this may not be workable in rural areas. If, for example, you are detained at a birth or someone goes into labor on a clinic day, mothers already en route to see you may be quite unhappy to have come so far only to find you gone when they arrive. Rural midwives often end up doing a lot of care at their clients' homes, unless they have an extra assistant or backup from other midwives.

In fact, what rural midwives seem to miss most is contact with others in practice. Midwifery is, after all, an interactive profession, not just a bunch of skills. Midwives need regular opportunities to share experiences in peer review or with continuing education. If these opportunities are not available locally, the rural midwife may have to travel to an urban location or be content with periodic attendance at midwifery conferences.

In addition, good medical backup and consultation may be limited in rural areas; it can be very difficult to get a second or third opinion. And transport time may be considerable. Thus any midwife practicing more than half an hour from the nearest hospital will probably need advanced skills and equipment.

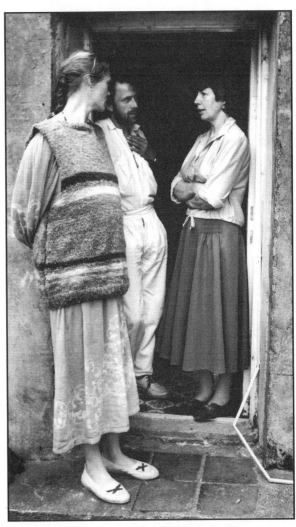

An Irish midwife responding to the call of a woman in early labor.

EQUIPMENT

Most beginning midwives take great pleasure and pride in their growing treasury of equipment. It is usually best to purchase equipment slowly, using the apprenticeship period to try out various brands and see which suit you best. Slow acquisition is also a lot easier on the pocketbook. A complete midwife's kit, including birth bag and oxygen system, can easily run around $3,000. Fortunately, birthing supply houses such as Cascade Health Care Products (see appendix B) cater to midwives and home-birth couples, reducing costs for those who buy in bulk.

Take a look at the supply list in appendix L ("The Midwife's Kit"). Certain basics like urine sticks, nonsterile exam gloves, Betadine antiseptic, sterile gauze pads, underpads, and bulb syringe can be purchased at your local drugstore.

When students ask which equipment to purchase first, I suggest they start with a fetascope. This tool for taking fetal heart tones can be your ticket to interaction with pregnant women and will give you the opportunity to develop a trained ear before you begin primary practice. Mothers in your childbirth classes or doula clients are usually eager to have you listen to the baby and may also want you to palpate for position, size, and so on. The best fetascope currently available is the Allen Series 10, which features an amplification unit in the horn (avoid Allen-type economy models). If you elect to purchase a Doppler, the most popular model is the Huntleigh, available in audio-only or audio-plus-digital display. Both come with water and shockproof 2 MHz probes and run around $500.

Other items, like your sphygmomanometer (blood pressure cuff), should be purchased by comparison shopping, your goal being quality without tinsel. Blood pressure cuffs are sporting some stylish colors of late, but apart from looks, the most important component is the gauge. The cuff, bladder, and tubing are readily and cheaply replaced, but the gauge should be built to last. Make sure it is constructed without an automatic pin stop, which keeps the gauge at zero even if it needs an adjustment. The unit should come with a warranty of at least three years, and the gauge should be certified (you can see a registered number stamped on the face of any decent gauge).

Although your lab will supply everything you need for doing blood draws, consider purchasing a hemoglobinometer for office use. These currently run about $200—much less expensive than a centrifuge. You might also wish to invest in a blood glucose monitor; Cascade Health Care Products sells a fully equipped model called Accu-Chek III for about $100.

Beyond what your lab provides, you should stock disposable items for urinalysis, pH assessment, and pregnancy testing. Your resuscitation equipment should include DeLee suction devices, pocket masks for mouth-to-mouth, oxygen tanks and regulator, adult oxygen mask for the mother, bag-mask unit for the baby, and, if you are trained to use them, laryngoscope and endotracheal tubes. The Spur Disposable bag-mask costs around $40 and may be a wise choice for the midwife with a small practice. For a more permanent investment, both the Hudson Lifesaver Infant Resuscitator and the Ambu Baby Resuscitator are excellent choices; the latter meets and exceeds all standards for neonatal resuscitation.

Make sure your hand instruments are 100 percent stainless steel. It is particularly important that your blunt scissors and curved hemostats be top quality, as you will use them repeatedly for cord-cutting. It is also wise to get a good needle-holder, as the precision work of suturing is best accomplished with a quality tool. The finest instruments are made in Germany by Medline and Miltex; they are lifetime guaranteed. A less expensive grade is entirely adequate for instruments like ring forceps or mosquito forceps that you will rarely use.

Last but not least are the restricted items: suture material and syringes. If you have authorization to purchase these items in your state, no problem. Otherwise, you may be able to enlist the help of a colleague with the proper credentials. The same goes for oxytocic drugs and other medications; if you are legally authorized to order these, count your blessings. Otherwise, if you must rely on a sympathetic physician or other midwives, stock up whenever you have the opportunity.

SETUP AND ADMINISTRATION

In terms of physical setup, you have a number of choices. You can see clients in your home, using a bedroom for exams and your living room for waiting. You can see clients in their homes (some midwives do this exclusively). Or if you elect to rent an office, you will need to find a facility with an exam room, waiting area, restroom, and storage area. If you set up a freestanding birth center, all of the above plus birth rooms should be housed under one roof.

Prenatal care by home visit would undoubtedly be the first choice of most clients. Midwives who give care this way report fewer transports than those working in an office setting, and for the most part, feel the driving is worth it. Being in a client's home repeatedly can shed light on household and relationship dynamics that might not otherwise be discovered until labor. Visits are more leisurely and often involve sharing meals—all in all, a more intimate type of caregiving experience.

Next to this, most clients would probably prefer to see you in your home rather than in an office. The obvious drawback with this is having to keep everything neat and clean on a regular basis. This can be especially challenging if you have just come in from a birth at 3 A.M., and appointments start in a few hours. Lack of privacy for family members is yet another issue—there may be strenuous objections from your partner if he or she needs extra sleep or solitude. If the cost of renting

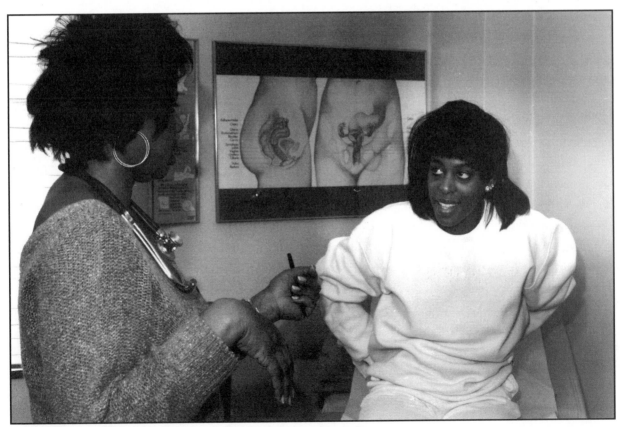

This midwife provides care in a comfortable office, in an informal manner.

an office is prohibitive, consider sharing office space with other midwives or health providers in your area.

Whatever you decide, your exam room should be arranged for comfort and efficiency. Most women prefer to be examined on a bed, rather than an exam table. Choose a firm mattress, large enough for you and your assistant to sit comfortably on either side of the mother. Another possibility is either a chaise lounge (if not too low) or antique "fainting sofa," with chairs on either side. Use a closet for storage, a corner of the room for lab equipment, and your exam room is ready to go.

In the waiting area, you need adequate seating, a water cooler, toys for small children, birth pictures (or art) on the wall, birth and parenting periodicals on end tables, and a bookcase with a lending library. Also post all pertinent documents, such as the WHO/UNICEF Breastfeeding Resolution, the WHO Resolution on Midwifery, the Patient's Bill of Rights in your state of practice, and so on.

In terms of clinic supplies, what will you need, and how much should you keep in stock? Besides your permanent essentials, various disposable items must be kept on hand. Underpads may be purchased in bulk for economy—the small, 17-inch-by-23-inch size is fine for doing internal exams. Exam gloves, lubricating jelly, urine testing strips, long-handled cotton swabs for cultures, cotton balls and Band-Aids for venipuncture, paper cups for urinalysis, and lots of toilet paper should be kept in stock at all times. Take inventory of these items weekly.

You must also keep tabs on your stock of forms, and make sure you have the necessary supplies for filing, bookkeeping, and correspondence. Have backup cartridges for your printer, disks or CDs for your computer, and so on. It never hurts to post a running list of needs, with highlighted priorities. No matter what your level of practice, keep it organized.

What about the actual structure of caregiving? How much time should you schedule for initial, follow-up, and routine visits? That depends on your style and volume of practice. If you assist four to six births per month, you can probably limit yourself to two clinic days per week. Schedule two hours for the initial visit and one-and-a-half hours for the visit immediately after, to allow for routine assessments plus medical history intake and review, consent to care, nutritional counseling, complete physical assessment, and/or pelvimetry. Routine checkups take forty-five minutes to an hour, allowing twenty-five minutes for physical assessment and at least twenty minutes for discussion.

If topics of conversation result in controversy or upset, or if physical findings are questionable, a visit may run over. This is why you need a well-stocked library in the waiting area and may also want to have tea and healthy snack foods available. When a visit is running over, make sure to notify the mothers waiting their turn, and if anyone is on a tight schedule, have your partner or apprentice begin their physical assessments. If possible, schedule mothers due around the same time so their appointments overlap, giving them opportunity to meet or even share in one another's checkups. This principle of overlap can also be used to bring partners/fathers together.

Some midwives have extended this concept of overlap to group prenatal care. This requires a large block of time, perhaps an entire day, when all your clients come together for prenatals. Women due at the same time love the opportunity to socialize and learn from each other and may choose to participate in one another's physical assessments. New mothers can also be invited to come with their babies and birth stories. If you decide to try group prenatal care, you may need assistance for either the clinical or discussion portion. Beloved California midwife June Whitson (who died of breast cancer some years ago) introduced this system as the best possible way to help new mothers find support and autonomy.

Apart from client visits, schedule weekly business meetings with your colleagues to go over finances, marketing, special events, and so on. This is also a good time to consider purchasing new reference books, supplies, or furnishings for your facility. Consider dividing weekly meetings into two segments: the first for business, the second for airing interpersonal concerns. The latter is critical to the psychological health of your practice. Occasionally, or perhaps initially, an outside facilitator may be helpful. Make separate time for case review.

Also plan a comprehensive annual review of all aspects of your business: facilities, organization, location, image, competition, finances, marketing strategies, as well as community and professional relationships. This provides an opportunity to create long-term goals for your organization, in contrast to the short term, problem-solving focus of weekly meetings. At this time, you should refer back to your basic premise of operation—your intention, as expressed in your philosophy of care. *Are all the components of your business still in keeping with this?* If not, your documents may need to be revised, or your practice restructured.

Be sure your filing system is at all times in order. Although the laws vary from state to state, medical records must be kept for many years (twenty-one years in California). Closed cases should be filed by year and kept in a fireproof container (for more on this, see the discussion on the HIPAA guidelines in the "Medical Records, Charting, Informed Choice, and Client Confidentiality" section later in this chapter). You may also need to hire an accountant, or consult an expert on tax laws and organizational options relevant to small business owners. Good references on this subject are *Small Time Operator,* by Bernard Kamoroff, and *Business Mastery,* by Cherie Sohnen-Moe.

GENERAL PRESENTABILITY AND PERSONAL HYGIENE

Most working women carefully plan their wardrobes for a variety of occasions, and there is no reason a midwife should not do the same. Clothes to wear to births should be readily washable; dark-colored pants are most practical. Tops should be layered, as the amount of warmth required upon arrival will be way too much once the birth room is adequately heated for delivery. Some midwives prefer to wear waterproof aprons in the final stages of labor. Apron or not, you should definitely have a change of clothes with you at all times.

One of the reasons there is less infection with home birth is that the mother has resistance to microorganisms in her environment. However, she may not have resistance to what you bring in from outside. This is why your clothes should be completely clean, and why you should always wash your hands upon arrival. This is important with postpartum home visits as well: wash your hands before examining the mother and again before handling the baby.

When doing prenatals in your office or home, observe proper aseptic technique and always wash your hands before and after each client. Clean, fresh-smelling clothes make a good impression. (In fact, pregnant women are exceedingly sensitive to smell, which is why you should avoid wearing perfume or cologne.)

To return to wardrobe, consider several highly presentable outfits for greeting the public. Midwives are increasingly called to political work in the legislature or the public arena, for which you will need a suit, heels, the whole bit. Don't be put off by the notion of dressing to fit the part. If life is a stage, then it pays to have your costumes in order.

FEES

A midwife's fee should be fair and reasonable, which should make it affordable for most parents. Beyond that, a sliding-scale policy makes way for exceptions. Many midwives have great success with this. For example, of a total fee of $3,500–$5,500, clients can be asked to pay anything in that range which is appropriate for their financial situation.

Once you have decided your fee, explain to your clients the services it includes and how you would like it to be paid. Some midwives work on a pay-per-visit basis. This may provide some protection against rip-offs but can be difficult for clients with erratic work and pay schedules. And too, if a mother is short of funds but feels pressed to bring money to her next pre-natal, she may cancel the visit, or if she does come, anxiety on this point may overshadow other impor-tant issues. If the mother is behind on her balance at twenty-eight weeks, firm up future payments more pre-cisely. Most midwives ask to be paid in full by thirty-six weeks.

A word now about outside work. Beginning mid-wives sometimes plan to supplement their income with another, part-time occupation. Well, never mind that idea, unless you have a highly flexible, home-based sideline. Regularly scheduled employment is really out of the question; no employer will tolerate an employee apt to run off at any moment and likely to phone in sick the next day. Midwifery practice is much more time and energy consuming than you might imagine. And it just won't do for you to be preoccupied with extra-neous, work-related concerns or wound up by ten-sions that disrupt your concentration on clients about to give birth.

Midwifery requires abundant energy and tremen-dous personal commitment. Try to take a realistic, long-term view of your needs right from the start, and then design your practice in a way that will keep you financially solvent and anxiety free. No one wants a tense, worried midwife to assist her. It is up to you to set up a practice that suits your style, reflects your beliefs, and accommodates your personal needs.

PUBLIC RELATIONS AND EDUCATION

The first step in public relations is to become visible. Begin with the obvious and list your services with birth resource centers and women's switchboards. Then con-tact prominent, alternative health-care providers in your area, like homeopaths, acupuncturists, naturopaths, massage therapists, herbal practitioners, and woman-centered counselors, to announce your new practice. Some may want to contact your former clients for their opinions of your care. Once on file, client feedback may be made available to the general public, which can boost your professional profile and credibility.

Midwives occasionally have opportunity to com-bine a presentation on birth with an introduction to their services. Consider hosting a video and informa-tion night for the general public, with business cards or brochures ready for the taking. Even small, infor-mal video showings with clients and their friends will keep your name circulating and bring you business by word-of-mouth.

Public events featuring well-known speakers can be organized to focus on alternatives in childbirth, family participation in the birth process, breastfeed-ing, adjustment to parenthood, or other topics. Panel discussion is another format interesting to the public. These events take some effort to coordinate and require plenty of advance publicity to assure good attendance. Although sometimes profit generating, their main function is to expose a large, diverse audience to the benefits of midwifery and, more specifically, to your services.

You might also consider renting a booth at the county or city fair. Our local midwifery organization has done this for several consecutive years, with great suc-cess. We show birth videos right at the booth to draw people in, and have T-shirts, bumper stickers, flyers, and a directory of local midwives available. Jan Tritten, edi-tor of *Midwifery Today,* never misses a chance to run her amazingly profitable lemonade stand at the Oregon Country Fair, where you can bet there is midwifery talk going on!

Television and radio appearances can boost pub-lic awareness of midwifery (and your practice), but adequate preparation is essential. Have statistics on the tip of your tongue and anticipate questions you

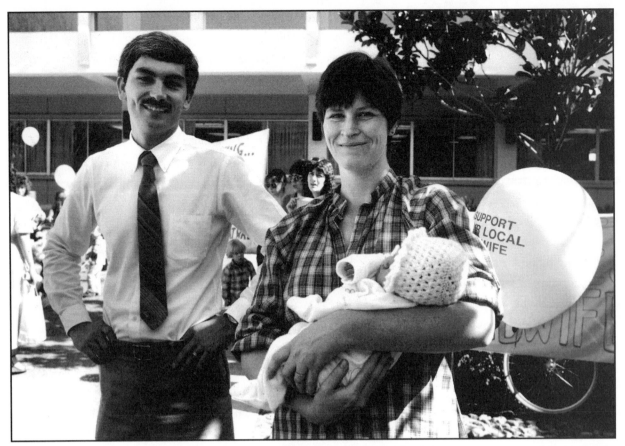

It pays to keep an updated client list, so support can be rallied in time of need.

are likely to be asked. And remember that you always have the option of responding to an unappealing question with one you would rather answer, as the media savvy do. For example, if your interviewer asks, "Is home birth safe?" you might respond with, "Well, who says hospital birth is all that safe?" and launch into a discussion of iatrogenic complications. If you are being taped for either radio or television, prepare a series of simple statements virtually impervious to an editor's distortion. The same goes for statements you make to journalists (although liability concerns increasingly prompt editorial departments to fact-check before they go to print). Do not let yourself be badgered, but if you are, don't get flustered—just calmly return to your key position statement, pose another question or raise a new issue more to your liking.

Midwife Diane Barnes claims that the remarkable success of her freestanding birth center was largely due to advertising spots on cable TV networks. She warns that results take time—in her case, calls started to pour in after six months or so. The obvious advantage of paying for advertising is that you get to say, and portray, exactly what you want the public to know about you and your services.

Whenever you go public for midwifery, remember that your words and appearance reflect on the entire profession. Consult with your colleagues, ask for feedback on other presentations you have made, prepare carefully, and dress the part. Promotional packets of information are often available from state midwifery organizations, or contact MANA for information.

MEDICAL BACKUP AND CONSULTATION

By grace, faith, or the law of averages, the midwife's first births usually go well. But with time, the unusual and unexpected begin to manifest, along with a desire for more in-depth medical consultation and assistance.

In areas where midwifery is illegal or unregulated, a new midwife may be hesitant to search out medical backup. But if transport becomes necessary, she clearly needs a working relationship with the local hospital if she hopes to safeguard her clients' well-being. Long before we became midwives, my first partner and I began working on getting backup. We gradually developed a relationship with a progressive hospital where we worked as birth assistants. Once in practice, we began transporting our clients there. We used the "iron fist in a velvet glove" approach, maintaining a low profile while persistently advocating our clients' wishes. We won the confidence of the staff physicians by being clearheaded and articulate and by presenting complete, well-organized client records. After several more drop-in transports, the head obstetrician called and asked if we would like his assistance on a continuing basis, and we formalized our backup relationship.

If you must transport a mother to a hospital where you do not have backup, maintain an open, adaptable, friendly attitude. The staff may be suspicious at first but may become accommodating if you act responsibly and present the details of your case intelligently. Although some physicians remain openly hostile, others are curious to learn just what midwives do, and so may give you opportunities to demonstrate your skills and knowledge.

Particularly if you have no official backup at your local hospital, it is crucial to appreciate the psychology of labor and delivery personnel. The nursing staff is overworked, underpaid, and underacknowledged, so why not offer assistance? Although nurses are legally responsible for routine assessments, you can certainly fetch drinking water, help your client to the bathroom, and change bedding. When the birth is over and you are preparing to leave, go out of your way to personally thank every nurse who participated.

If your local hospital trains residents, you have a challenging but promising situation on your hands. Fresh out of school, their heads crammed with information, medical residents are primed to answer questions. In fact, speculative discourse is their forte and your key to forging a connection. If you acknowledge the resident's authority in the realm of information as you project authority in action, you will be perfect complements. Pose a question on episiotomy, for example, and the resident may be only too happy to discuss the data as you provide perineal support. Suddenly, the baby is crowning and you are catching it together.

Residents are also hopelessly overworked and almost always exhausted. As a way of breaking the ice, one of my former apprentices would offer candy or gum to the resident on duty, followed by a vigorous shoulder rub as I went ahead and attended our client. Again, always remember to be generous with appreciation and praise before you leave, as an appreciative colleague.

In contrast, the attending obstetrician may be in and out of the room before you have a chance to say a word. If so, immediately step out in the hall to converse. Establish your authority by asking whether he or she has reviewed the chart or would like to see it, and then ask his or her opinion on the case. Listen respectfully, chime in agreement whenever you can, but assume a collegial air as you discuss your client as technically as possible. If the physician suggests a course of action you do not agree with, never confront him or her directly. Reiterate his or her recommendations so it is clear that you understand, then offer to present these to the mother. Once alone with her, let her know her options. You will, of course, express your opinion if requested. When she has decided what she wants to do, present her decision to the physician. Thus you avoid direct confrontation with the physician, while upholding principles of woman-centered care. Even if the physician is entirely disinterested in you and your ideas, fear of liability will prompt him or her to at least consider the mother's wishes.

If you are in very good standing at a particular hospital, you may link up with several doctors, and if problems arise in the future you can choose your consult at will. But in the early stages of establishing backup, consider distributing your clients among various practitioners so as not to overwhelm anyone in particular. Decide on whom to consult according to what is required. For example, if you need an ultrasound for suspected twins, order it through the obstetrician most likely to support vaginal twin birth. You need not be so picky with an ultrasound for third-trimester bleeding. But if you are trying to establish dates on a latecomer with uncertain menstrual history, you might have a general practitioner do the authorization to avoid involving an obstetrician in what might later be construed as a postdates pregnancy. Minor questions can be referred to a friendly resident.

If you are legally licensed or certified to practice in your state, your backup arrangement will probably be defined by law. In some states, the midwife must have a relationship with a particular physician, who usually has a cap on how many midwives he or she may assist. Sometimes the midwife and physician must work under mutually agreed upon written practice guidelines, which, due to malpractice concerns, can make formal backup almost impossible to obtain. Still, a progressive local hospital may be receptive to your transports.

Another approach to is to have mothers find their own backup. This may be your only option if you practice in a conservative area. In other words, a physician unwilling to back you personally might feel more comfortable backing your client as his or her private patient. Advantages of this arrangement are: (1) the midwife is free to practice according to midwifery guidelines; (2) the mother is free to choose her own physician; and (3) liability for the physician, professionally and politically, is reduced. (This approach is also in keeping with the original *MANA Standards and Qualifications for the Art and Practice of Midwifery* statement, which states that requiring the midwife to have a relationship with a particular physician is at odds with a mother's right to self-determination; see appendix A.)

In areas where the political climate is very oppressive and the "old boys" are out to get you, getting backup may seem impossible. Nevertheless, explore each and every inroad. For example, if you can't find a sympathetic doctor, perhaps you can find a progressive labor and delivery nurse who might give advice and then put in a good word for you. This takes time and is more than a little humiliating, but you owe it to your clients. The ideal is to have backup at every hospital where client insurance might necessitate transport.

Here is a story of acquiring backup on the spot (before midwifery was legalized in California). This was a first birth, and after many hours of ineffective labor resulting in maternal exhaustion, we all agreed on transport. Our usual backup doctor was not available, so we were forced to take "OB potluck." As the mother curled up contentedly on her hospital bed, it was obvious that she had deep ambivalence about home birth that was only now coming to the surface. But after forty-eight sleepless hours, my partner and I felt only relief. Our rapport with the nurses had always been great, and that night, even the head nurse (who was usually a bit disapproving) seemed sympathetic and supportive.

Progress with pitocin was much more rapid than anyone expected. Braving disapproval, my partner donned a glove and checked the mother, who was fully dilated. By the time the head nurse came back, the head was beginning to show, and I was doing perineal massage/support. She paused and took it all in before going to get the doctor. As the doctor (a woman) came in and the nurses gathered around, the head was close to crowning. My partner took heart tones as I attended to the perineum. When a nurse brought the instrument tray and asked the doctor where she wanted it, she said, motioning to us, "Ask them, I don't have anything to do with it." The tray was placed at the end of the bed, and after an awkward moment, someone unwrapped it for us. Good thing, too, for just then, a sweet baby girl was born. The doctor stepped up to help me check for tears; the perineum was intact but there was an internal muscle split. "She may need a few stitches there," she commented.

"No," I said, "just press down with some gauze and it will stop bleeding." She did so and watched, waited a moment, and concurred as I told her, "Those little tears heal fine if the mother keeps her legs together."

After some time had passed, she motioned me to step outside the room. "Uh oh," I thought, "This is it. I'm busted." Instead, she held up the birth certificate and asked me uncertainly, "Do you sign this, or should I?"

In my amazement, I uttered, "I consider it a privilege to be able to work here, so just do whatever works best for you."

"Then I'll sign it," she said. "You know, this is the first time I've ever done this." Then came a marvelous exchange of warmth and appreciation, with good feelings all around.

Whatever the genesis of your consulting relationship, you must continue to cultivate good communication. Periodic chart review, and disclosure of any revisions in your practice protocol, is critical to maintaining a solid working relationship. Friendly lunch dates are a good idea too. Trust and openness between you and your backup associates make all the difference in crisis situations.

MEDICAL RECORDS, CHARTING, INFORMED CHOICE, AND CLIENT CONFIDENTIALITY

This section will focus on the midwife's responsibility to document all aspects of caregiving. Accurate and appropriately detailed medical records are essential for professional practice. The forms in the appendix are intended not as models, but as samples you may freely adapt to your own needs.

As her training nears completion, it is a good idea for the apprentice to begin evaluating the forms of various midwives so she can decide what suits her. The Medical Health History form varies most dramatically, depending on whether it is formatted for take-home use or for interview. Patch appealing sections or components of various forms together to create your own.

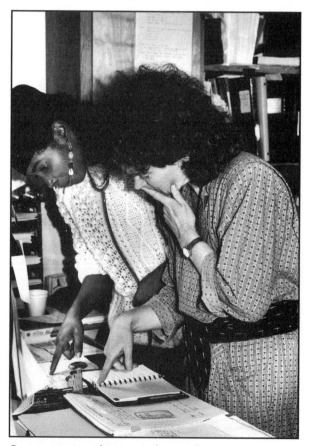

Partners review their records together.

And plan to revise your forms periodically, perhaps with your annual review of practice.

Since a medical chart is a legal document, the importance of complete and accurate charting cannot be overemphasized. In the event of a civil or malpractice lawsuit, your chart may be your only witness to thorough and responsible caregiving. For this reason, you must record everything you say and do, every assessment and recommendation, as well as all pertinent discussions between you and the mother, you and other health-care providers, you and your backup physician(s), and you and hospital staff.

Certain styles of charting are considered the most legally defensible. For example, all your commentary should be on lined paper, and your notes should be continuous, broken only by your initials and the date and time of each assessment. (Occasionally, you will need to end an entry with both your initials and the mother's, for example, in the event she declines a routine procedure.) Do not leave any part of a line blank; in fact, if your forms are designed with areas that could be left partially empty, a court could find your entire chart invalid because you could easily have gone back and added to your notes at any time. Also, take care not to cross out information so it is unintelligible: put a straight line through it, write "error" above it, and date and initial it (by the same token, do not use white-out either).

There is a particular format for note-taking that is commonly taught to medical students, called **SOAP charting.** These initials respectively stand for subjective, objective, assessment, and plan, all of which are crucial aspects of caregiving essential to document.

For example, say you are confronted with a client at twenty-six weeks complaining of middle back pain. Start with S (subjective), which is the mother's report. Then note your O (objective) determination based on exam or observation, for example, CVAT present. Your A (assessment) would probably be suspected kidney infection, and your P (plan) would consist of urinalysis, consultation with your backup physician, follow-up appointment, and so on. In some cases, SOAP may be extended to SOAPIER charting: I (implementation) refers to steps the mother will take to enact the plan; E (evaluation) is your follow-up determination; and R (reassessment) includes any recommended modifications to the plan, based on evaluation.

And yet, even SOAPIER charting does not cover everything. Remember that you must also chart every interaction between you and the mother, your backup associates, hospital staff, and other health professionals, including not only personal interactions, but phone or email consultations (which should be printed out and placed in the chart).

Also be sure to chart not only the mother's response to recommended procedures or tests, but all information you provided regarding respective benefits and risks. For example, if you recommend a nonstress test, inform the mother of risks and benefits, and chart. Next, chart her response. If she declines the test, and you recommend fetal kick-counts as an alternative, chart this too, along with her response to this new suggestion. Then ask her to review your notes and sign to verify that your notes are accurate. Some midwives work with special forms for this purpose (see the discussion below on informed consent).

When doing prenatals, be sure to make notes during, rather than after, the visit. Yes, this can be distracting in the midst of a passionate discussion, but unless you stop and make notes in the moment, you may forget important details later on.

Keeping up with note-taking can be even more difficult during labor. There is usually a point in second stage when it is virtually impossible to continue charting. Midwife Tish Demmin suggests putting strips of masking tape on your pants, jotting notes there, and then transferring them to the chart as soon as possible. It is particularly important to note both time and results of all fetal heart rate assessments.

In the event of transport, make certain to update the chart completely before arriving at the hospital.

Your chart will be carefully scrutinized, possibly photocopied and made part of the woman's hospital record. It also serves as a testament to your professionalism, or lack thereof. Protect yourself by noting when you first contacted the hospital, to whom you spoke, and what they recommended. And continue to make notes once you arrive: you cannot assume the hospital's charting system to be unbiased or as accurate and complete as your own. Again, this is for your protection, though it will also be important to the mother later for purposes of debriefing her experience.

As mentioned earlier, **informed consent** is the cornerstone of charting. When decisions must be made regarding complex issues like vaginal birth after cesarean (VBAC) or group B streptococcus (GBS) screening, it makes more sense to use a form specifically outlining the procedure rather than trying to get everything in your notes. Your form should include: (1) risks and benefits of the test or procedure; (2) alternatives, with risks and benefits of each; (3) a place for the mother to indicate her response and plan; and (4) a place for her signature. Yes, this is complicated, especially for a beginner. But in our increasingly litigious society, even birth assistants have begun charting in hopes of protecting themselves.

If you remain unconvinced that this is necessary, imagine yourself in court, facing the parents of a stillborn, postmature baby as they claim, "She told us we needed a nonstress test, but didn't tell us what could happen if we said no." Of course, none of us want to think that we might be sued. We tell ourselves that we screen more carefully or maintain higher standards for communication and caregiving than the "average" midwife. But I have seen it happen to the most experienced, dedicated, and competent midwives, and the effects, both professionally and personally, can be devastating.

The statute of limitations runs three years for criminal charges, much longer for civil and malpractice suits. People change, so be prepared. To this end, most midwives have parents sign a Professional Disclosure and Consent to Care form at the onset of the caregiving relationship (see chapter 2, "The Initial Interview," for details).

However, lest we dismiss midwifery wisdom entirely, cultivating the best possible relationships with our clients *does* make a difference, especially if we put them in charge of decision-making right from the start. This is common knowledge in medical circles now, and medical textbooks increasingly allude to the importance of good practitioner-patient relations in avoiding litigation.

Another critical principle of professional practice is to uphold client **confidentiality** at all times. This can be challenging if one of your clients hears that another had a difficult birth and asks you to talk about it. Particularly if there is some question of why you handled the case as you did, the temptation to explain or defend your actions may be very strong. But nothing is worse for a woman than having her birth discussed at large! The only ethical response is to refer the curious client directly to the mother, who can tell her whatever she chooses. Midwifery students or other associates in the practice must also agree to uphold your confidentiality policy.

There are, in fact, new legal strictures in this regard, via the **Health Insurance Portability and Accountability Act (HIPAA)**. HIPAA guidelines apply to all health practitioners that bill insurance. The guidelines are a bit overwhelming, but a good place to start is at the website of the administrative agency, the U.S. Department of Health and Human Services (www.hhs.gov/ocr/hipaa).

As HIPAA guidelines ultimately concern client confidentiality, many midwives report a new level of care taken with client records, which must be secure at all times. For example, if doing a home visit, charts for other clients should not be brought along (they may be locked, out of view, in the car). Similarly, the file cabinet must be kept locked unless under the midwife's direct supervision. All inactive files must be stored in locked, fireproof containers. See appendix N for a summary of the guidelines.

PARTNERSHIP

No matter where you are located, working with a partner is usually the best way to practice. Midwives who work alone are rare. If such is their style, they must instruct the mother's partner or other attendant in how to assist in the event of an emergency. With partnership opportunities available, I cannot imagine why a midwife would choose to work alone unless for financial reasons.

Partnership is a safer way of practicing. A normal labor and birth can be managed by one person, but if certain complications arise, an extra pair of skilled hands is essential. Long or difficult labors, for example, often produce a mildly depressed baby, a tired mother, and a tired uterus predisposed to hemorrhage. How can a solitary midwife deal with all of these complications simultaneously? How can she possibly do resuscitation on the baby and bimanual compression on the mother at the same time?

Other benefits of partnership include increased comfort and ease in practicing. Partners can spell one another at births, they can fill in emotionally for each other in times of personal crisis, and they can give each other days or weeks off once in a while. Best of all, they have the opportunity to share their mutual passion for midwifery. Working in collaboration with a partner you know and trust gives you confidence in your abilities and also helps you identify areas where you have difficulty being assertive.

Of course, partners do not always agree. One may become passionately involved with a mother that the other considers at risk. Ironing out these disagreements will teach each of you about your blind spots

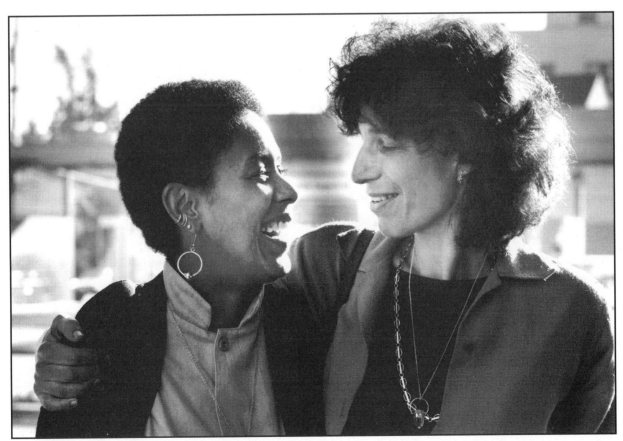

Much like a successful marriage, partnership is nourishing.

and will help keep humility a constant for you both. Evolving and implementing creative responses to problematic situations is the great pleasure and power of partnership.

Partners need humor and good judgment to make it together. They need to respect one another's intimacies with various clients, and take pleasure in both high- and low-profile roles. In a successful partnership, midwives truly enjoy one another's company—not unlike a successful marriage.

Partnership can be timesaving, particularly if an apprentice assists with prenatals so that partners need not attend each one. As the apprentice becomes increasingly skilled, she can accompany one partner to births, with the other coming near the end. Alternating full-time attendance at births can help keep partners vital.

Another possibility is to work collectively, using principles of partnership in a group of individual practices. In my locale, the Bay Area Homebirth Collective is a good example. These five midwives take their own clients, and each has at least one assistant or apprentice. At the beginning of pregnancy, clients have the opportunity to meet other available partners and choose one as second midwife for their birth. This midwife will come to a few prenatals—definitely to the home visit with the entire birth team—but is not expected at the birth until delivery approaches. Payment is received by the primary midwife, who pays the second midwife about $600 for her assistance.

Financial benefits of this collective structure are obvious. And think of the possibilities for taking time off. However, communication can be challenging with more partners, not to mention the diversity of practice styles. Regular meetings are essential in order to air grievances, clear up misunderstandings, and make decisions by consensus.

TRAINING THE STUDENT OR APPRENTICE

Why bother with the added responsibility of training an apprentice? There are several reasons, the most obvious being help with the work. An apprentice can save you time and energy by monitoring early labor, assisting at prenatals, running errands, doing bookkeeping and filing, and keeping the office clean and tidy. With her studies fresh in mind, she can offer new, interesting bits of information to you and your clients. And when you are tired or worn thin, she can lend you some of her beginner's stamina and passion. With just a little guidance on your part, her enthusiasm can revitalize your practice.

Other benefits are less tangible but more personally affecting. Deep satisfaction can be found in transmitting knowledge. And it can be exciting to tailor information to a student's degree of readiness while observing her growth. Above all, training an apprentice allows you to play a pivotal role in preserving this traditional entry route to our profession. Those of us trained by apprenticeship know of its many advantages over other educational models. The learning process is integrated and therefore more complete. If the apprentice trains in a community where she will one day practice, she is well prepared to field the health needs and issues of her future clientele. And too, the interdependency of teacher and student fosters an intimacy that can be a great pleasure.

Taking on an apprentice can also be a challenge. It requires top-notch communication, based on an understanding of normal stages in the process. Not to condescend, but the stages of parent-child relationship are remarkably similar to those of the midwife-apprentice configuration. They are (1) infancy—the time of being one, (2) childhood—the time of being together, (3) adolescence—the time of breaking away and being separate, and (4) adulthood—the time of being together again. For the apprentice, the stages of falling in love are also relevant: (1) infatuation, (2) disillusionment and struggle, (3) communication and compromise, and (4) mature love.

In the beginning, both teacher and student are pleased with the promise and excitement of their new relationship. But gradually, differences arise. The apprentice may be disappointed that her teacher does not have all the answers, or seem open to experimentation or willing to give her as much responsibility as she thinks she can handle. The midwife may feel that her student lacks humility, expects too much too soon, or has lost interest in the basic tasks she did so willingly in the beginning. Then power struggles can threaten the relationship.

The ensuing adolescent phase is the most difficult. The apprentice may openly contradict the midwife in the presence of clients, and if the midwife responds by limiting privileges, the apprentice may threaten to leave. But if the two can hold to their original commitment while articulating their disappointments, expectations, and needs, the relationship may mature into one of mutual respect and understanding. Many a former apprentice of mine has phoned in the early months of independent practice to say that she finally understood the degree of responsibility I carried, and why I was so conservative at times. With this, teacher and student begin a new relationship as equals.

Unfortunately, many apprenticeships do not survive the adolescent phase and reach maturity. As a mother of teens, I was repeatedly advised that no matter how defiant and insulting they became, I should do everything in my power to keep communication channels open. I also learned how important it is to help adolescents find appropriate outlets for their fulminating energies. When your apprentice reaches this stage, give her new responsibilities—perhaps just a bit beyond her immediate grasp—to inspire her to work harder and come to terms with her limits.

At the same time, you might consider taking another, junior apprentice. The senior apprentice can teach the junior what she has learned, testing her wings while still being supervised. The dynamics of this arrangement work quite well. At births, the midwife is in charge, with the senior apprentice directing the junior in basic tasks and responsibilities. Then, as the senior apprentice begins doing catches under supervision, the junior assists. This gives the midwife a well-deserved rest.

This break is unfortunately short-lived, as the junior apprentice must soon begin working directly with the midwife. Once the senior apprentice has completed her training, you may need to set a graduation date to encourage her to get out on her own. Plan to celebrate with her when she passes her licensing/certification exam. And once she is in practice, refer a few clients to her to help her get started. Or, if she decides to relocate, recommend her to other midwives or health workers in her new locale.

Growing pains are natural in the apprenticeship process, but if emotional problems become overwhelming, create more structure. The National Midwifery Institute offers a blueprint to help midwife and apprentice develop realistic timelines for skills and knowledge acquisition, with guidelines for communication and feedback. The NARM Certified Professional Midwife (CPM) process also provides a blueprint for learning. If your apprentice is not enrolled in a program, give her reading and research assignments relevant to the NARM process. Have her write up analyses of particularly difficult cases. Test her by oral or practical examination. Your student must have ample opportunity to demonstrate her learning, and you, a chance to evaluate the effectiveness of your teaching style.

In the document *Qualifications and Competencies of Midwifery Teachers*, the International Confederation of Midwives states that effective midwifery teachers:

1. Understand their own values related to teaching and learning, and provide an environment for values clarification among learners related to working with a variety of clients.

2. Promote the professional and ethical aspects of midwifery care.

3. Understand that individuals learn at different rates and in different ways.

4. Use a variety of teaching methods to facilitate learning with a progression from a very directive style to a coaching style with more independent learners.

5. Create a learning environment based on mutual trust and respect.

6. Are always well prepared for each theory and clinical session.

7. Arrange appropriate experiences for the level of learner.

8. Provide appropriate feedback on learner progress in collaboration with the learner's self-appraisal using both formative and summative evaluation strategies appropriately.

9. Understand that teaching methods are different for promoting learning in the psychomotor, cognitive, and affective domains of learning.

10. Understand that some individuals may need extra help in theory or practice, and provide this within the constraints of a given program.

11. Are guardians of safe, competent, respectful midwifery care.

Regarding points 3, 4 and 9, every midwifery instructor should be familiar with the various learning styles and types of intelligences she may encounter in her students. As author Howard Gardner has revealed in his book *Frames of Mind,* we tend to approach learning by employing one or more of seven intelligences. These are:

1. **Verbal/linguistic.** Learning through written and spoken language.

2. **Logical mathematical.** Deductive reason, recognition of abstract patterns.

3. **Intrapersonal.** Learning based on self-awareness, meta-cognition, intuition.

4. **Interpersonal.** Learning in relationship to others, based on communication.

5. **Musical/rhythmical.** Learning based on sound, tonal patterns, rhythm.

6. **Body/kinesthetic.** Body-based knowing, learning through movement.

7. **Visual/spatial intelligence.** Learning based on sight, and an ability to visualize.[1]

With this in mind, consider presenting material to your apprentice in a variety of ways. For example, when teaching fetal heart tone patterns common during labor, provide her with written information, use diagrams to illustrate as you explain, sound out various rhythms, and suggest that she tap along to feel the beat while listening. Interpersonal learning is facilitated by group discussion (with other apprentices), and assignments involving self-reflection stress intrapersonal learning. To better delineate the faculties of reason, intuition, and compassion, and to help your apprentice see the interplay of these in midwifery work, read *Emotional Intelligence,* by David Goleman.[2]

Instruction should be as student-centered as possible, considering the weighty responsibilities attendant to midwifery practice. From the beginning, do whatever it takes to put your apprentice in charge of her learning process. Ask her how she learns best, and whether she needs more or less structure to meet her learning objectives. Continually give her opportunities for self-evaluation. And get her hands-on as soon as possible. Remember that your apprentice is there to learn, not to practice. Her responsibilities should change continuously so she can achieve proficiency in all areas.

Also thoroughly debrief your apprentice after caregiving, and especially after births, by asking for her experience of the event. Was there anything that occurred that she didn't understand, or felt should have been handled differently? Challenge her to think as your equal (this may greatly abbreviate the adolescent phase), and take the time to carefully provide both factual information and context for her learning.

As mentioned earlier, the structure of a practice impacts the learning dynamic. There are a variety of possible practice arrangements; here is a sampling, with pros and cons of each:

1. **One midwife, one apprentice.** It is undeniably cost saving for a midwife to practice solo, counting on an apprentice for assistance and paying her a nominal sum concomitant to her level of responsibility. But this arrangement is quite stressful in the early stages, especially if the apprentice is inexperienced.

2. **One midwife and two apprentices (one senior and one junior).** This arrangement has been discussed already as per its value in helping the senior apprentice consolidate her learning by teaching the junior. The downside is that the two may occasionally conspire against the midwife. Training two students at once is ultimately more work and more responsibility than training just one, even though there is more opportunity to receive assistance.

3. **Two midwives and one apprentice.** This can be a confusing arrangement if the midwives have major differences in how they work. Then again, the contrast can be instructive for the apprentice, and may keep her from getting locked in to one way of thinking or practicing. A distinct benefit of this setup is that the apprentice is strictly a student. The midwives have the support of one another and need not saddle her with responsibilities she may not be ready to handle. By the same token, they must be careful to see she has ample opportunity to demonstrate her learning and to advance at a reasonable pace.

4. **Two midwives and two apprentices.** This arrangement is optimal in several respects. The apprentices not only have opportunity to observe different styles of practice, but they can also compare notes. As there are two of them, they have a stronger voice in the practice. The midwives also benefit from the opportunity to compare notes

and double-check their evaluations. The main drawback is the complex interpersonal dynamic inherent in a practice this size. It may be best for each midwife to take primary responsibility for one apprentice.

If you have a solo practice, you can enhance your apprentice's learning experience by asking another midwife to take her to a few births. This is particularly appropriate if you have a small practice. Once arranged, you and your apprentice should periodically discuss her goals and accomplishments with the other midwife, so everyone knows what to expect.

Training an apprentice is a lot of work, but well worth it. Once you experience the joy of teaching this way, you will probably want to continue. In so doing, you will make an invaluable contribution to the international effort to keep community-based apprenticeship alive and growing.

PEER REVIEW

Peer review provides a mechanism for midwives to meet and review their work. In a larger sense, peer review promotes quality assurance for consumers by encouraging safe and responsible caregiving. Exposure to the standards and practices of others motivates participants to continually upgrade their knowledge and skill. Participants thus become accountable to one another, and ultimately to the profession at large.

Peer review is also known as chart review because it revolves around the discussion of difficult or challenging cases. Besides debriefing troubling outcomes, unusual cases in progress are also discussed. In the event of a tragic occurrence like fetal death, emergency peer review may also serve to forestall litigation or a damaging spread of rumors throughout the community.

All it takes to begin peer review is a group of midwives committed to meeting every six to eight weeks.

Five participants minimum, ten maximum, is ideal. Here is a description of how each midwife participates:

1. She states the number of normal births attended since the last meeting.

2. She reports fully on any births with complications, including her assessment of what might have been done differently.

3. She mentions all prenatal cases with risk factors, including those referred to another provider.

4. She takes feedback from the group.

Since quality assurance is a major goal of peer review, educational workshops should be arranged as follow up.

The greatest benefit of peer review is that it promotes midwifery as an independent and self-regulating profession. It is a required part of the CPM process, and many states offering midwifery licensing or certification either require peer review or recommend it on an ongoing basis. Peer review has become increasingly popular with physician groups, in response to the malpractice crisis. It is one way to weed out incompetent or irresponsible providers.

Peer review may also help defend a midwife who has been unjustly accused of wrongdoing. On one occasion, my local group called an emergency meeting to address a case where the parents were dissatisfied with their care and threatened to sue the midwife. After receiving written testimony from both sides, we found in favor of the midwife, at the same time making recommendations to help her avoid this sort of situation in the future. We then drafted a statement supporting her management of the case, and the parents took no further action. This process is particularly efficacious if dissatisfied clients are talking around town.

On the other hand, lack of consumer participation in peer review may be seriously at odds with principles of woman-centered caregiving. New Zealand midwife and political activist Joan Donnely was the first to espouse the merits of involving consumers in virtually every aspect of midwifery regulation, including the annual review of standards, chart and peer review, conflict resolution, and disciplinary proceedings. She claims this is essential to counteract the historical tendency of professions that self-regulate to become self-serving and elitist.

It takes some courage to participate in peer review at first, especially if you have been isolated in your work. It is normal to fear that no other midwife thinks or does as you do, when in fact most midwives operate from a common base of knowledge and experience. Peer review will improve your practice and your communication with other midwives and, most likely, your self-esteem.

Notes

1. Howard Garner, *Frames of Mind: The Theory of Multiple Intelligences* (New York: Basic Books, 1993).

2. David Goleman, *Emotional Intelligence: Why It Can Matter More Than IQ* (New York: Bantam Books, 1997).

Chapter 9

THE LONG RUN

This final chapter focuses on the midwife again, this time in terms of the many adaptations involved in continued practice. No doubt about it, midwifery is a way of life, both grueling and transformative. The intensive and unpredictable nature of this work soon persuades the novice that midwifery is much more than the joy of catching babies. It works a woman on all levels, either disintegrating her or bringing her to essence.

In optimal caregiving, the midwife is not the only one making assessments. Before entrusting herself to care, the mother will scrutinize the midwife carefully: her appearance, personality, and character. At the same time, the midwife encourages this by being candid and forthcoming. Thus each prenatal visit provides an opportunity to deepen communication and develop trust. But this does not afford the midwife much privacy, and so can be draining at times.

On the other hand, beginning midwives may be so carried away by the thrill of practicing that they overwhelm clients with their energy. This contradicts the definition of care, which is based on receptivity and discretion. In order to truly be of service, the midwife must be sensitive enough to pick up her cues and respond without ego. Take this a step further and observe the difference between making assessments and passing judgment. It is easy to pass judgment at the threshold of our limitations, particularly on one

who inadvertently reveals them by leaving our expectations unmet. In contrast, the ability to make assessments has no strings attached and is the key to a sane and enduring practice.

What most beginners fail to realize is that midwifery will work them on every level. There may be major upheavals in love, especially if the midwife's partner is unable or unwilling to communicate as deeply as a midwife must to practice effectively. Men in particular may feel this intensity as pressure to be more than they are. Some partners feel jealous or threatened if their way of making a living seems less principled or dynamic. This may necessitate a joint review of personal and professional goals, both long and short term. It has been said that midwifery is the acid test of a relationship, which is absolutely true.

Conversely, it is important that the midwife acknowledge the demands her work places on her intimate relationships. Abruptly running off to births can be hard on small children and really rough on the nursing baby. Not to mention the obvious; more than once I have been interrupted by "the call" in the middle of lovemaking. Occasionally I find myself saying as I pick up the phone, "Don't let this be a heavy one," or even, "I hope no one's in labor." Usually this is because my children or relationship need attention, I have shopping, cleaning, or paperwork to do, or I want simply to relax without interruptions. Being on-call means

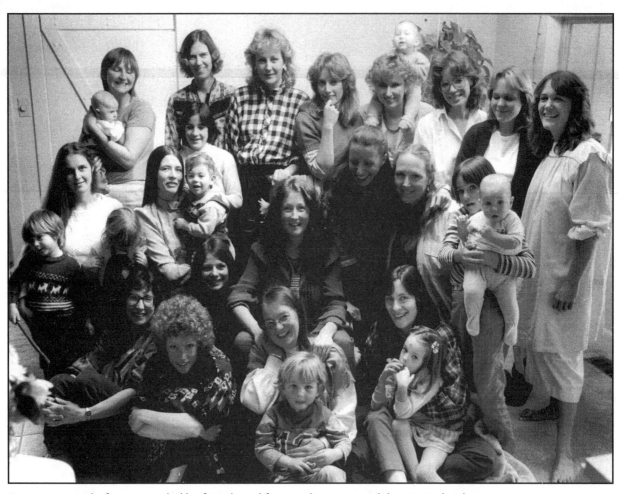

A pregnant midwife, surrounded by friends and former clients at a celebration in her honor.

keeping one's self, home, and family in a constant state of readiness. All midwives should consider getting household help as necessary and must strive to keep their practice at a workable level. If doing home birth, this is around four to six births a month, which generally allows for time to integrate each birth experience, catch up on sleep, get the family back in order, and rejuvenate before going on.

It is interesting to note how principles of smooth labor and birth also apply to smooth practice. The frustration of trying to make labor fit a preconceived pattern is similar to what a midwife may experience if she tries to make her practice develop too quickly, or be of a certain size. And just as there comes a time in birth when the mother must stop bearing down in order to ease her baby out, the midwife must also know when to ease up and let life happen. Even though birth offers potent lessons in this regard, impatience versus forbearance are often at play in the midwife's psyche.

Anne Frye has offered the following exercise to help midwives explore their beliefs about caregiving. See if any of these apply to you:

- A competent midwife can handle anything.

- A competent midwife always knows what is going on.

- A competent midwife can always trust her judgment.

- A compassionate midwife always acquiesces to the mother's wishes.

- A competent midwife never transports.

- A competent midwife transports at the first hint of a problem.

- A competent midwife never has a mother or baby die under her care.

She then suggests the following healthier beliefs:

- As a midwife, I support each woman to have the most healthy and healing birth experience possible.

- As a midwife, I must remember that what is most healthy and healing is different for every woman and may differ from what might be so for me.

- As a midwife, I need to recognize complications that require care I cannot provide and deal with them appropriately.

- As a midwife, I understand that birth, by its very nature, cannot be completely understood or predicted.

- As a midwife, I need appropriate and healthy professional limitations and boundaries regarding the types of situations I am willing and competent to handle.

- As a midwife, I cannot control whether someone lives or dies. I can control only how I prepare myself to take on the responsibility of being a primary attendant and how I respond to the situation in the moment.[1]

Every midwife must be willing to get help when she is floundering. This means learning to take as well as give, humbling herself to wise counsel, being receptive to her intimates, and listening well to the experience of other midwives. In short, she needs to access her recuperative powers.

Intrinsic to this is development of her intuition. At first, she may feel somewhat uncomfortable as hunches and precognitions play themselves out in her work and life. But this is part of a long tradition of women's ways of knowing, crucial for handling the challenges of comprehensive and safe care.

Part of the task of nurturing psychic faculties and protecting the delicacy in oneself as these emerge is to make time to relax and reflect every day. This can be difficult with young children, but easier to manage if incorporated from the beginning. Along these lines, a student of mine recalled that her mother routinely sent both her and her sister for naps after lunch each day. They never slept though, and eventually she realized that her mother knew this and didn't care. But she learned to treasure this time of privacy with the freedom to do whatever she wanted. Meanwhile, her mother was reading, relaxing, and otherwise taking care of herself.

In the same vein, midwifery practice requires the art of energy conservation. Otherwise, the midwife may find herself in tough situations where the appropriate course of action is perfectly clear, yet she lacks the strength to carry it out. Yaqui shaman Don Juan says that for all humans, power is our natural enemy; in midwifery practice, it is power derived from increasing clarity that may lead us beyond our capacity.[2] Overextension, even when the calling is clear, leads to burnout. To avoid this, delegate responsibility to students, apprentices, and other midwives. Learn to work to your maximum, and then say no.

Another way to conserve energy is to pass clients on whenever you find yourself at capacity. Be aware that the number of clients you can handle will vary from time to time, depending on your other obligations. Learn to recognize signs of burnout, such as faulty communication, general distraction or absent-mindedness, or in progressed cases, borderline hysteria. Without exception, midwives need regular vacations. In order to get away, you must create a support system strong enough to allow for your absence. This may require a new form of practice. Particularly if you have been working with an assistant only, a partnership or group practice may free you up to take better care of yourself.

Speaking of which, midwives often forget to apply their knowledge of health promotion to their own lives. For example, nutrition should be optimal on clinic days and in the midst of a long labor watch. Mental deliberations concerning a complicated pregnancy or pending labor may take so much energy that extra sleep is required. Stress reduction techniques, herbal remedies for relaxation, massage therapy, and regular exercise all have an important place in the midwife's daily life. She must also take care to separate the threads of her own problems from those of her clients. This happens less by rational process than by contemplative reflection, which brings us to the crux of the matter: midwives need to "bottom out" and get down to essence periodically. Emptying yourself makes room for insight and new direction. This is so important!

Although midwifery should marry service and self-expression, the high-stress demands of practice tend to interfere with healthy narcissism. Developing personal interests, new skills, and latent talents is an essential counterbalance to the selfless dedication required by this work. The midwife's primary gift to her clients is her ability to think creatively and independently, and to keep this alive it must be nourished. She should make time to find pleasure in many things, to expand her horizons, to be not just the changer but also the changed.

It is also important that she continue to nurture her professional identity by joining and participating in local, state, and national midwifery organizations. Particularly if she works in a hostile community, con-tact with a larger circle of midwives can help her rise above petty concerns and recall her original dedication to this work. I still recall the first time I attended a national midwifery convention—what a powerful awakening of identity and purpose! Regular attendance at conferences also helps the midwife stay current with the latest research, which can inspire her to try new approaches in practice.

In this respect, take care not to become jaded as you become seasoned. Just when you think you have seen it all, some new configuration occurs to set you back on your heels and teach you humility all over again. Tune up your sensitivities so intuitive directives keep coming through, and be grateful for higher intelligence.

Time and again, we come full circle to the heart of our work. What keeps us coming back for more? Pure and simple, it is the transformative power of love. No matter where midwifery takes you, do not forget this. Be who you are, and do what you can to keep your love alive.

Notes

1. Anne Frye, *Holistic Midwifery (Volume II)* (Portland, Oreg.: Labrys Press, 2004), manuscript pages.
2. Carlos Casteneda, *The Teachings of Don Juan* (New York: Pocket Books, 1968), 82–87.

For Parents: Support Your Local Midwife!

Here are some suggestions for keeping midwifery alive in your community:

1. Because the midwife's fee is usually modest, give her a bonus if you can possibly afford it. Consider the astronomical amount charged by physicians. Particularly if your midwife assisted you above and beyond her usual duties, pay her accordingly.

2. If you cannot afford more than the basic fee, perhaps you can help with clerical work or child care. In the past, midwives were fully supported by their community, all their personal and material needs completely met. Traditionally, midwives have been older women, past childbearing and unburdened with family responsibilities. But today, due to the practice's recent resurgence, midwives are coming from the younger generation. This is why help with child care is so important. Even if you are only able to volunteer once, it will be greatly appreciated.

3. Understand that in many states, midwives are under fire politically and may need support for legislative efforts. Contact your local or state midwifery association to see how you can help. Perhaps you can send a letter or email to your local legislator, make a donation, write a letter to the editor of your newspaper, or help organize a public event. Let everyone know how much having a midwife meant to you!

4. Tell your friends all about midwifery and out-of-hospital birth. Refer them to books or articles. Solicit their questions and inspire them with your passion. Move them to investigate alternatives and make informed decisions. With your help, midwifery will not only survive, but flourish! ■

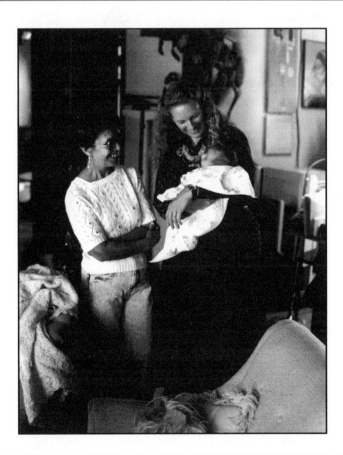

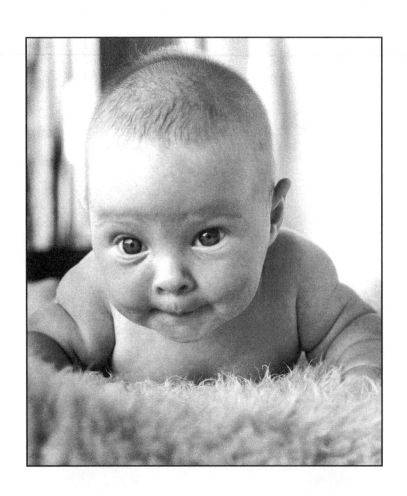

THE MANA STATEMENT OF VALUES AND ETHICS

We, as midwives, have a responsibility to educate ourselves and others regarding our values and ethics and to reflect them in our practices. Our exploration of ethical midwifery is a critical reflection of moral issues as they pertain to maternal/child health on every level. This statement is intended to provide guidance for professional conduct in the practice of midwifery, as well as for MANA's policy making, thereby promoting quality care for childbearing families. MANA recognizes this document as an open, ongoing articulation of our evolution regarding values and ethics.

First, we recognize that values often go unstated, and yet our ethics (how we act) proceed directly from a foundation of values. Since what we hold precious, that is, what we value, fuses and informs our ethical decisions and actions, the Midwives Alliance of North America wishes to explicitly affirm our values[1] as follows:

I. Woman as an Individual with Unique Value and Worth

A. We value women and their creative, life-affirming and life-giving powers which find expression in a diversity of ways.

B. We value a woman's right to make choices regarding all aspects of her life.

II. Mother and Baby as Whole

A. We value the oneness of the pregnant mother and her unborn child; an inseparable and independent whole.

B. We value the birth experience as a rite of passage; the sentient and sensitive nature of the newborn; and the right of each baby to be born in a caring and loving manner, without separation from mother and family.

C. We value the integrity of a woman's body and the right of each woman and baby to be totally supported in their efforts to achieve a natural, spontaneous vaginal birth.

D. We value the breastfeeding relationship as the ideal way of nourishing and nurturing the newborn.

III. The Nature of Birth

A. We value the essential mystery of birth.[2]

B. We value pregnancy and birth as natural processes that technology will never supplant.[3]

C. We value the integrity of life's experiences; the physical, emotional, mental, psychological and spiritual components of a process are inseparable.

D. We value pregnancy and birth as personal, intimate, internal, sexual, and social events to be shared in the environment and with the attendants a woman chooses.[4]

---

1. The membership largely agrees with the values that follow. However, some may word them differently or may leave out a few. This document is intended to prompt personal reflection and clarification, not to represent absolute opinions.

2. Mystery is defined as something that has not or cannot be explained or understood, the quality or state of being incomprehensible or inexplicable; a tenet which cannot be understood in terms of human reason.

3. Supplant means to supersede by force or cunning; to take the place of.

4. In this context internal refers to the fact that birth happens within the body and psyche of the woman; ultimately she and only she can give birth.

E. We value the learning experiences of life and birth.

F. We value pregnancy and birth as processes which have lifelong impact on a woman's self esteem, her health, her ability to nurture, and her personal growth.

IV. The Art of Midwifery

A. We value our right to practice the art of midwifery. We value our work as an ancient vocation of women which has existed as long as humans have lived on earth.

B. We value expertise which incorporates academic knowledge, clinical skill, intuitive judgment and spiritual awareness.[5]

C. We value all forms of midwifery education and acknowledge the ongoing wisdom of apprenticeship as the original model for training midwives.

D. We value the art of nurturing the intrinsic normalcy of birth and recognize that each woman and baby have parameters of well-being unique unto themselves.

E. We value the empowerment of women in all aspects of life and particularly as that strength is realized during pregnancy, birth and thereafter. We value the art of encouraging the open expression of that strength so women can birth unhindered and confident in their abilities and in our support.

F. We value skills which support a complicated pregnancy or birth to move toward a state of greater well-being or to be brought to the most healing conclusion possible. We value the art of letting go.[6]

G. We value the acceptance of death as a possible outcome of birth. We value our focus as supporting rather than avoiding death.[7]

H. We value standing for what we believe in in the face of social and political oppression.

V. Woman as Mother

A. We value a mother's intuitive knowledge of herself and her baby before, during and after birth.[8]

B. We value a woman's innate ability to nurture her pregnancy and birth her baby; the power and beauty of her body as it grows and the awesome strength summoned in labor.

C. We value the mother as the only direct care provider for her unborn child.[9]

D. We value supporting women in a non-judgmental way, whatever their state of physical, emotional, social or spiritual health. We value the broadening of available resources whenever possible so that the desired goals of health, happiness and personal growth are realized according to women's needs and perceptions.

E. We value the right of each woman to choose a care giver appropriate to her needs and compatible with her belief systems.

F. We value pregnancy and birth as rites of passage integral to a woman's evolution into mothering.

G. We value the potential of partners, family and community to support women in all aspects of birth and mothering.[10]

---

5. An expert is one whose knowledge and skill are specialized and profound, especially as the result of practical experience.

6. This addresses our desire for an uncomplicated birth whenever possible and recognizes that there are times when it is impossible. That is to say, a woman may be least traumatized to have a cesarean and a live birth, but a spontaneous vaginal birth, in this case, is not possible. We let go of that goal to achieve the possibility of a healthy baby. Likewise, the situation where parents choose to allow a very ill, premature or deformed infant to die in their arms rather than being subjected to multiple surgeries, separations, and ICU stays. This too, is letting go of the normal for the most healing choice possible within the framework of the parent's ethics given the circumstances. What is most healing will, of course, vary from individual to individual.

7. We place the emphasis of our care on supporting life (preventative measures, good nutrition, emotional health, etc.) and not pathology, diagnosis, treatment of problems, or heroic solutions in an attempt to preserve life at any cost of quality.

8. This addresses the medical model's tendency to ignore a woman's sense of well-being or danger in many aspects of health care, but particularly in regard to her pregnancy.

9. This acknowledges that the thrust of our care centers on the mother, her health, her well-being, her nutrition, her habits, her emotional balance and, in turn, the baby benefits. This view is diametrically opposed to the medical model which often attempts to care for the fetus/baby while dismissing or even excluding the mother.

10. While partners, other family members, and a woman's larger community can and often do provide her with vital support, in using the word potential we wish to acknowledge that many women find themselves pregnant and mothering in abusive and unsafe environments.

VI. The Nature of Relationship

A. We value relationship. The quality, integrity, equality and uniqueness of our interactions inform and critique our choices and decisions.

B. We value honesty in relationship.

C. We value caring for women to the best of our ability without prejudice against their age, race, religion, culture, sexual orientation, physical abilities, or socioeconomic background.

D. We value the concept of personal responsibility and the right of individuals to make choices regarding what they deem best for themselves. We value the right to true informed choice, not merely informed consent to what we think is best.

E. We value our relationship to a process larger than ourselves, recognizing that birth is something we can seek to learn from and know, but never control.

F. We value humility in our work.

G. We value the recognition of our own limits and limitations.

H. We value direct access to information readily understood by all.

I. We value sharing information and our understanding about birth experiences, skills, and knowledge.

J. We value the midwifery community as a support system and an essential place of learning and sisterhood.

K. We value diversity among midwives; recognizing that it broadens our collective resources and challenges us to work for greater understanding of birth and each other.

L. We value mutual trust and respect, which grows from a realization of all of the above.

Making Decisions and Acting Ethically

These values reflect our feelings regarding how we frame midwifery in our hearts and minds. However, due to the broad range of geographic, religious, cultural, political, educational and personal backgrounds among our membership, how we act based on these values will be very individual. Acting ethically is a complex merging of our values and these background influences combined with the relationship we have to others who may be involved in the process taking place. We call upon all these resources when deciding how to respond in the moment to each situation.

We acknowledge the limitations of ethical codes which present a list of rules which must be followed, recognizing that such a code may interfere with, rather than enhance, our ability to make judgments, and we must have adequate information; with all of these an appeal to a code becomes superfluous. Furthermore, when we set up rigid ethical codes we may begin to cease considering the transformations we go through as a result of our choices as well as negate our wish to foster truly diversified practice. Rules are not something we can appeal to when all else fails. However, this is the illusion fostered by traditional codes of ethics.[11] MANA's support of the individual's moral integrity grows out of an understanding that there cannot possibly be one right answer for all situations.

We acknowledge the following basic concepts and believe that ethical judgments can be made with these thoughts in mind:

• Moral agency and integrity are born within the heart of each individual.

• Judgments are fundamentally based on awareness and understanding of ourselves and others and are primarily derived from one's own sense of moral integrity with reference to clearly articulated values. Becoming aware and increasing our understanding are on-going processes facilitated by our efforts at personal growth on every level. The wisdom gained by this process cannot be taught or dictated but one can learn to realize, experience and evaluate it.

---

11. Hoagland, Sarah, paraphrased from her book *Lesbian Ethics*.

- The choices we can or will actually make may be limited by the oppressive nature of the medical, legal or cultural framework in which we live. The more our values conflict with those of the dominant culture, the more risky it becomes to act truly in accord with our values.
- The pregnant woman and midwife are both individual moral agents unique unto themselves, having independent value and worth.
- We support ourselves and the women and families we serve to follow and make known the dictates of our own conscience as our relationship begins, evolves and especially when decisions must be made which impact us or the care being provided. It is up to all of us to work out a mutually satisfactory relationship when and if that is possible.

It is useful to understand the two basic theories upon which moral judgments and decision making processes are based. These processes become particularly important when one considers that in our profession, a given woman's rights may not be absolute in all cases, or in certain situations the woman may not be considered autonomous or competent to make her own decisions.

One of the main theories of ethics states that one should look to the consequences of the act (i.e. the outcome) and not the act itself to determine if it is appropriate care. This point of view looks for the greatest good for the greatest number. The other primary ethical theory states that one should look to the act itself (i.e., type of care provided) and if it is right, then this could override the net outcome. This is a more process oriented, feminist perspective. As midwives we weave these two perspectives in the process of making decisions in our practices. Since the outcome of pregnancy is ultimately an unknown and is always unknowable, it is inevitable that in certain circumstances our best decisions in the moment will lead to consequences we could not foresee.

In summary, acting ethically is facilitated by:

- Carefully defining our values.
- Weighing our values in consideration with those of the community of midwives, families, and culture in which we find ourselves.
- Acting in accord with our values to the best of our ability as the situation demands.
- Engaging in ongoing self-examination and evaluation.

There are both individual and social implications to any decision making process. The actual rules and oppressive aspects of a society are never exact, and therefore conflicts may arise and we must weigh which choices or obligations take precedence over others. There are inevitably times when resolution does not occur and we will be unable to make peace with any course of action or may feel conflicted about a choice already made. The community of women, both midwives and those we serve, will provide a fruitful resource for continued moral support and guidance.

Bibliography

Star Cross, MANA Ethics Chair (unpublished draft of MANA Ethics code, 1989).
Mary Daly, *GynEcology: The Metaethics of Radical Feminism* (Boston: Beacon Press, 1978).
Sarah Lucia Hoagland, *Lesbian Ethics: Toward New Value* (Palo Alto, CA: Institute of Lesbian Studies, 1988).
Sonia Johnson, *Going Out of Our Minds: The Metaphysics of Liberation* (Berkeley, CA: The Crossing Press, 1987).

MANA Core-Competencies for Midwifery Practice

Guiding Principles of Practice

The midwife provides care according to the following principles:

A. Midwives work in partnership with women and their chosen support community throughout the care-giving relationship.

B. Midwives respect the dignity, rights and the ability of the women they serve to act responsibly throughout the care-giving relationship.

C. Midwives work as autonomous practitioners, collaborating with other health and social service providers when necessary.

D. Midwives understand that physical, emotional, psychosocial and spiritual factors synergistically comprise the health of individuals and affect the childbearing process.

E. Midwives understand that female physiology and childbearing are normal processes, and work to optimize the well-being of mothers and their developing babies as the foundation of care-giving.

F. Midwives understand that the childbearing experience is primarily a personal, social and community event.

G. Midwives recognize that a woman is the only direct care provider for herself and her unborn baby; thus the most important determinant of a healthy pregnancy is the mother herself.

H. Midwives recognize the empowerment inherent in the childbearing experience and strive to support women to make informed decisions and take responsibility for their own well-being.

I. Midwives strive to ensure vaginal birth and provide guidance and support when appropriate to facilitate the spontaneous processes of pregnancy, labor and birth, utilizing medical intervention only as necessary.

J. Midwives synthesize clinical observations, theoretical knowledge, intuitive assessment and spiritual awareness as components of a competent decision making process.

K. Midwives value continuity of care throughout the childbearing cycle and strive to maintain continuous care within realistic limits.

L. Midwives understand that the parameters of "normal" vary widely and recognize that each pregnancy and birth is unique.

General Knowledge and Skills

I. The midwife provides care incorporating certain concepts, skills and knowledge from a variety of health and social sciences, including but not limited to:

A. Communication, counseling and teaching skills.

B. Human anatomy and physiology relevant to childbearing.

C. Community standards of care for women and their developing infants during the childbearing cycle, including midwifery and bio-technical medical standards and the rationale for and limitations of such standards.

D. Health and social resources in her community.

E. Significance of and methods for documentation of care through the childbearing cycle.

F. Informed decision making.

G. The principles and appropriate application of clean and aseptic technique and universal precautions.

H. The selection, use and care of the tools and other equipment employed in midwifery care.

I. Human sexuality, including indications of common problems and indications for counseling.

J. Ethical considerations relevant to reproductive health.

K. The grieving process.

L. Knowledge of cultural variations.

M. Knowledge of common medical terms.

N. The ability to develop, implement and evaluate an individualized plan for midwifery care.

O. Woman-centered care, including the relationship between the mother, infant and their larger support community.

P. Knowledge of various health care modalities[12] as they apply to the childbearing cycle.

Care during Pregnancy

II. The midwife provides health care, support and information to women throughout pregnancy. She determines the need for consultation or referral as appropriate. The midwife uses a foundation of knowledge and/or skill which includes the following:

A. Identification, evaluation and support of maternal and fetal well-being throughout the process of pregnancy.

B. Education and counseling for the childbearing cycle.

C. Preexisting conditions in a woman's health history which are likely to influence her well-being when she becomes pregnant.

D. Nutritional requirements of pregnant women and methods of nutritional assessment and counseling.

E. Changes in emotional, psychosocial and sexual variations that may occur during pregnancy.

F. Environmental and occupational hazards for pregnant women.

G. Methods of diagnosing pregnancy.

H. Basic understanding of genetic factors which may indicate the need for counseling, testing or referral.

I. Basic understanding of the growth and development of the unborn baby.

J. Indications for, and the risks and benefits of bio-technical screening methods and diagnostic tests used during pregnancy.

K. Anatomy, physiology and evaluation of the soft and bony structure of the pelvis.

L. Palpation skills for evaluation of the fetus and uterus.

M. The causes, assessment and treatment of the common discomforts of pregnancy.

N. Identification of, implications of and appropriate treatment for various infections, disease conditions and other problems which may affect pregnancy.

O. Special needs of the Rh– woman.

Care during Labor, Birth, and Immediately Thereafter

III. The midwife provides health care, support and information to women throughout labor, birth and the hours immediately thereafter. She determines the need for consultation or referral as appropriate. The midwife uses a foundation of knowledge and/or skill which includes the following:

A. The normal processes of labor and birth.

B. Parameters and methods for evaluating maternal and fetal well-being during labor, birth and immediately thereafter, including relevant historical data.

C. Assessment of the birthing environment, assuring that it is clean, safe and supportive, and that appropriate equipment and supplies are on hand.

D. Emotional responses and their impact during labor, birth and immediately thereafter.

E. Comfort and support measures during labor, birth and immediately thereafter.

F. Fetal and maternal anatomy and their interactions as relevant to assessing fetal position and progress of labor.

G. Techniques to assist and support the spontaneous vaginal birth of the baby and placenta.

H. Fluid and nutritional requirements during labor, birth and immediately thereafter.

---

12. Health care modalities may include but are not limited to such practices as bio-technical medicine, homeopathy, naturopathy, herbology, Chinese medicine, chiropractic, etc.

I. Assessment of and support for maternal rest and sleep as appropriate during the process of labor, birth and immediately thereafter.

J. Causes of, evaluation of and appropriate treatment for variations which occur during the course of labor, birth and immediately thereafter.

K. Emergency measures and transport procedures for critical problems arising during labor, birth or immediately thereafter.

L. Understanding of and appropriate support for the newborn's transition during the first minutes and hours following birth.

M. Familiarity with current bio-technical interventions and technologies which may be commonly used in a medical setting.

N. Evaluation and care of the perineum and surrounding tissues.

Postpartum Care

IV. The midwife provides health care, support and information to women throughout the postpartum period. She determines the need for consultation or referral as appropriate. The midwife uses a foundation of knowledge and/or skill which includes but is not limited to the following:

A. Anatomy and physiology of the mother during the postpartum period.

B. Lactation support and appropriate breast care including evaluation of, identification of and treatment for problems with nursing.

C. Parameters of and methods for evaluating and promoting maternal well-being during the postpartum period.

D. Causes of, evaluation of and treatment for maternal discomforts during the postpartum period.

E. Emotional, psychosocial and sexual variations during the postpartum period.

F. Maternal nutritional requirements during the postpartum period including methods of nutritional evaluation and counseling.

G. Causes of, evaluation of and treatment for problems arising during the postpartum period.

H. Support, information and referral for family planning methods as the individual woman desires.

Newborn Care

V. The entry-level midwife provides health care to the newborn during the postpartum period and support and information to parents regarding newborn care. She determines the need for consultation or referral as appropriate. The midwife uses a foundation of knowledge and/or skill which includes the following:

A. Anatomy, physiology and support of the newborn's adjustment during the first days and weeks of life.

B. Parameters and methods for evaluating newborn wellness including relevant historical data and gestational age.

C. Nutritional needs of the newborn.

D. Community standards and state laws regarding indications for, administration of and the risks and benefits of prophylactic bio-technical treatments and screening tests commonly used during the neonatal period.

E. Causes of, assessment of, appropriate treatment and emergency measures for newborn problems and abnormalities.

Professional, Legal, and Other Aspects

VI. The entry-level midwife assumes responsibility for practicing in accord with the principles outlined in this document. The midwife uses a foundation of knowledge and/or skill which includes the following:

A. MANA's documents concerning the art and practice of midwifery.

B. The purpose and goal of MANA and local (state and provincial) midwifery associations.

C. The principles and practice of data collection as relevant to midwifery practice.

D. Laws governing the practice of midwifery in her local jurisdiction.

E. Various sites, styles and modes of practice within the larger midwifery community.

F. A basic understanding of maternal/child health care delivery systems in her local jurisdiction.

G. Awareness of the need for midwives to share their knowledge and experience.

Well-Woman Care and Family Planning

VII. Depending upon education and training, the entry-level midwife may provide family planning and well-woman care. The practicing midwife may also choose to meet the following core competencies with additional training. In either case, the midwife provides care, support and information to women regarding their overall reproductive health, using a foundation of knowledge and/or skill which includes the following:

A. Understanding of the normal life cycle of women.

B. Evaluation of the woman's well-being including relevant historical data.

C. Causes of, evaluation of and treatments for problems associated with the female reproductive system and breasts.

D. Information on, provision of or referral for various methods of contraception.

E. Issues involved in decision-making regarding unwanted pregnancies and resources for counseling and referral.

MANA Standards and Qualifications for the Art and Practice of Midwifery

The midwife recognizes that childbearing is a woman's experience and encourages the active involvement of family members in her care.

1. **Skills:** Necessary skills of a practicing midwife include the ability to:
   - Provide continuity of care to the woman and her family during the maternity cycle, continuing interconceptionally throughout the childbearing years;
   - Assess and provide care for healthy women in antepartal, intrapartal, postpartal and neonatal periods;
   - Identify and assess deviations from normal;
   - Maintain proficiency in life-saving measures by regular review and practice; and
   - Deal with emergency situations appropriately.
   - In addition, a midwife may choose to provide well-woman care.

   It is affirmed that judgment and intuition play a role in competent assessment and response.

2. **Appropriate equipment:** Midwives are equipped to assess maternal, fetal and newborn well-being; to maintain a clean and/or aseptic technique; to treat maternal hemorrhage; and to resuscitate mother or infant.

3. **Records:** Midwives keep accurate records of care provided for each woman such as are acceptable in current midwifery practice. Records shall be held confidential and provided to the woman on request.

4. **Data collection:** Midwives collect data for their practice on a regular basis. It is highly recommended that this be done prospectively, following the guidelines and using the data form developed by the MANA Statistics and Research Committee.

5. **Compliance:** Midwives will inform and assist parents regarding the Public Health requirements of the jurisdiction in which the midwifery practice will occur.

6. **Medical consultation and referral:** All midwives recognize that there are certain conditions when medical consultations are advisable. The midwife shall make a reasonable attempt to assure that her client has access to consultation and/or referral to a medical care system when indicated.

7. **Screening:** Midwives respect the woman's right to self-determination within the boundaries of responsible care. Midwives continually assess each woman regarding her health and well-being relevant to the appropriateness of midwifery services. Women will be informed of this assessment. It is the right and responsibility of the midwife to refuse or discontinue services in certain circumstances. Appropriate referrals are made in the interest of the mother or baby's well-being, or when the required or requested care is outside the midwife's legal or personal scope of practice as described in her protocols.

8. **Informed choice:** Each midwife will present accurate information about herself and her services, including but not limited to:
   - Her education in midwifery
   - Her experience level in midwifery
   - Her protocols and standards
   - Her financial charges for services
   - The services she does and does not provide
   - The responsibilities of the pregnant woman and her family

9. **Continuing education:** Midwives will update their knowledge and skills on a regular basis.

10. **Peer review:** Midwifery practice includes an on-going process of case review with peers.

11. **Protocols:** Each midwife will develop protocols for her services that are in agreement with the basic philosophy of MANA and in keeping with her level of understanding. Each midwife is encouraged to put her protocols in writing.

(Revised October, 1996)

References

American College of Nurse-Midwives' documents.

ICM membership and joint study on maternity, FIGO, WHO, etc. revised 1972.

New Mexico regulations for the practice of lay midwifery, revised 1982.

North West Coalition of Midwives Standards for Safety and Competency in Midwifery.

Helen Varney, *Nurse Midwifery* (Boston: Blackwell Scientific Pub., 1980).

RESOURCES

Alliance for Transforming the Lives of Children
901 Preston Ave., Suite 400
Charlottesville, VA 22903-4491
www.atlc.org

American College of Nurse-Midwives (ACNM)
8403 Colesville Rd., Suite 1550
Silver Spring, MD 20910
(240) 485-1800
www.acnm.org

Association for Pre- and Perinatal Psychology
and Health
P.O. Box 1398
Forestville, CA 95436
(707) 887-2838
www.birthpsychology.com

Association of Labor Assistants and Childbirth
Educators (ALACE)
P.O. Box 390436
Cambridge, MA 02139
(617) 441-2500; (888) 222-5223
www.alace.org

Association of Radical Midwives (ARM)
62 Greetby Hill
Ormskirk, Lancashire, L39 2DT
United Kingdom
www.radmid.demon.co.uk

The Birth Gazette
42-MT The Farm
Summertown, TN 38483
(931) 964-3798

Birthing From Within, Inc.
P.O. Box 4528
Albuquerque, NM 87196
(505) 254-4884
www.birthingfromwithin.com

Birth With Love Midwifery Supplies
Ollie Anne Hamilton
513 27th St. N.
Great Falls, MT 59401
(800) 434-4915
www.birthwithlove.com

Birth Works®, Inc.
P.O. Box 2045
Medford, NJ 08055
(888) 862-4784
www.birthworks.com

The Bradley Method®
P.O. Box 5224
Sherman Oaks, CA 91413-5224
(818) 788-6662; (800) 4-A-BIRTH
www.bradleybirth.com

Canadian Association of Midwives
http://members.rogers.com/canadianmidwives

Cascade Health Care Products, Inc.
1826 NW 18th Ave.
Portland, OR 97209
(503) 595-1720; (800) 443-9942
www.1cascade.com

Childbirth Graphics
www.childbirthgraphics.com

Citizens for Midwifery (CFM)
P.O. Box 82227
Athens, GA 30606-2227
(316) 267-7236
www.cfmidwifery.org

Coalition for Improving Maternity Services (CIMS)
P.O. Box 2346
Ponte Vedra Beach, FL 32004
www.motherfriendly.org

Compleat Mother
5703 Hillcrest
Richmond, IL 60071
(815) 678-7531
www.compleatmother.com

Doulas of North American (DONA)
P.O. Box 626
Jasper, IN 47547
(888) 788-DONA
www.dona.org

Doula World
www.doulaworld.com

Foundation for the Advancement of Midwifery
1779 Wells Branch Pkwy, #110B-284
Austin, TX 78728
www.formidwifery.org

Global Maternal/Child Health Association, Inc.
Waterbirth International
P.O. Box 1400
Wilsonville, OR 97070
(503) 673-0026; (800) 641-2229
www.waterbirth.org

HypnoBirthing® Institute
P.O. Box 810
Epsom, NH 03234
(877) 798-3286
www.hypnobirthing.com

Informed Birth and Parenting
P.O. Box 1733
Fair Oaks, CA 95628
IHIBP@sbcglobal.net

In His Hands Birth Supplies
(800) 247-4045
www.homebirthsupplies.com

International Association for Infant Massage (IAIM)
1891 Goodyear Ave., Suite 622
Ventura, CA 93003
(805) 644-8524
www.iaim-us.com

International Center for Traditional Childbearing
 (ICTC)
P.O. Box 11923
Portland, OR 97217
(503) 460-9324, ext. 3
www.blackmidwives.org

International Cesarean Awareness Network, Inc.
 (ICAN)
1304 Kingsdale Ave.
Redondo Beach, CA 90278
(310) 542-6400; (800) 686-ICAN
www.ican-online.org

International Childbirth Educators Association (ICEA)
P.O. Box 20048
Minneapolis, MN 55420
(952) 854-8660
www.icea.org

International Confederation of Midwives (ICM)
Eisenhowerlaan 138
2517 KN The Hague
The Netherlands
+ 31 70 3060520
www.internationalmidwives.org

La Leche League, Int.
P.O. Box 4079
Schaumburg, IL 60168-4079
(847) 519-7730
www.lalecheleague.org

Lamaze International
2025 M St., Suite 800
Washington, D.C. 20036-3309
(202) 367-1128; (800) 368-4404
www.lamaze.org

MIDIRS
9 Elmdale Rd.
Clifton, Bristol BS8 1SL
England
www.midirs.org

Midwifery Education Accreditation Council (MEAC)
318 W. Birth, Suite 5
Flagstaff, AZ 86001
(928) 214-0997
www.meacschools.org

Midwifery Today, Inc.
P.O. Box 2672
Eugene, OR 97402-0223
(800) 743-0974
www.midwiferytoday.com

Midwives Alliance of North American (MANA)
4805 Lawrenceville Hwy., Suite 116-279
Lilburn, GA 30047
(888) 923-MANA (6262)
www.mana.org

Midwives Model of Care
www.midwivesmodelofcare.org

Moon Dragon Birth Supply
0 Boardman St.
Salem, MA 01970
(978) 744-5583
www.moondragon.org/pregnancy/birthkits.html

Mothering
P.O. Box 1690
Santa Fe, NM 87504
(800) 984-8116
www.mothering.com

National Association of Childbearing Centers (NACC)
3123 Gottschall Rd.
Perkiomenville, PA 18074
(215) 234-8068
www.birthcenters.org

National Association of Parents and Professionals for
   Safe Alternatives in Childbirth (NAPSAC)
Rt. 4, Box 646
Marble Hill, MO 63764
(573) 238-2010
www.napsac.org

National Association of Postpartum Care Services
   (NAPCS)
800 Detroit St.
Denver, CO 80206
(800) 453-6852
www.napcs.org

National Organization of Circumcision Information
   Resource Centers (NOCIRC)
P.O. Box 2512
San Anselmo, CA 94979
(415) 488-9883
www.nocirc.org

National Organization of Mothers of Twins Club, Inc.
P.O. Box 438
Thompsons Station, TN 37179-0438
(615) 595-0936; (877) 540-2200
www.nomotc.org

North America Registry of Midwives (NARM)
Applications
P.O. Box 420
Summertown, TN 38483
http://narm.org

Perinatal Education Associates, Inc.
www.birthsource.com

Safe Motherhood Quilt Project
P.O. Box 30955
Bethesda, MD 20824
http://131.103.210.241

SLC Birth Supplies
P.O. Box 1225
Oakhurst, CA 93644
(888) 683-2678
www.birthsupplies.com

Yalad Birthing Supply
P.O. Box 8111
Canton, OH 44711-8111
(330) 493-3050
www.yalad.com

MEDICAL/HEALTH HISTORY

Please fill out this medical and personal history very carefully. When you come for your next visit we will go over the history together and discuss any questions that you might have. Just leave blank any technical terms or questions with which you are not familiar.

Personal Information

Your name _____

Address _____

Date of Birth _____ Height _____

Partner's name _____

Address _____

Emergency contact person _____

Who referred you to me? _____

Insurance _____

Do you have any drug allergies or sensitivities? _____

Date _____

Phone _____

Occupation _____

Usual Weight _____

Date of Birth _____

Phone _____

Pediatrician _____

Menstrual History

When do you think you may have conceived? _____

How long is your menstrual cycle? _____

LMP—last menstrual period _____

○ Yes   ○ No   Was it normal in length and heaviness of flow?

○ Yes   ○ No   Did you have a pregnancy test?

○ Yes   ○ No   Was this a planned pregnancy?

PMP—previous menstrual period _____

Were you using birth control when you conceived?

○ Yes   ○ No   What kind? _____

Any complications after abortion or miscarriage?

○ Pain   ○ Infection   ○ Incomplete   ○ Emotional trauma

If Rh negative, did you receive RhoGAM? ○ Yes   ○ No

Please list information about your previous births:

Obstetrical History

Total pregnancies: _____

Full term: _____

Premature: _____

Abortion: _____

Ectopic: _____

Miscarriage: _____

Twins: _____

Living children: _____

Cesarean section: _____

VBAC: _____

Date Mo/Yr.	# of Weeks	Length Labor	Sex M/F	Place of Birth	Comments/Complications

Medical History

Please check if you have had any of the following conditions. In the space below, record date, treatment, and any follow-up you received. Also feel free to list any other important conditions/concerns.

- ○ Kidney disease
- ○ Diabetes
- ○ Hypertension
- ○ Epilepsy
- ○ Heart disease
- ○ Thyroid problems
- ○ Blood clotting problems
- ○ Asthma
- ○ Hepatitis

- ○ Liver problems
- ○ Tuberculosis
- ○ Urinary tract surgery
- ○ Pelvic/back injuries
- ○ Stomach problems
- ○ Bowel problems
- ○ Skin problems
- ○ Bladder infection
- ○ Anemia

- ○ Hospitalizations
- ○ Seizures
- ○ Surgeries
- ○ Hemorrhage
- ○ Allergies
- ○ Severe headaches
- ○ Dental problems
- ○ Phlebitis/Varicosities
- ○ Hemorrhoids

_____

_____

_____

_____

_____

Is there any hereditary disease or condition in your family such as diabetes, cancer, heart disease, hypertension? (List, and indicate in which relative.)

_____

_____

_____

Lab Work (please leave blank)

INITIAL LABS	DATE	RESULT
BLOOD TYPE	/ /	A B AB O
D (Rh) TYPE	/ /	
ANTIBODY SCREEN	/ /	
HCT/HGB	/ /	_____% _____g/dL
PAP TEST	/ /	NORMAL/ABNORMAL/_____
RUBELLA	/ /	
VDRL	/ /	
URINE CULTURE/SCREEN	/ /	
HBs Ag	/ /	
HIV COUNSELING/TESTING	/ /	❑ POS. ❑ NEG. ❑ DECLINED
PPD	/ /	
CHLAMYDIA	/ /	
GC	/ /	
TAY-SACHS	/ /	
OTHER	/ /	

8–18-WEEK LABS	DATE	RESULT
AFP	/ /	
AMNIO/CVS	/ /	
24–28-WEEK LABS	DATE	RESULT
HCT/HGB	/ /	_____%_____g/dL
DIABETES SCREEN	/ /	1 HOUR_____
GTT (IF SCREEN ABNORMAL)	/ /	___FBS ___1 HOUR ___2 HOUR ___3 HOUR
D (Rh) ANTIBODY SCREEN	/ /	
32–36-WEEK LABS	DATE	RESULT
HCT/HGB	/ /	____%___g/dL
GROUP B STREP (35–37 WKS.)	/ /	

○ Yes   ○ No   Have you or the father of your baby ever had a baby with a birth defect or mental retardation?

○ Yes   ○ No   Do you or the father of your baby have any family members with birth defects or conditions diagnosed as genetic or inherited?

○ Yes   ○ No   Are you and the father of your baby related by blood? (e.g. cousins)

○ Yes   ○ No   Certain genetic problems may occur in the following ethnic/racial groups. Are you or the father of your baby:

    ○ Jewish   ○ Black/African   ○ Asian   ○ Aleutian   ○ Mediterranean

How many times was your mother pregnant? _____ How many children did she have? _____

Did she have any miscarriages? _____ How long were her labors? _____

Were there any complications in any of her pregnancies? _____ How much did you weigh at birth? _____

What did your mother tell you about birth? _____

_____

_____

○ Yes   ○ No   Do you suffer from recurrent anxiety or depression?

○ Yes   ○ No   Have you ever had anorexia, bulimia, or eating problems?

○ Yes   ○ No   Have you ever been in an abusive relationship, including now, or been abused in the past (physically and emotionally intimidated, beaten, or injured)?

○ Yes   ○ No   Have you ever had non-consensual sex?

○ Yes   ○ No   Do you think, or has anyone ever told you, that you have used drugs/alcohol excessively?

○ Yes   ○ No   Have you ever used any drug intravenously (IV)?

○ Yes   ○ No   Have you ever had a blood transfusion?   Year ____

○ Yes   ○ No   Do you think you are at increased risk for HIV/AIDS?

○ Yes   ○ No   Do you want information about safer sex practices?

Gynecological/Contraceptive History

When was your last Pap smear? _____

Have you ever had an abnormal Pap? If so, when? _____ How was it resolved? _____

Do you do self breast exam? _____

Please check if you've ever had any of the following:

- ○ Yeast
- ○ Bacterial vaginosis
- ○ Syphilis
- ○ Genital herpes
- ○ Cervicitis
- ○ Ovarian cyst
- ○ Abnormal bleeding
- ○ Breast surgery
- ○ Trichomonas

- ○ Chlamydia
- ○ PID
- ○ Oral herpes
- ○ Cervical surgery
- ○ Fibroids
- ○ Uterine surgery
- ○ Infertility
- ○ Gardnerella
- ○ Gonorrhea

- ○ Genital sores
- ○ Condyloma (warts)
- ○ HPV (human papilloma virus)
- ○ Cervical polyp
- ○ Endometriosis
- ○ Breast lumps
- ○ Other reproductive problems/conditions

○ Yes   ○ No   Have you ever used birth control? If so, what kind? Problems/complications?

_____

_____

Current Pregnancy

What prenatal care have you had up to the present? Please list doctors, clinics, and hospitals where you have had care, what was done, and especially if you have had any lab work or special testing done.

_____

_____

Please check if you've had any of the following problems during this pregnancy:

- ○ Nausea
- ○ Headache
- ○ Leg cramps
- ○ Swelling
- ○ Urinary problems
- ○ Vaginal discharge
- ○ Indigestion
- ○ Vomiting

- ○ Dizziness
- ○ Fever
- ○ Rash
- ○ Bleeding gums
- ○ Constipation
- ○ Hemorrhoids
- ○ Abdominal/pelvic pain
- ○ Vaginal bleeding/spotting

- ○ Varicose veins
- ○ Backache
- ○ Diarrhea
- ○ Family problems
- ○ Loneliness
- ○ Relationship problems
- ○ Depression
- ○ Work problems

Have you used or been exposed to any of the following in this pregnancy?

- ○ Tobacco
- ○ Caffeine
- ○ Alcohol
- ○ Marijuana
- ○ Cocaine
- ○ Street drugs

- ○ Viruses
- ○ Measles
- ○ Cats
- ○ Vaccinations
- ○ Ultrasound
- ○ X-rays

- ○ Herbs
- ○ Vitamins
- ○ Non-prescription drugs
- ○ Prescription drugs
- ○ Fumes/sprays
- ○ Other environmental hazards

How would you describe your usual diet? _____

What do you generally do for exercise? _____

How do you feel about this pregnancy? _____

_____

How does your partner feel about this pregnancy? _____

_____

Do you feel that your sexual relationship has changed appreciably since you became pregnant? _____

_____

Do you plan to breast feed this baby? If so, for how long do you think you'll nurse? _____

_____

Are there any particular ethnic, cultural, or religious preferences for your care that you'd like to discuss?

_____

_____

Do you feel you have adequate resources, i.e., food, shelter, money, for this pregnancy? _____

_____

Do you have a car seat for the baby yet? _____

Please list the people you plan to invite to your birth _____

_____

Have you faced any opposition to your plans for home birth? _____

_____

In general, how do you cope with stress? How do you cope with pain? _____

_____

_____

_____

Please give some thought to the following questions and write your ideas. If you and your partner are together, each of you should answer. Read all questions before answering.

Why do you want to have this baby at home? _____

_____

_____

Partner: _____

_____

_____

What do you see as the duties or responsibilities of your midwife? _____

_____

_____

Partner: _____

_____

_____

There are some things that can go wrong without previous warning during labor and birth and after. If you are a low risk woman, the chances of unpredictable complications are low. However, if such complications should occur, you or your baby might be at greater risk because of being at home. There are risks involved with childbirth just as there are with driving a car. Some of these risks will probably never be eradicated no matter what our state of technology. There is a certain subset of risks involved in having your baby in a hospital as well as in your home (or in an alternative birth center or birthing house). If you opt for the risks involved in birthing at home you need to find out what they are and how they can be dealt with. Please comment on what you know about risks and complications and how you feel about them:

_____

_____

_____

Partner: _____

_____

How do you feel about going to the hospital to deliver if your midwife feels that complications are arising?

_____

_____

Partner: _____

_____

How do you think you might deal with the problem of a baby or mother who suffered permanent injury or died at home? _____

_____

_____

Partner: _____

_____

What do you think are the benefits of having your baby at home? _____

_____

_____

Partner: _____

_____

Please add any comments or thoughts that you think might be important for your midwife to know about you:

_____

_____

_____

_____

_____

_____

_____

_____

_____

_____

_____

_____

_____

_____

_____

_____

_____

_____

Prenatal Care Record

Name _____ Phone _____

LMP _____ EDD _____

Visit	Date	Weeks Gestation	Urine	Weight	Pulse/ BP	FHR	Presentation/ Position	Fundal Height	Internal Exam	Next Appt.	Provider (Initials)

PRENATAL CARE PROGRESS NOTES

Name _____ EDD _____

_____
_____
_____
_____
_____
_____
_____
_____
_____
_____
_____
_____
_____
_____
_____
_____
_____
_____
_____
_____
_____
_____
_____
_____
_____
_____
_____
_____
_____
_____
_____
_____
_____
_____
_____
_____
_____
_____
_____
_____

LABOR RECORD

Name _____ Date _____

Labor onset: Latent _____ Active _____

Baby's position _____ EDD _____

Membranes _____ Usual FHT _____

Concerns _____ Midwife _____

Observations on arrival _____

Time	BP/Pulse	Fetal Heart Tones	Urinalysis	Contractions	Internal Exam

LABOR PROGRESS NOTES

Name _____ Date _____

_____
_____
_____
_____
_____
_____
_____
_____
_____
_____
_____
_____
_____
_____
_____
_____
_____
_____
_____
_____
_____
_____
_____
_____
_____
_____
_____
_____
_____
_____
_____
_____
_____

Appendix F

Transport Record from Home Delivery

Midwife _____ Date/Time _____
Mother's Name _____ Partner's Name _____
Address _____
EDD _____ Mother's Age _____ Gravida _____ Para _____

Prenatal History
Gestational age 1st visit _____ Weight gain _____ Usual BP _____
Urine _____ Edema _____ Pelvimetry _____ Fundus _____
HCT/HGB _____ ABO & Rh _____ GBS _____ at _____ weeks HBsAg _____
Comments _____
_____

Labor History
Began labor _____ Initial events _____ Midwife arrived at _____
General observations _____ Vaginal exam _____
Comments _____
_____

Course of Labor
Inactive labor _____ Active labor _____ Pushing _____
Ruptured membranes _____ How? _____ Meconium? _____
Fetal response to labor _____
_____

Comments _____
_____

Reasons for Transport
_____
_____
_____
_____
_____
_____
_____
_____
_____
_____
_____

Birth Record: Mother

Name _____ Date of Birth _____
Phone (home) _____ (work) _____ Age _____
Address _____
Gravida _____ Para _____ EDD _____ Date of Birth _____ Time _____
GBS _____ at _____ weeks

Labor Summary
Latent _____ hrs.
1st stage _____ hrs.   2nd stage _____ mins.   3rd stage _____ mins.
Membranes ruptured at _____ Spontaneously _____ Surgically _____ Clear _____ Stained _____
Estimated blood loss _____ Treatment _____
Comments/problems _____

Placenta
Size _____ Adherent clot _____
Method of delivery _____ Missing cotyledons _____
Infarcts _____ Calcifications _____ Succenturiate lobe _____
Time cord cut _____ Number of vessels in cord _____

Perineum
Lacerations _____ Repairs _____

Immediate Postpartum
BP _____ Pulse _____ Fundus _____
Shower _____ Urination _____ Food/drink _____
Stable at _____

Birth Record: Baby

Name _____ Sex _____ Weight _____ Length _____ Chest _____ Head _____
Apgar _____ 1 minute _____ 5 minutes _____ Suctioning _____
Resuscitation _____
Molding, Caput, Hematoma _____ Eye medication _____ Vitamin K _____
Nursing _____
Unusual behavior problems or abnormalities _____
_____
_____

If problems develop and you call in, give time of birth, sex, weight, Apgar, respirations per minute, temperature, heart rate and describe symptoms.

Newborn Examination

DATE _____

APGARS (one minute _____)   (five minutes _____)

SEX _____ WT. _____

AXILLARY TEMPERATURE

_____

TOTAL LENGTH _____

HEAD (O.F.) _____

CHEST _____

APGAR	0	1	2
Heart rate	Absent	Under 100	Over 100
Respirations	Absent	Slow (Irr.)	Good (cry)
Muscle tone	Limp	Some flexion	Active
Color	Blue/white	Blue hands or feet	Pink totally
Response to nasal catheter	None	Grimaces	Sneeze or cough

1. GENERAL APPEARANCE _____
   (Activity, tone, cry)
2. SKIN _____
   (Polycythemia, jaundice, desquamation, lanugo, birth marks)
3. HEAD, NECK _____
   (Molding, caput, bruising, cephalhematoma, fontanelles)
4. EYES _____
   (Red spots, jaundice, pupils, tracking, medication instilled)
5. ENT _____
   (Ear shape, ear placement, reactivity to sound, lips, palate, frenulum)
6. THORAX _____
   (Retractions)
7. ABDOMEN _____
   (Cord, masses)
8. HEART _____
   (Heart rate, femoral pulses)
9. GENITALS _____
   (Testes descended, edema, clitoris)
10. REFLEXES _____
   (Sucking, swallowing, palmar, Moro, Babinkski, plantar, step)
11. SPINE/ANUS _____
   (Sinuses, anus patent)
12. LUNGS _____
   (Respirations, all quadrants clear)
13. EXTREMITIES _____
   (Fingers, toes, clavicles, hip creases or abduction)
COMMENTS_____
_____
_____
_____

CLINICAL ESTIMATION OF GESTATIONAL AGE

PATIENT'S NAME _____

⬆ Examination First Hours

CLINICAL ESTIMATION OF GESTATIONAL AGE
An Approximation Based on Published Data*

PHYSICAL FINDINGS		20	21	22	23	24	25	26	27	28	29	30	31	32	33	34	35	36	37	38	39	40	41	42	43	44	45	46	47	48
																			WEEKS GESTATION											
VERNIX			APPEARS				COVERS BODY, THICK LAYER														SCANT IN CREASES		NO VERNIX						
BREAST TISSUE AND AREOLA				AREOLA & NIPPLE BARELY VISIBLE NO PALPABLE BREAST TISSUE												AREOLA RAISED		1-2 MM NODULE		3-5 MM	5-6 MM		7-10 MM			112 MM				
EAR	FORM					FLAT, SHAPELESS										BEGINNING INCURVING SUPERIOR		INCURVING UPPER 2/3 PINNAE			WELL-DEFINED INCURVING TO LOBE									
	CARTILAGE					PINNA SOFT, STAYS FOLDED								CARTILAGE SCANT RETURNS SLOWLY FROM FOLDING			THIN CARTILAGE SPRINGS BACK FROM FOLDING				PINNA FIRM, REMAINS ERECT FROM HEAD									
SOLE CREASES					SMOOTH SOLES 1 CREASES								1-2 ANTERIOR CREASES		2-3 AN-TER-IOR CREA-SES		CREASES ANTERIOR 2/3 SOLE		CREASES INVOLVING HEEL			DEEPER CREASES OVER ENTIRE SOLE								
SKIN	THICKNESS & APPEARANCE		THIN, TRANSLUCENT SKIN, PLETHORIC, VENULES OVER ABDOMEN EDEMA												SMOOTH THICKER NO EDEMA			PINK		FEW VESSELS		SOME DES-QUAMATION PALE PINK		THICK, PALE, DESQUAMATION OVER ENTIRE BODY							
	NAIL PLATES		AP-PEAR											NAILS TO FINGER TIPS									NAILS EXTEND WELL BEYOND FINGER TIPS							
HAIR					APPEARS ON HEAD	EYE BROWS & LASHES			FINE, WOOLLY, BUNCHES OUT FROM HEAD										SILKY, SINGLE STRANDS LAYS FLAT						RECEDING HAIRLINE OR LOSS OF BABY HAIR SHORT, FINE UNDERNEATH						
LANUGO			AP-PEARS		COVERS ENTIRE BODY											VANISHES FROM FACE			PRESENT ON SHOULDERS				NO LANUGO						
GENITALIA	TESTES										TESTES PALPABLE IN INGUINAL CANAL							IN UPPER SCROTUM			IN LOWER SCROTUM							
	SCROTUM											FEW RUGAE						RUGAE, ANTERIOR PORTION			RUGAE COVER		PENDULOUS						
LABIA & CLITORIS											PROMINENT CLITORIS LABIA MAJORA SMALL WIDELY SEPARATED				PROMINENT CLITORIS LABIA MAJORA LARGER NEARLY COVERED CLITORIS					LABIA MINORA & CLITORIS COVERED							
SKULL FIRMNESS					BONES ARE SOFT					SOFT TO 1" FROM ANTERIOR FONTANELLE					SPONGY AT EDGES OF FON-TANELLE CENTER FIRM			BONES HARD SUTURES EASILY DISPLACED			BONES HARD, CANNOT BE DISPLACED							
POSTURE	RESTING		HYPOTONIC LATERAL DECUBITUS				HYPOTONIC				BEGINNING FLEXION THIGH		STRONGER HIP FLEXION		FROG-LIKE	FLEXION ALL LIMBS			HYPERTONIC				VERY HYPERTONIC					
RECOIL - LEG						NO RECOIL				NO RECOIL			PARTIAL RECOIL			BEGIN FLEXION NO RE-COIL		PROMPT RECOIL MAY BE INHIBITED			PROMPT RECOIL		PROMPT RECOIL AFTER 30" INHIBITION					
	ARM																									
		20	21	22	23	24	25	26	27	28	29	30	31	32	33	34	35	36	37	38	39	40	41	42	43	44	45	46	47	48

POSTPARTUM CARE

Mother _____ Baby _____ Phone _____

Date	Temp/Pulse	B/P	Nipples Breastfeeding	Uterus	Lochia	Perineum	Baby's Cord	Baby's Color/Behavior

Date	Uterus	Lochia	Breastfeeding	Cervix	Vaginal/Abdominal Tone	Parenting
3 weeks						
6 weeks						

POSTPARTUM CARE PROGRESS NOTES

Mother _____ Baby _____

_____

_____

_____

_____

_____

_____

_____

_____

_____

_____

_____

_____

_____

_____

_____

_____

_____

_____

_____

_____

_____

_____

_____

_____

_____

_____

_____

_____

_____

Appendix K

POSTPARTUM INSTRUCTIONS

1. Let us know if you soak more than one pad in 20 minutes—massage your uterus firmly to re-contract it, and if bleeding doesn't stop, contact us at once or seek emergency care.
2. Change your pad with each trip to the bathroom, and rinse perineum with warm water.
3. Check your uterus for firmness and/or tenderness several times a day, for 3 days at least.
4. Notice if your flow has any bad odor (it should smell like your menses)—and report to us.
5. Take your temperature twice daily for at least four days.
6. Drink lots of water (about three quarts daily to establish milk flow) and make one quart of that a mixture of shepherd's purse and comfrey tea (for healing and bleeding control).
7. If you've had stitches, soak them in (or use compresses of) comfrey, goldenseal, and ginger tea—three or four times daily. Air dry immediately after (in sunlight if possible). Report any pain.
8. Clean your baby's cord stump carefully with hydrogen peroxide or alcohol every few hours (or at each diaper change). Pay special attention to the folds where cord joins skin.
9. Nurse as much as the baby wants (usually every 2 to 3 hours; do not go more than 4 hours without nursing).
10. If the baby begins to look yellow within the first 24 hours, call us immediately.
11. Don't hesitate to call us if the baby seems disinterested in nursing, listless, or irritable.
12. Get lots of rest, sleep when the baby sleeps, eat lots of good food with plenty of iron to replenish lost blood, and visitors for real help—like doing your dishes or laundry. Work into activity slowly, and you won't have any sudden breakdowns later.
13. Try to take the parenting one day at a time—call if you feel upset, sad, or depressed.
14. Special instructions: _____

_____
_____
_____
_____
_____
_____
_____
_____
_____
_____
_____
_____
_____
_____

THE MIDWIFE'S KIT

fetascope

Doppler (optional)

watch, with second hand

blood pressure cuff

stethoscope

3 curved hemostats (Rochester-Pean)

1 pair scissors with blunt points

1 pair scissors with sharp points

1 pair umbilical scissors

1 Averbach cord bander

2 needleholders

3 mosquito forceps

1 ring forceps

stainless steel cord clamps (Hazeltine)

stainless steel instrument tray with cover

sterile gloves (elbow-length and wrist-length)

regular exam gloves

vinyl gloves (for use with oil)

disposable underpads

lubricating jelly

5cc syringes

3cc syringes

1^1/2-inch, 21-gauge needles (injections)

^{1}/2-inch, 23-gauge needles (suturing)

suture material (3-0 chromic)

lidocaine anesthetic

pitocin

methergine

tetracycline or erythromycin eye drops

vitamin K for baby

nitrazine paper

urine testing sticks

pregnancy tests

plastic disposable amnihooks

DeLee mucus traps

cord blood tubes

bulb syringe

Betadine solution

alcohol prep pads

4 x 4 sterile gauze pads, or topper sponges

water bottle

heating pad

stamp pad

light (and extension cord) for suturing

plasticized or fiberglass tape measure

infant scales (hanging fish-scale type)

oxygen system with infant resuscitation unit
    (Hudson Lifesaver or Ambu Baby Resuscitator)

pocket masks for resuscitation (newborn and adult)

IV equipment (optional)

blood draw equipment (optional)

hemoglobinometer (optional)

blood glucose monitor (optional)

herbs and tinctures

homeopathic remedies

Care and Preparation of Instruments

Most of the instruments require no special care, except for those which must be scrubbed and sterilized repeatedly. Careful cleansing immediately after use is a good idea; dried blood cakes up the hinges and is difficult to remove. Use scouring pads to clean blood from the grooved blades of the forceps and needleholder.

The first method for sterilizing your instruments is by boiling. Boil instruments and instrument tray in a large pot of water for 25 minutes. Be sure to remember to sterilize the tongs that you will use for removing instruments from the water, and be sure to place them in the water with handles up. Once the 25 minutes have passed, let the pot cool off a bit and then remove the tray with your tongs. Open some packets of sterile gauze, put on a sterile glove, and line your tray with the gauze. Then use the tongs once again to place the instruments in the tray, and cover (either drip-dry the cover as it's removed or blot with sterile gauze). Place in a doubled paper bag, wrap it up snugly, tape and date it.

A simpler method is the baking method. All you have to do is bake your double-wrapped package of tray, liner, and tools for one hour in a 250-degree oven. Be sure to add a pan of water so the bag doesn't scorch. Simply remove, cool, and store.

Repeat sterilization every two weeks.

PARENT'S SUPPLY LIST

Betadine solution
olive oil
bulb syringe (rubber ear type, 3 oz.)
4 x 4 sterile gauze pads (two dozen)
cotton balls
hydrogen peroxide
oral/axillary thermometer
bendable straws
plastic drop cloth and tape, or plastic sheet
bleach

flashlight with extra batteries
plastic trash bags
disposable underpads (at least 20)
sanitary napkins (heavy and mini-pads) plus belt
4 sheets, cases for all pillows, 4 washcloths, 4 towels,
    8 receiving blankets—all dried in hot dryer for ten
        extra minutes and bagged in plastic, then taped shut
herbs: shepherd's purse, comfrey, ginger root, etc.
plastic eye dropper

MIDWIFERY PROGRAMS AND INSTITUTIONS

MEAC Approved Direct-Entry Programs

Bastyr University
Department of Naturopathic Midwifery
14500 Juanita Dr. NE
Kenmore, WA 98028
(425) 602-3130
mmartin@bastyr.edu
www.bastyr.edu/academic/naturopath/midwifery

Miami Dade College
Midwifery Sciences Department
950 NW 20th St.
Miami, FL 33127-4693
(305) 237-4234
jclegg@mdcc.edu
www.mdc.edu/north/academic_programs.asp

MEAC Approved Direct-Entry Institutions

Arkansas Midwives School and Services
4528 E. Huntsville Rd.
Fayetteville, AR 72701
(479) 571-2229
info@midwifearmss.org
www.midwifearmss.org

Birthingway College of Midwifery
12113 S.E. Foster Rd.
Portland, OR 97266
(503) 760-3131
birthing@teleport.com
www.birthingway.org

Birthwise Midwifery School
24 S. High St.
Bridgton, ME 04009
(207) 647-5968
birthwise@ime.net
www.birthwisemidwifery.org

Florida School of Traditional Midwifery
P.O. Box 5505
Gainesville, FL 32627-5505
(352) 338-0766
info@midwiferyschool.org
www.midwiferyschool.org

Manna School of Midwifery and Health Sciences
P.O. Drawer 2248
Bonita Springs, FL 34133
(239) 992-1211
www.mannaschoolofmidwifery.org

Maternidad La Luz
1308 Magoffin St.
El Paso, TX 79901
(915) 532-5895
www.maternidadlaluz.com

Midwives College of Utah
(Formerly Utah College of Midwifery)
560 S. State St., Suite B2
Orem, UT 84058
(801) 764-9068; (888) 489-1238
office@midwifery.edu
www.midwifery.edu

National College of Midwifery
#209 State Rd. 240
Taos, NM 87571
(505) 758-1216
elizabet@taosnet.com
www.midwiferycollege.org

National Midwifery Institute
P.O. Box 128
Bristol, VT 05443-0128
(802) 453-3332
santon@nationalmidwiferyinstitute.com
www.nationalmidwiferyinstitute.com
Includes Heart & Hands Midwifery course work.
Also contact:
edavis@heartandhandsmidwifery.com
www.heartandhandsmidwifery.com

Seattle Midwifery School
2524 16th Ave. S. #300
Seattle, WA 98144-5104
(206) 322-8834; (800) 747-9433
info@seattlemidwifery.org
www.seattlemidwifery.org

Nonaccredited Direct-Entry Programs
(may be state recognized)

Ancient Arts Midwifery Institute
P.O. Box 788
Claremore, OK 74018-0788
(918) 342-2926
www.ancientartmidwifery.com

Association of Texas Midwives Training
401 E. Front, Suite 143
Tyler, TX 75702
(903) 592-4220
www.texasmidwives.com

Casa de Nacimiento
1511 E. Missouri Ave.
El Paso, TX 79902-5615
(915) 533-4932

Delphi Center for Midwifery Studies
3716 W. Swann Ave.
Tampa, FL 33609
(813) 873-7135
www.delphicenter.org

The Farm Midwifery Workshops
42 The Farm
Summertown, TN 38483
(931) 964-2472
www.midwiferyworkshops.org

Hygieia College
40 N. State St.
Joseph, UT 84739
www.freestone.org/hygieia

International School of Midwifery
140 N.E. 119th St.
Miami Beach, FL 33161
(305) 754-2354

Iowa School of Classical Midwifery
P.O. Box 614
Kalona, IA 52247
(319) 656-3962
www.angelfire.com/ia/russianbirthproject/ISCM.htm

Michigan School of Traditional Midwifery
P.O. Box 162
Mikado, MI 48745
(989) 736-6583
www.traditionalmidwife.com

ACNM Approved Post-Baccalaureate
Certificate Programs

Baystate Health Systems
Midwifery Education Program
689 Chestnut St.
Springfield, MA 01199
(413) 794-4448
barbara.graves@bhs.org
www.baystatehealth.com

Institute of Midwifery at Philadelphia University
Hayward Hall, Room 222
Schoolhouse Lane and Henry Ave.
Philadelphia, PA 19144
(215) 951-2525
instituteofmidwifery@philau.edu
www.instituteofmidwifery.org

Parkland School of Nurse-Midwifery
UT Southwestern Medical School
2330 Butler, Suite 103
Dallas, TX 75235
(214) 905-2129
mary.brucker@utsouthwestern.edu

University of Medicine and Dentistry of New Jersey
School of Health Related Professions
Nurse-Midwifery Program
65 Bergen St.
Newark, NJ 07107-3001
(973) 972-4298
diegmaek@umdnj.edu
www.umdnj.edu/shrpweb/programs/midwife

ACNM Approved Master's Programs

Baylor College of Medicine (MS)
Nurse-Midwifery Education Program
6550 Fannin, Suite 954
Houston, TX 77030
(713) 793-8895
sbarry@bcm.tmc.edu
www.bcm.tmc.edu/midwifery

Boston University (MPH)
School of Public Health
Nurse-Midwifery Education Program T-5W
Department of Maternal and Child Health
715 Albany St.
Boston, MA 02118
(617) 638-5012
mbarger@bu.edu
www.bumc.bu.edu/sph/mc/nmep

California State University, Fullerton (MSN)
Nurse-Midwifery Specialty
Department of Nursing
800 N. State College Blvd., EC199
Fullerton, CA 92834
(714) 278-2973
bjsnell@fullerton.edu

Case Western Reserve University (MSN or ND)
Frances Payne Bolton School of Nursing
Nurse-Midwifery Program
10900 Euclid Ave.
Cleveland, OH 44106-1712
(216) 368-2532
ggm@po.cwru.edu
http://fpb.cwru.edu

Charles R. Drew University of Medicine
  and Science (MS)
Nurse-Midwifery Education Program
College of Allied Health Sciences
1731 E. 120th St.
Los Angeles, CA 90059
(213) 563-4912
jacrowde@sbcglobal.net
www.cdrewu.edu/coah2002/academic/master/
  nurse.asp

Columbia University (MS)
School of Nursing
Midwifery Program
630 W. 168th St., Box 49
New York, NY 10032
(212) 305-5887
lzl108@columbia.edu
http://cpmcnet.columbia.edu/dept/nursing/

East Carolina University (MSN)
Nurse-Midwifery Program
School of Nursing
E. 5th St.
Greenville, NC 27858-4353
(252) 328-4302
www.nursing.ecu.edu

Emory University (MSN or MSN/MPH)
Nell Hodgson Woodruff School of Nursing
Atlanta, GA 30322
(404) 727-6961
jmashbu@nurse.emory.edu
www.nurse.emory.edu/Admissions/
    AcademicPrograms.asp

Frontier School of Midwifery
    and Family Nursing (MSN)
Community-Based Nurse-Midwifery
    Education Program (CNEP)
195 School St.
P.O. Box 528
Hyden, KY 41749
(606) 672-2312
CNEP@midwives.org
www.midwives.org

Georgetown University (MS)
Graduate Program in Nurse-Midwifery
School of Nursing and Health Studies
Box 571107
3700 Reservoir Road N.W.
Washington, D.C. 20007
(202) 687-4772
eg83@georgetown.edu
http://snhs.georgetown.edu/
    /content.cfm?objectID=1467

Marquette University (MSN)
College of Nursing
Nurse-Midwifery Program
P.O. Box 1881
Milwaukee, WI 53201-1881
(414) 288-3842
leona.vandevusse@marquette.edu
www.mu.edu or www.wi-cnm.net

Medical University of South Carolina (MSN)
Nurse-Midwifery Program
College of Nursing
99 Jonathan Lucas St.
Charleston, SC 29403
(843) 792-5857
hortonl@musc.edu
www.musc.edu/nursing/programs/msn.htm

New York University (MA)
Midwifery Education Program
Division of Nursing
Steinhardt School of Education
246 Greene St.
New York, NY 10003-6677
(212) 998-5895
patricia.burkhardt@nyu.edu
www.nyu.edu/education/nursing

Ohio State University (MS or PhD)
Nurse-Midwifery Graduate Program
College of Nursing
1585 Neil Ave.
Columbus, OH 43210-1289
(614) 292-4041
nursing@osu.edu
www.con.ohio-state.edu

Oregon Health and Science University (MS)
School of Nursing
Nurse-Midwifery Program
3181 S.W. Sam Jackson Park Rd.
Portland, OR 97201
(503) 494-3114, 3822
howec@ohsu.edu

San Diego State University (MS)
Nurse-Midwifery Graduate Education Program
San Diego State University
School of Nursing
5500 Campanile Drive
San Diego, CA 92182-4158
(619) 594-2540
lhunter@mail.sdsu.edu
http://nursing.sdsu.edu

Shenandoah University (MSN)
Nurse-Midwifery Education Program
Division of Nursing
1775 N. Sector Court
Winchester, VA 22601
(540) 678-4382
jfehr@su.edu
www.su.edu/nursing/mas_mid.html

State University of New York–
   Downstate Medical Center (MS)
Health Sciences Center at Brooklyn
College of Health Related Professions
Midwifery Education Program
Box 1227, 450 Clarkson Ave.
Brooklyn, NY 11203
(718) 270-7742
ronnie.lichtman@downstate.edu
www.hscbklyn.edu/CHRP/Midwif

State University of New York–Stony Brook (MS)
School of Nursing
Health Sciences Center
Stony Brook, NY 11794-8240
(631) 444-2867
peter.johnson@stonybrook.edu
http://sonce1.nursing.sunysb.edu/nursingweb.nsf/
   AboutMidwifery

University of California–San Francisco
San Francisco General Hospital (MS)
Interdepartmental Nurse-Midwifery Education Program
SFGH, 6D21
1001 Porter Ave.
San Francisco, CA 94110
(415) 206-5106
ennisl@obgyn.ucsf.edu; holly.kennedy@nursing.ucsf.edu
http://nurseweb.ucsf.edu/www/speclist.htm

University of Cincinnati (MSN)
Nurse-Midwifery Education Program
College of Nursing and Health
P.O. Box 210038
Cincinnati, OH 45221-0038
(513) 558-5512
nancy.moss@uc.edu
http://nursing.uc.edu

University of Colorado (MS)
Health Sciences Center
School of Nursing
Box C288
Nurse-Midwifery Option
4200 E. 9th Ave.
Denver, CO 80262
(303) 315-0150
Pam.Spry@UCHSC.edu
www.uchsc.edu/nursing

University of Florida (MSN or MN)
Nurse-Midwifery Program
UFHSC-J College of Nursing 653 W. 8th St.
Bldg 1, 2nd Floor
Jacksonville, FL 32209-6561
(904) 244-5174
poeah@nursing.ufl.edu
http://con.ufl.edu

University of Illinois–Chicago (MS or PhD)
College of Nursing M/C 802
Nurse-Midwifery Program
845 South Damen Ave.
Chicago, IL 60612
(312) 996-1867
engstrom@uic.edu
www.nurs.uic.edu

University of Indianapolis (MSN)
Nurse-Midwifery Program
Graduate Programs
School of Nursing
1400 E. Hanna Ave.
Indianapolis, IN 46227
(317) 962-0750
bwinningham@uindy.edu
http://nursing.uindy.edu

University of Kansas (MS)
Nurse-Midwifery Education Program
3901 Rainbow Blvd.
Kansas City, KS 66160-7502
(913) 588-1683
gbreedlove@kumc.edu
www2.kumc.edu/midwife

University of Maryland (MS)
Nurse-Midwifery Education Program
School of Nursing, Suite 575
655 W. Lombard St.
Baltimore, MD 21201
(410) 706-8625
stom@son.umaryland.edu
http://nursing.umaryland.edu

University of Miami (MSN)
School of Nursing
5801 Red Rd.
P.O. Box 248153
Coral Gables, FL 33124-3850
(305) 284-6256
jgottlieb@miami.edu
www.miami.edu/nur

University of Michigan (MS/PhD)
Nurse-Midwifery Program
School of Nursing
400 N. Ingalls, Room 3320
Ann Arbor, MI 48109-0482
(734) 763-5985; (800) 458-8689
umnursing@umich.edu
www.nursing.umich.edu/academics/masters/
    midwifery.html

University of Minnesota (MS/PhD)
School of Nursing
6-101 Weaver-Densford Hall
308 Harvard St., S.E.
Minneapolis, MN 55455
(612) 624-6494
avery003@tc.umn.edu
www.ahc.umn.edu/ahc_content/colleges/
    nursing/index.cfm

University of New Mexico (MSN)
Nurse-Midwifery Program
College of Nursing
Nursing/Pharmacy Building
Albuquerque, NM 87131-1061
(505) 272-4125
http://hsc.unm.edu/consg/Graduate_splash.shtml

University of Pennsylvania (MSN)
School of Nursing
Nursing Education Building
420 Guardian Dr.
Philadelphia, PA 19104-6096
(866) 867-8677
MSNadmissions@nursing.upenn.edu
www.nursing.upenn.edu/midwifery

University of Puerto Rico (MPH)
Nurse-Midwifery Education Program
Graduate School of Public Health
Medical Sciences Campus
P.O. Box 5067
San Juan, PR 00936-5067
(787) 281-7355; (787) 758-2525 ext. 2401
irene.delatorre@gte.net

University of Rhode Island (MSN)
Graduate Program in Nurse-Midwifery
College of Nursing
Kingston, RI 02881-0814
(401) 874-5323
debeo@uri.edu
www.uri.edu/nursing/programs/msmidwife.html

University of Texas–El Paso/TexasTech University
    Health Sciences Center (MSN)
Nurse-Midwifery Program
Texas Tech University HSC
Department of OB/GYN
4800 Alberta Ave.
El Paso, TX 79905
TTUHSC (915) 545-6490

University of Texas–El Paso/TexasTech University
    Health Sciences Center
Nurse-Midwifery Education Program
1101 N. Campbell Ave.
El Paso, TX 79902-0581
(915) 747-7263
midwifery@ttmcelp.ttuhsc.edu
www.nurse.utep.edu/nursing/degree.programs/
    midwife.htm

University of Texas Medical Branch–Galveston
Collaborative Nurse-Midwifery
    Education Program
School of Nursing
301 University Blvd., Route 1029
Galveston, TX 77555-1029
(409) 772-8347
bcamune@utmb.edu
www.utmb.edu

University of Utah (MS)
College of Nursing
Nurse-Midwifery Program
10 S. 2000 E. Front
Salt Lake City, UT 84112-5880
(801) 587-7605
jane.dyer@nurse.utah.edu
www.nurs.utah.edu

University of Washington (MN)
School of Nursing
Nurse-Midwifery Program
Box 357262
Seattle, WA 98195-7262
(206) 543-8241
midwife@u.washington.edu
www.son.washington.edu/eo/midwifery/

Vanderbilt University (MSN)
Nurse-Midwifery Program
School of Nursing
102 Godchaux Hall
Nashville, TN 37240-0008
(615) 322-3800
vusn_admissions@mcmail.vanderbilt.edu
www.mc.vanderbilt.edu/nursing/

Wayne State University (MSN)
College of Nursing
Nurse-Midwifery Concentration
5557 Cass Ave., Room 346
Detroit, MI 48202
(313) 577-1798
dswalker@wayne.edu
www.nursing.wayne.edu/programs.htm

Yale University (MSN)
School of Nursing
Nurse-Midwifery Specialty
100 Church St. S., Box 9740
New Haven, CT 06536-0740
(203) 785-2389
maryellen.rousseau@yale.edu
http://nursing.yale.edu

Appendix N

HIPAA GUIDELINES

This is a summary of the Health Insurance Portability and Accountability Act (HIPAA) guidelines as applied to midwifery practice which can be used to develop a Notice of Privacy Practices statement for clients to read and sign. (Personalize this document by changing the word midwife to "my" or "I," and the word client to "you" or "your.")

Midwife's Legal Duty
1. To maintain privacy of client's health information.
2. To provide clients written notice about midwife's privacy practices and their rights concerning their health information.
3. To change privacy practices according to applicable law and make new written notice available to clients.

Uses and Disclosures of Health Information
1. **Treatment.** The midwife may disclose health information to other health care providers providing client treatment.
2. **Payment.** The midwife may use or disclose information to obtain payment for services.
3. **Health-care operations.** The midwife may use and disclose health information in connection with quality assessment and improvement activities, reviewing the competence or qualifications of the midwife and her associates, or conducting training, accreditation, certification, or licensing activities.
4. **Client authorization.** The client may give the midwife written authorization to use or disclose her health information to anyone for any purpose. Authorization may also be revoked, in writing, at any time.
5. **To family and friends.** The midwife will disclose information to family and friends only with the client's written consent.
6. **Persons involved in care.** In the event of emergency or client incapacity, the midwife may use or disclose health information to notify, or assist in notifying, a family member, personal representative, or other person responsible for client's care, of client's location and general condition, disclosing only the health information directly relevant to that person's involvement in client's care.
7. **Marketing services.** The midwife will not use client information for marketing operations without the client's written authorization.
8. **Required by law.** The midwife may disclose the client's health information when required to do so by law.
9. **Abuse or neglect.** The midwife may disclose the client's health information to appropriate authorities if it reasonably appears the client is a possible victim of abuse or domestic violence, to the extent necessary to avert a threat to the client's health or safety.

Client Rights
1. **Access.** The client has the right to look at or get copies of her health information.
2. **Disclosure accounting.** The client has a right to receive a list of occasions in which the midwife has disclosed her information for purposes other than treatment, payment, or health-care operations for the past six years, but not before April 14, 2003 (the date HIPAA guidelines became effective).

3. **Restriction.** The client has the right to request that additional restrictions be placed on the use and disclosure of her health-care information. The midwife is not required to abide by these but may agree to do so (except in emergency).

4. **Alternative communication.** The client has a right to request that the midwife communicate with her by alternative means or at alternative locations, as necessary to maintain confidentiality (request must be in writing).

5. **Amendment.** The client has the right to request that the midwife amend her health information (request must be in writing, and must explain why the information should be amended). Under certain circumstances, the midwife may deny this request.

6. **Questions.** The client may contact the midwife for information about privacy practices at any time.

7. **Complaints.** If the client has complaints about the midwife's use or disclosure of her health information, or the midwife's response to her request to amend health information or communicate with her by alternative means or at alternative locations, she may complain to the midwife and to the U.S. Department of Health and Human Services.

ABOUT THE AUTHOR

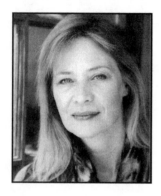

A renowned expert on women's issues, Elizabeth Davis has been a midwife, women's health-care specialist, educator, and consultant for more than twenty-five years. She is active internationally in women's rights and lectures widely on midwifery, sexuality, and women's spirituality.

She has served as a representative to the Midwives Alliance of North America (MANA) for five years and as president of the Midwifery Education Accreditation Council (MEAC) for the United States. She is cofounder and director of the National Midwifery Institute, a three-year, MEAC-accredited, apprenticeship-based midwifery program leading to licensure in California. She holds a degree in holistic maternity care from Antioch University and is certified by the North American Registry of Midwives (NARM).

In addition to writing several books on women's sexuality, intuition, and pregnancy, Davis is widely quoted in women's periodicals and is a popular radio and television guest. Her hobbies are gardening, snorkeling, hiking, and metaphysical studies. She lives in Sebastopol, California, and is the mother of three children. Contact her at www.elizabethdavis.com.

INDEX

Color
of baby's scalp, 123
of baby's skin, 82, 85, 134, 193, 195
cyanosis, 82, 134, 180, 201, 202
shoulder dystocia and, 159
Colostrum, 22, 137
Comfrey, 46, 200
Comfrey tea compresses, 200
Complaints common in pregnancy, 42–50
Complete blood count (CBC), 35–36, 163
The Complete Book of Pregnancy and Childbirth (Kitzinger), 219
Complete breech, 80
Complete cord prolapse, 154
Complete mole, 71
Composition of Foods (USDA), 32
Compound presentation (nuchal arm), 157, 158
Compresses
for breasts, 195, 200
for hemorrhoids, 49, 207
hot, 122–123, 150
for perineum, 119, 122–123, 192
Concerned United Parents, 93
Condom, 37, 46, 82, 216
Condyloma accuminata, 36
Cone biopsy, 15
Confidentiality, client, 242
Conjugate
diagonal, 24, 26
obstetrical, 24
Consent to care, 13–14, 242
Constipation, 34, 49
herbs for, 45
mother's, 45, 206–207
Consultation, medical, 231, 238–240
Continuity of care, 11, 41, 217
Contraception, 15–16, 197, 216
Contraceptive history, 15–16
Contractions
blowing through (pant with), 120
Braxton-Hicks, 88
danger signs in, 104
early labor and, 105, 107, 108
incoordinate, 36, 56, 66, 78, 146, 150, 164, 165
pitocin and, 7
premature birth and, 104
second stage, 120
transition, 114
See also Labor
Contraindications for home birth, preexisting, 14, 19–20
See also Screening out
Contraindications for suturing, 172
Contreras, Dona Queta, 150
Controlled traction of umbilical cord, 130
Cooper, Margaret, 219
Copper 7 IUD, 208

Cord. *See* Umbilical cord
Core areas of study (checklist), 225
Core-Competencies for Midwifery Practice (MANA), 259–262
Coronal suture, 115
Coroner notification, 181
Costovertebral angle tenderness (CVAT), 44
Cotyledon, 130–131
Counseling
genetic, 40
for history of abuse, 101
for hypertension, 75
nutritional, 33, 67, 79
for postpartum depression, 213, 214
techniques, 50
CPD. *See* Cephalopelvic disproportion (CPD)
CPM (Certified professional midwife), 4, 218, 245, 248
CPR (cardio-pulmonary resuscitation), 176, 179
infant, 128, 179
mother, 163
neonatal advanced life support (NALS) and, 176
Cradle cap, 206
Cranberry juice, 46
Cranial-sacral therapy, 205
Crepitus, 136
Cretinism, 19
Crying baby, 196, 205
sound of, 193
Cryosurgery, 15
CVAT (costovertebral angle tenderness), 44
Cyanosis, 82, 134, 180, 201, 202
Cystocele, 192, 195
Cytomegalovirus, 14, 16, 20
Cytotec (labor stimulant), 14, 163

D

D & C, 14, 166, 170
Dandelion, tea/tincture, 44, 48
Danger Signs in Pregnancy (checklist), 104
Davis-Floyd, Robbie, 219
Day-one visit, postpartum, 191–194
Day-seven visit, postpartum, 196–197
Day-three visit, postpartum, 194–196
Death
of baby, 68, 104, 181, 182–188
of mother, 163
Death certificate, baby, 181
Deep transverse arrest, 146, 148
Deflexion, in CPD, 145
Dehydration
checking baby's, 193
homeopathic remedies for, 127
hyperemesis gravidarium and, 44
and oligohydramnios, 78

and postdatism, 86
and prematurity, 82
with prolonged labor, 141
DeLee suction device, 121, 124, 125, 232
Delivery, 122–126
assisting, 122–126
baby's scalp color during, 123
bradycardia during, 123
checking for umbilical cord, 124–125
episiotomy and, 123
hands-and-knees position, 122
maintaining flexion of head during, 123
meconium aspiration and, 124
mother's access to baby, 126
placental, 130–133
positions for, 122
precipitous, 121–122
of shoulders and body, 125
signs of stress in baby, 124
stabilizing the newborn, 125–126
tear prevention, 122–123
See also Cesarean section; Labor
Delivery Self Attachment (video), 126
Demmin, Tish, 241
Denominator, 28, 30
Depo-Provera, 208
Depression, postpartum, 66, 190, 196, 210, 212–214
Descent of baby, 56, 115–116, 117, 142
Desquamation, 85, 134
Dextrostix, 198–199
Diabetes
as contraindication for home birth, 14, 19
gestational, 40, 72–74
jelly bean test for, 73
LGA and, 85
polyhydramnios and, 77
treatment for, 74
Diagonal conjugate, 24, 26
Diaper rash, 206
Diarrhea remedies, 49
Diastolic pressure, 21, 74, 75, 77.
See also Blood pressure
DIC (disseminated intravascular coagulation), 69
Dick-Read, Grantly, 223
Diet
active labor and, 113
anemia and, 65–67
counseling for, 33–34
early labor and, 107
for hypertension, 75
malnutrition, 14, 20, 68, 76
postpartum, 198
preeclampsia and, 76
prenatal, 32–34
supplements, 32
for vaginal infection, 45
Dilation of cervix
in active labor, 116
checking, 109, 116

I

ICAN (International Cesarean Awareness Network), 15, 266
ICM (International Confederation of Midwives), 4–5, 245–246, 266
In Case of Transport (checklist), 171
Incoordinate uterine action, 36, 56, 66, 78, 146, 150, 164, 165
Indigestion, 44, 60, 66, 210
Induction of labor
  biophysical profile and, 88
  condition of the cervix and, 86
  methods for, 86
  postdatism and, 86–88
  prolonged rupture of the membranes and, 155
  See also Labor
Inevitable abortion, 69
Infant. *See* Baby
Infection
  after circumcision, 204
  bladder, 17
  breast, 200, 210
  eye, baby, 37
  hematoma and, 207
  hepatitis, 37
  kidney, 17, 38, 44
  neonatal, 16, 202–203
  ruptured membranes and, 155
  thrush, 206
  urinary tract, 17, 21, 38, 82, 193
  uterine, 37, 45, 82, 106, 155–156, 193, 195, 207–208
  vaginal, 45–46
  viral, 14, 16, 20, 68
  See also Herpes
Informed Birth and Parenting (organization), 266
Informed consent, 81, 242
Initial interview, 12–14
Injection technique, 166, 174
Inlet disproportion, 146, 148
Insomnia, 68, 91. *See also* Sleep difficulties
Internal examination, 22–23, 54, 109, 115, 116, 197
Internal monitoring, 152, 153
Internal pressure catheter, 152
Internal rotation, 117, 146
International Cesarean Awareness Network (ICAN), 15, 266
International Confederation of Midwives (ICM), 4–5, 245–246, 266
International Definition of a Midwife, 4
International Federation of Gynecologists and Obstetricians (FIGO), 4
Interspinous diameter, 25
Intertuberous diameter, 25, 29
Intrahepatic cholestasis, 44
Intrauterine growth restriction (IUGR), 74, 77, 78, 79, 83–85

Intuition, 101,167, 220, 246, 251, 252, 256, 259
Inverted uterus, 130, 170
Iorillo, Maria, 40
Iron, 32, 65–66
Iron deficiency anemia, 65, 66, 198, 211
Ischial spines, 24–25, 27, 121, 146, 148
Ischial tuberosity, 25, 29, 57, 143, 148
Isoimmunization, 38
IUD (intrauterine device), 15–16, 216
IUGR (intrauterine growth restriction), 83–85

J

Jaundice
  ABO incompatability, 203
  breast milk, 203, 204
  from hepatitis B, 37
  herbs for, 200
  inspecting for, 134, 193, 195
  pathological, 203
  physiologic, 203, 204
  polycythemia and, 85
  treatment for, 200, 203–204
Jelly bean test for diabetes, 73
Jones, Ricardo Herbert, 169

K

Kalman, Janice, 90, 199
Kamoroff, Bernard, 235
Kangaroo care, 83
Kelp, 48
Kernicterus, 203
Ketoacidosis, 141
Ketonuria, 21, 108, 113, 141
Kick-counts, fetal, 84, 87
Kidney infection, 17, 38–39, 44
Kitzinger, Sheila, 119
Klaus, Phyllis, 100
Knee-chest position, 120, 152

L

Labial tears, 172
Labor, 105–138
  active, 108, 109, 111–116
  bath during, 112
  checking dilation, 109, 115
  checking for tears, 133, 172
  delivery, 122–126
  early, 105–109
  endorphins in, 107, 111
  environment during, 108, 111, 112–113, 144
  false, 56, 106
  herbs during, 127–128
  homeopathy during, 127–128
  incoordinate, 36, 56, 66, 146, 164, 150, 165

induction by castor oil, 86
induction by herbs, 86
induction by homeopathy, 49
length of time for, 140–141
movements of baby during, 117
newborn exam, 133–136
partner's participation, 138
plateau phenomenon, 114, 141
postpartum watch, 136–137
premature, 49, 79, 82–83
relaxation during, 107
role of midwife versus birth assistant, 108
second stage, 119–122
sexual nature of, 91, 99, 126
transition, 116–119
true, 107, 141
urination after, 128, 193
urination during, 119
warm-up,106
when to attend, 107–108
See also Arrest; Delivery; Induction of labor; Prolonged labor
Labor-aide formula, 113
The Labor Progress Handbook (Simkin and Ancheta), 219
Labor Record
  form, 276–277
  starting the, 108
Lab work, prenatal, 35–41
  alpha-fetoprotein screening, 39
  amniocentesis, 39
  antibody screen, 38
  blood type, 38
  chorionic villus sampling, 39
  complete blood count, 35–36
  gestational diabetes screening, 40
  group B streptococcus screening, 40–41
  hepatitis screening, 37
  Pap smear, 36
  rubella titre, 38
  syphilis screening, 36
  triple screen, 39
  HIV screening, 37–38
  tuberculosis screening (PPD), 39
  urinalysis, 38
  See also Prenatal care
Lacerations
  cervical, 164, 165
  with compound presentation, 157
  healing, 192–193, 197, 198, 199
  repair, 172, 173–176
  vaginal, 165, 172
  See also Suture/suturing technique; Tears (muscle)
Lactation. *See* Milk; Nursing
Lactiferous ducts, 208
Lactiferous sinus (ampulla), 208
Lactiferous tubules, 208
La Leche League, 92, 266
Lambdoidal suture, 115